What You Think
ADD/ADHD Is, It Isn't

Symptoms and Neuropsychological
Testing Through Time

What You Think ADD/ADHD Is, It Isn't

Symptoms and Neuropsychological Testing Through Time

Barbara C. Fisher, PhD

Edited by
Kristine Holton Dulapa

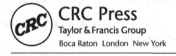

CRC Press
Taylor & Francis Group
Boca Raton London New York

CRC Press is an imprint of the
Taylor & Francis Group, an **informa** business

CRC Press
Taylor & Francis Group
6000 Broken Sound Parkway NW, Suite 300
Boca Raton, FL 33487-2742

© 2013 by Taylor & Francis Group, LLC
CRC Press is an imprint of Taylor & Francis Group, an Informa business

No claim to original U.S. Government works

Printed on acid-free paper
Version Date: 20130313

International Standard Book Number-13: 978-1-4398-3996-6 (Hardback)

Visit the Taylor & Francis Web site at
http://www.taylorandfrancis.com

and the CRC Press Web site at
http://www.crcpress.com

This book is dedicated with love to my mother, Audrey L. Fisher

Contents

Preface

This book is unique in that it is the first of its kind to provide scientific evidence of clinical population reporting data gathered over a period of 20 years. More importantly, this book provides documentation of 20 years of neuropsychological evaluation: the art form of diagnosing an attention disorder by using brain behavior measures to systematically record attention symptoms of slow cognitive or thinking speed, distractibility, information processing and input, as well as the pattern of visuospatial problems found to lead to reading comprehension difficulties and dislike of reading. We have used the same measures to document the presence of ADD/ADHD (Attention Deficit Disorder/Attention Deficit Hyperactivity Disorder) over time. The accuracy of these measures has been demonstrated through concurring diagnoses by other professionals as well as documentation of the same patterns (sometimes the same scores) obtained almost 15 years later on re-testing. Neuropsychological assessment is complemented by numerous self-report measures completed by parents and teachers as well as by the individual. The data is enormous, and in an effort to make reading easier, we have included graphs demonstrating the finding for each question for the self-report measures and individual test finding. We hope this is helpful to you in bringing some clarity to a disorder that has been too often misunderstood and misdiagnosed.

Acknowledgment

This book was conceived in January of 2010 when I decided to trek through 6000 files to separate out over 3000 cases that met the criteria for the research underpinning this book. It took a year to gather the data and generate the percentiles that you see today. There are two research articles in preparation and a number of abstracts presented at various conferences based upon the information presented here. This book represents the sum total of all of the data including numerous checklists and neuropsychological testing gathered over a period of 20 years. Once the statistical analysis was complete; then it took over 1½ years to write the text, and configure all of the data into the format that you see today. I hope that you find the graphs helpful. I have added these for easier reading and comprehension of the data.

This book was clearly an arduous process and one that I put aside for many years when it was suggested by various professional colleagues, specifically my mentor Dr. Art Walters, to publish this data. The enormity of this project was rather daunting at times. For this reason, the book is dedicated to my mother who in and of herself is a rather miraculous individual. She keeps on going even when she is in pain, and her mind is running faster than her body. It is because of my mother that I never give up no matter how difficult things become. At 91 years, her tenacity has allowed her to circumvent the odds and emerge successful no matter what life brings to her. Her strength and her courage through life have been a wonderful beacon for me to emulate. Bravo for you, mom!

I would like to first acknowledge the main person who made this book possible, completing both the editing and the graphs, Kristine Dulapa. Next, Danielle Garges, the researcher who worked on the data and provided all of the frequencies that you see today. Then there is Dee Bradley, who worked on the math computations for the percentages. Maria Gambino is the person who helped to start the project, organizing the people as well as the data. Dr. Stephany Fulda was instrumental in directing the research to prepare for publication.

Finally, I wish to thank my son, Jeff Fortuna, for all of his support and Bob Booth for his understanding. I could not close without thanking the original team who worked on the data: Maria Gambino, Katie Maguire, Danielle Zipay, and Lori Tabor. And of course, my friend Art Walters, who encouraged me to write this book almost ten years ago.

Introduction

The impetus to write this book sprang from a need to offer a truly authentic look at the ADD/ADHD disorder from the basis of many years of clinical experience and testing. This disorder is not as easily diagnosed or clear cut as many believe; in fact it very often acts as a masking agent for other underlying, contributing disorders. It's important that we understand ADD/ADHD better and by sharing the years of clinical experience and testing that I've accumulated, I hope to do just that.

This book is the result of a research study compiling 20 years of testing for ADD/ADHD. My research assistants and I started with 6000 files, paring them down to a little over 3000 to provide the initial sample of children, adolescents, and adults who were tested in an outpatient clinical setting to rule in or rule out ADD/ADHD. The group was further separated into two groups: ADHD inattentive type and ADHD plus an additional disorder. All subjects were de-identified and IRB approval was obtained. All 3000 cases were diagnosed with ADD/ADHD. Generally those referred for testing had already been screened by the referral sources (teachers, doctors, and other professionals) resulting in the majority referred for ADD/ADHD testing being diagnosed with the disorder.

The ruling in of an additional disorder, ADHD plus, was the result of neuropsychological evaluation that revealed a more severe picture on testing than would typically be seen accompanying the genetic disorder of ADHD. We have derived from this significant amount of testing that the inattentive subtype is actually more predominant in the general population. It would make sense that a less severe disorder is the one seen more often. From there, testing revealed that the ADHD combined subtype or ADIID hyperactivity subtype is the result of symptoms manifested by issues or underlying conditions that are in addition to ADHD.

What I propose to show you in the data gathered using both neuropsychological evaluation and self-report measures is that more often than not we are really seeing symptoms of inattention. Less often seen is the presence of the combined subtype or hyperactivity subtype. Many in the field of psychology and psychiatry would not disagree with that point. They would argue with the contention that anxiety masks itself as hyperactivity (shown in our research) and symptoms of the combined subtype are actually symptoms of ADHD plus an additional disorder such as sleep-disorder or the result of any type of impact of injury to the brain. Anxiety is often misread as overactivity or impulsivity.

The ADHD disorder frequently brings to light the presence of executive reasoning symptoms; although this is not always the case. In the past, before the *DSM-IV*, we had ADD without hyperactivity and ADHD. When everything changed to ADHD the theory of executive reasoning and ADD was born. In my opinion, supported by years of testing, when predominant symptoms of executive reasoning or memory exist, then the diagnosis is actually ADHD plus an additional disorder. We do not see memory problems associated with the genetic disorder of ADD/ADHD. In fact, memory is often a primary tool to compensate for attention deficits. We do not see executive reasoning deficits unless there is an additional disorder affecting the frontal processes, which could be due to anything from a brain injury to severe sleep disorders. Whenever a research study tries to measure executive reasoning in a population diagnosed with ADHD, they may find planning problems, but deficits related to the frontal processes remain elusive and generally inconclusive.

ADD/ADHD has too often become a universal label to attach to a symptom or group of symptoms that could just as easily be attributed to an underlying disorder. Using labels becomes a problem when we get caught up in trying to make the label fit something that does not always match what the brain is doing. This creates differences between what we see outwardly as symptoms and what we measure in testing, because what we see outwardly as symptoms can be the result of many different things. This is why neuropsychological testing is so helpful in providing a more conclusive picture.

While labels help us to talk the same language using a universally agreed upon concept, they can also be restrictive, leading to misdiagnosis.

Here is an example that has to do with sleep. Is ADHD a product of lack of sleep or a standalone disorder? To what degree does poor sleep and/or lack of sleep contribute to the symptoms of ADHD? In our experience using neuropsychological test data, lack of sleep impacts performance of about one standard deviation. A standard deviation is a measurement that we use to tell us how far the score is above or below the average. This means that lack of sleep results in the decline from above average to average or average to below average. Sleep apnea, however, especially when severe and ongoing for some time, can create more severe test results of two standard deviations for attention, resulting in above average declining to below average and average to well below average. So an adult reports attention symptoms that are now becoming out of control and he or she seeks evaluation as a result. However, it could be that sleep is driving the attention problems to become worse or sleep apnea over time has created a condition that is well beyond attention affecting memory and executive reasoning processes. In other words, sleep may be the driving force for attention symptoms having enough of an effect upon a person's life that he or she seeks evaluation. This is a different picture from the more natural process of life becoming more complicated and attention symptoms having a greater effect.

So what is the problem with labeling everything ADHD? Well, to use the aforesaid example, if sleep apnea is the driving force behind attention symptoms (that created the decision for evaluation and seeking help), then testing and symptoms may fit the criteria of attention and executive reasoning effects. The diagnosis of ADHD combined subtype is given. The person is placed on stimulant medication and no one asks about sleep because the criteria for the diagnosis of ADHD were met.

You can substitute the same scenario with a head injury, a car accident that everyone thought was not a problem, an undiagnosed seizure disorder, a cardiovascular problem, and the list goes on. Because we look beyond attention when there is not the typical pattern of inattention, we find these other disorders working jointly within the medical field. The diagnosis and treatment of these additional comorbid disorders have made huge differences in the lives of children, adolescents, and adults. Researchers in the field of ADHD agree that this is a complex disorder; neuropsychological testing is a critical component. ADHD is not a convenient catch-all to see as responsible for a wide variance and range of behaviors. It is complex because often there are many other disorders in addition to that involving attention. It becomes our job to separate out the issues; hence the reason for this book.

In labeling everything as ADHD—inattentive, combined, or overactive—we are actually doing a disservice to individuals who end up being placed on medications (which generally results in numerous medication changes), chasing down the treatment of an attention disorder when the medication is not totally successful because an underlying disorder remained undiagnosed and therefore not treated. In this regard, the child population data had an almost equal number of ADHD inattentive and ADHD plus, suggesting the overlap of undiagnosed disorders of sleep and brain. In fact, the plus label was given when there was an additional sleep disorder and/or brain disorder that was subsequently diagnosed as a result of the original testing for ADD/ADHD. Although it is fine that ADHD is the first diagnosis to explore to explain the problems a child may be having academically or behaviorally, it is not fine that this is the last diagnosis given when there are problems that remain and are not explained totally by a genetic disorder of attention.

Attention by definition means cognitive thinking; it does not mean behavior. However, most of the time ADD is diagnosed by behavioral checklists and not by testing. When testing is done, it is completed using achievement measures and an intellectual assessment. Rarely is the testing neuropsychological to measure the attention processes in the brain, which is what this disorder supposedly represents.

The enormity of this research is that it represents the largest clinical study of its kind, that there is no other research that has been done that utilized a full battery of neuropsychological testing for a period of 20 years with a significant number of self-report measures. The combination of symptoms reported and testing measured allows me to say that clearly ADHD is typically the inattentive type and there is no combined or hyperactivity subtype; it is actually ADD and something additional such as a sleep or brain disorder. The amount of sleep symptoms reported from 1989 to 2009 was significant for all ages. Children and adolescents, as well as adults, all reported being sleepy. The sleep problems increased with age as did the comorbid symptoms of anxiety and depression.

So I ask you: What is ADD? My belief is that there is a genetic attention disorder that has specific cognitive symptoms and seems to run together accompanied by anxiety, and the two increase cyclically over time. Just like any other population, ADD individuals are also prone to develop sleep disorders (although some sleep disorders are more often associated with ADD than others) and/or brain issues. These are represented by the wild child at 3 and 4 years of age, the argumentative, pot-smoking adolescent, and the anxious, avoidant adult. If you have ever been in the position of knowing children and then seeing them 15 and 20 years later, you know that what you see in childhood is not the same thing in adulthood.

I give you the example of Robert, who was seen at age 18 years for ADD testing. He was already on stimulant medication and had been since 5 years of age. There was evidence of more severe problems on testing, and sure enough, he had an undiagnosed seizure disorder. But we were too late. The result was grand mal seizures at age 21, complete loss of memory at age 23, and declined functioning since. Then there was Timothy, who at age 9 presented to us already diagnosed with Asperger's syndrome and ADHD, and taking several different medications. He was nonresponsive to his parents, who eventually ended up taking everything out of his room. Today, at age 21, he is running his father's company with a fast talking pace and heavy hand, negotiating with his customers. He has many friends and certainly does not appear anything like he did at 9 years of age. The essential question is: How well do we really understand ADD/ADHD? What I ask is that you keep an open mind, enough to think beyond what you think you see. As in so many things in life, do not be too quick to label. Not everything is as it first appears. I will tell you the first thing I learned when I took basic neurology with the medical school: "What you know today is a lie tomorrow."

This book is the result of rather painstaking research that has taken years to complete and place into written form. It is about sharing the voluminous information gathered from the neuropsychological testing and the self-report measures that hopefully will be helpful to you in shedding light upon what this disorder truly means for people as well as what it does not. For ease of reading, we have divided it into sections: children, adolescents, and adults. We have also included numerous graphs to help make the information more visually accessible.

Author

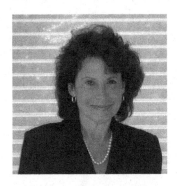 **Dr. Barbara C. Fisher, PhD**, is the author of three prior books on ADD/ADHD. Trained as a neuropsychologist, she has been involved in the diagnosis of ADD/ADHD for over 20 years. She speaks nationally and internationally on topics involving the brain as well as sleep. She is continually involved in research on ADD/ADHD as well as traumatic brain injury and dementia. Pediatrics and the aging population have been her focus of specialization in order to understand the impact of the brain upon behavior and thinking processes. On the cutting edge of assessing ADD/ADHD with neuropsychological testing and not relying upon self-report measures for diagnosis, she has systematically through time isolated a population with disorders in addition to attention problems, which has resulted in more positive effects for treatment. She continually hears from parents and adults about how their lives have been changed by a clear diagnosis and treatment. Dr. Fisher is board certified in behavioral sleep medicine. She did her sleep fellowship at the JFK Neuroscience Center in Edison, New Jersey. She has participated in several research projects identifying the relationship of restless leg syndrome and periodic limb movements in sleep to the ADHD population of children and adults. Dr. Fisher has developed a program for insomnia based upon principles of cognitive behavioral therapy. She developed a school, the Fisher Academy, with the goal of encouraging learning based upon frontal lobe principles to help children diagnosed with autism and frontal lobe disorders. She also operated a camp for several years that provided education in social skills and the development of "emotional intelligence" in order to develop positive peer interactions to children who struggled to connect socially.

Dr. Fisher is clinic director for United Psychological Services, which offers cutting-edge diagnostic assessment and treatment for ADD/ADHD as well as additional disorders involving the brain. Treatment has been highly successful due to accurate diagnosis.

1 Common Definition of ADD/ADHD as We Know It Today

DSM-IV-TR

Attention deficit disorder or ADHD as defined in the DSM-IV-TR must meet the following five criteria:

1. A "persistent pattern of inattention and/or hyperactivity–impulsivity that is more frequently displayed and more severe than typically observed in individuals at a comparable level of development."
2. "Some hyperactive–impulsive or inattentive symptoms that cause impairment must have been present before age 7 years."
3. "Some impairment from the symptoms must be present in at least two settings" (home, school, or work).
4. There must be "clear evidence of interference with developmentally appropriate social, academic, or occupational functioning."
5. The disturbance cannot be explained by another disorder.

The basic symptoms of inattention are as follows:

- Not giving close attention to details or making careless mistakes.
- Work is messy, poor sustained attention, and difficulty persisting to task completion.
- Often appear as if they are not listening.
- Shifts from one activity to another; lack of follow-through.
- Tasks that require sustained mental effort are avoided and not seen as pleasant. The avoidance is due to inattention and not being oppositional.
- Disorganized work habits; items necessary for task completion are lost or scattered.
- Easily distracted by irrelevant stimuli and interrupt tasks to attend to trivial noises and events.
- Forgetfulness in daily activities.
- Inattention expressed as shifts in attention occurring in social conversation.

Basic symptoms of hyperactivity:

- Fidgeting or squirming in the seat
- Not remaining seated when expected to
- Excessive running or climbing when inappropriate for environment
- Appearing to be on the go
- Talking excessively

- There are three different symptoms for developmental ages:
  - *Toddlers and preschoolers*: Constantly on the go and into everything, darting back and forth.
  - *School age children*: Less intensity; they tend to get up frequently, squirm in their seat, and fidget with objects.
  - *Adolescents and adults*: Symptoms take on the form of restlessness and difficulty engaging in sedentary activities.

Basic symptoms of impulsivity:

- Impatience, difficulty delaying responses, and blurting out answers
- Frequently interrupting and intruding on others
- Initiating conversations at inappropriate times
- Talking excessively
- Fidgety or squirming in the seat
- Not remaining seated when expected

There are three subtypes:

- *Attention deficit/hyperactivity disorder, combined subtype*: Six or more symptoms of inattention and six or more of hyperactivity–impulsivity persisting for at least 6 months.
- *Attention deficit/hyperactivity disorder, predominantly inattentive type*: Six or more symptoms of inattention, but fewer than six symptoms of hyperactivity–impulsivity have persisted for at least 6 months.
- *Attention deficit/hyperactivity disorder, predominantly hyperactive–impulsive type*: Six or more symptoms of hyperactivity–impulsivity and fewer than six symptoms of inattention that has persisted for at least 6 months.

It is difficult to diagnose in children younger than 4 or 5 years of age. The diagnosis for adults should not be made solely on the basis of their recollection of behavior as a child (American Psychiatric Association, 2000).

REFERENCE

American Psychiatric Association. (2000) *Diagnostic and Statistical Manual of Mental Disorders*, 4th edn., text rev. American Psychiatric Association, Washington, DC, pp. 85–87.

2 Description of the Population

The information and data presented in this book are the result of a process that began in January of 2010. At that time, we took approximately 6000 files or cases and sorted out those that met the criteria for having all of the checklists or self-report measures as well as the testing. Included in the study were only those cases where all of the neuropsychological testing and the self-report measures had been completed. If the primary referral was for something other than ADHD (such as a brain injury or psychological evaluation), then it was not included in this sample. Cases that were referred for ADHD testing were excluded if neuropsychological testing established a brain dysfunction as primary as opposed to secondary to the ADHD diagnosis or if there was a prominent genetic emotional disorder (bipolar, schizophrenia, major depression). When the primary referral was ADHD and there was evidence of an additional significant disorder that would have compromised or impacted the ADD testing, then the file was labeled "ADHD plus".

ADHD plus referenced the presence of an additional disorder that was thought to have impacted performance on the neuropsychological testing mostly involving sleep (such as sleep apnea), more extensive psychological problems (such as severe depression), or a mild brain injury (due to sports concussion or birth complications such as delayed labor, prematurity, meconium, cord wrapped two or three times, slightly lowered Apgar score, or emergency Caesarean section).

Included were all individuals tested from 1989 to 2009. We have additional data and cases that remain ongoing at this time. Time did not permit recording of cases since 2009; however, the patterns described in the following pages continue to be seen from 2010 onward. Some of the numbers for the responses or respondents varied on the self-report measures, given that individuals were allowed to provide more than one response to a specific item and some did not respond to a particular item.

Adolescents from the ages of 15 to 17 years were included in the adult group when the only measures they completed were the adult checklists. When the adolescent completed some adolescent checklists in addition to the adult measures, they were included in the adolescent sample.

TOTAL SAMPLE SIZE

ADULTS

The total sample size for the adults was 1296 individuals from the ages of 15 to 80 years. Thirty-six percent were males compared to 64% females. Seventy-five percent were diagnosed with ADHD inattentive type and 25% with ADHD plus. Percentiles of adults tested for specific ages are noted in the following:

- 14% were 15–19 years.
- 23% were 20–29 years.
- 25% were 30–39 years.
- 24% were 40–49 years.
- 11% were 50–59 years.
- 2% were 60–69 years.
- 0.002% were 70–80 years.

ADOLESCENTS

The total sample size was 402 adolescents from the ages of 12 to 17 years. Sixty-eight percent were males compared to 32% females. Seventy-four percent were diagnosed with ADHD inattentive type and 26% with ADHD plus an additional disorder. Percentiles of adolescents tested for specific ages are noted in the following:

- 15% were 12 years.
- 18% were 13 years.
- 20% were 14 years.
- 19% were 15 years.
- 12% were 16 years.
- 15% were 17 years.

CHILDREN

The total sample size was 833 children from the age of 5 to 11 years. Seventy-one percent were males compared to 29% females. Fifty-six percent were diagnosed with ADHD inattentive type and 44% with ADHD plus an additional disorder. Percentiles of children tested for specific ages are noted in the following:

- 7% were 5 years.
- 14% were 6 years.
- 17% were 7 years.
- 18% were 8 years.
- 18% were 9 years.
- 14% were 10 years.
- 11% were 11 years.

AGE AT THE TIME OF TESTING AND REASON FOR TESTING

CHILDREN

Testing by Age
- Highest percentage by age was for the following:
  - 7 years
  - 8 years
  - 9 years
- Lowest percentage by age was 5 years

Reasons for Testing

Parents initiated the child testing, as a result of a conversation with a teacher, other professionals or primary care physician. Parents sought testing to address either behavioral problems in school such as distractibility or constant movement, hyperactivity, or resistance to academic work. Testing was also initiated as a result of concerns with regard to reading and skill development. Probable reasons for testing at these ages are as follows:

- Ages 7, 8, and 9 years revealed a higher percentage (or greater numbers of children tested) as a result of increased school difficulties with reading comprehension. Math generally becomes more problematic in the later elementary and junior high grades.
- Need for more independent work and increased homework and overall school work output.
- Writing and reading were primary referral complaints.

- Many children were referred due to either not liking school or being more hyperactive (anxious) in the classroom or more outwardly inattentive and distracted.
- Dislike of school would tend to relate to difficulty with reading, not enjoying reading, and difficulty comprehending what they have read. The tendency was to have more problems with decoding whereby reading becomes too effortful to recall what one has read. Handwriting is poor and usually hard to read.
- There were additional, undiagnosed disorders creating more problems resulting in the almost equal numbers of ADHD and ADHD plus.
- Issues of missing assignments including work not completed in class, not wanting to study or finish homework, and overall dislike of school.
- Age 5 was the lowest percentage; symptoms of inattention were not sufficiently disruptive to require testing and, in the mind of their parents, the possible introduction of medication. The children in this study tended to come in as medication naïve or not on any medication. Parents were hesitant about getting testing, thinking that evaluation equaled the need for medication intervention.

ADOLESCENTS

Testing by Age
- Highest percentage by age was for the following:
  - 13 years
  - 14 years
  - 15 years
- Lowest percentage by age was for the following:
  - 6 years

Reasons for Testing
Much of the adolescent testing was parent initiated. Parents sought testing to try to help their child who was struggling in school and subsequently making poor choices of friends. Some of the adolescents had already been tested and medication already trialed as an intervention. When there was no previous testing, generally, attention had been suspected for some time dating back to earlier grades. Poor grades were becoming more prevalent and school was more difficult. Probable reasons for testing for these ages are as follows:

- Ages 13, 14, and 15 years revealed a higher percentile related to the transition from elementary school to junior high and junior high to high school.
- Increased school demands in terms of reading, writing, and completion of research papers as well as increased homework.
- Homework is no longer being monitored by the teacher, and parents remained unaware of what homework is due (power school was just starting), resulting in assignments not being turned in.
- Grade decline is higher due to missing assignments given the increased consequence of the child needing to be responsible for their own work.
- Homework becomes more important and affects the grade to a greater degree. Poorer grades prompt parents to seek help.
- Continued poor grades despite medication intervention would prompt parents to go to a clinic setting to revisit the diagnosis of ADHD and/or to see what changes can be made in their child's life.
- Age 16 years was the lowest percentage as adolescents have made it through the transition to high school and are not yet concerned about college.

ADULTS

Testing by Age
- Highest percentage by age was for the following:
  - 20–29 years
  - 30–39 years
  - 40–49 years
- Lowest percentage by age was 60–80 years

Reasons for Testing

Generally, people only look to be tested when they are struggling in their life or needing to make changes in their life. Probable reasons for testing for these ages are as follows:

- The percentage was higher for ages 40–49 years as a result of a life review period, changing career or need to change careers, and/or the career has become more demanding and performance is suffering as a result.
- The percentage was higher for ages 30–39 years due to a return to school, the need to foster their career and attain upward mobility, the addition of children and increased life demands, as well as stress.
- The higher percentage for ages 20–29 years related to college difficulties and poor grades, too much partying and not enough time spent on school, problems in the first year of college, in process of establishing a career, and looking toward graduate work.
- Attention is not a typical reason for testing ages 60–80 years unless ruling out dementia, and individuals are thinking that attention is their primary problem, which may be exacerbating or masking memory or other types of cognitive decline.

DESCRIPTION OF THE CHILD POPULATION

Descriptions of the child and family background were recorded on two checklists. The Developmental History Checklist was the measure used until 2006. In 2006, the Child Neuropsychological History was used to record basic data on the child. The Sleep Evaluation Questionnaire was another measure that we began to use in 2008.

RESULTS OF THE DEVELOPMENTAL HISTORY CHECKLIST

The Developmental History Checklist is a general measure providing basic information that the parents provided regarding their child. There were 496 parents who completed this measure. This measure was replaced in 2006. Questions in this checklist addressed reasons for the evaluation, severity of the problem, school and academic issues, pregnancy and birth, health history, family relationships, emotions, and overall behavior. Percentages were computed for the individual questions from this measure, resulting in the following findings.

Reason for Evaluation

The main reason for bringing the child to our clinical setting was the presence of academic and behavior problems in school, followed by behavior problems at home. The problem was more often indicated as moderate to severe, meaning that the parents did not bring their child to be tested until forced to do so as a result of escalating problems. We see the same pattern today where parents are fearful of bringing their child in for testing, laboring under the belief that if diagnosed with an attention disorder, this will result in medication being prescribed. Often that was the fear expressed directly by the parent, or the parent would indicate without prompting that "they do not believe in medication."

Another important caveat that emerged with the percentages is that the majority of the children evaluated had the problem for the past 2 years or for several years, meaning that again this was not a new phenomenon and instead a problem that had built up sufficiently to compel parents to bring the child in for evaluation.

Problem Areas

Primary problem areas reported more often by parents were the child's academic performance and, secondarily, the child's behavior. A greater percentage had not had their child in for evaluation (63%) before. Nineteen percent were seeking help due to the lack of success of intervention trialed thus far, which typically was stimulant medication.

The problems reported by parents that the child was having revolved around being not able to think clearly (26%), arguments with parents (32%), academic problems (36%), and behavior problems at home (45%).

Education and Socio-Economic Background

The majority of the children were in regular classes (77%) and in grades first through fifth (81%) attending public (80%) or parochial school (10%).

Ninety-one percent of the children lived in a house and were either the youngest (34%) or the oldest (37%).

Parents of the children were educated and had either graduated from high school (23%), had some college (31%), or graduated from college (24%). Fathers were mostly employed, doing skilled work (19%), business management (13%), or working as a health professional (14%). Sixty-eight percent of the fathers indicated that this was their first marriage.

Mothers were similar, having graduated from high school (22%), attended some college (33%), or were a college graduate (28%). Mothers were working in clerical positions (10%) or military service (24%) or not working outside the home (20%). Sixty-six percent of the mothers indicated that this was their first marriage.

In half of the sample, the father's job was primary (52%) as the main source of income. Parents with equal incomes were seen in 30% of the population. Eighty-four percent of the population defined themselves as middle class. Parents were mostly between the ages of 20 and 30 years when their child was born (98% for fathers and 90% for mothers).

Pregnancy

The mother's condition while pregnant was primarily normal (66%) without complication of bleeding, threatened miscarriage, or high blood pressure (93%–94%). Fifty-eight percent indicated no use of alcohol, and only 1% drank alcohol frequently. However, 52% smoked cigarettes (keep in mind that this study dates back to 1989), but only 3% reported smoking more than one pack of cigarettes per day. Sixty-four percent indicated no use of illegal drugs, and only 1% reported use of illegal drugs as a past event and not the result of current behavior. Forty-nine percent did not take prescription drugs, and only 11% reported current use.

Half of the births were reported as normal (57%). Long labor was indicated for 13%, prematurity for 9%, and Caesarian section for 24%. The child's physical condition following birth was indicated as normal in 75% of the sample. Difficulty breathing was 5% and low birth weight was 6%.

Temperament

Parents responded to descriptors about their child's temperament before the age of 2 years and from the ages of 2 to 5 years. Parents were able to respond to several descriptors describing their child.

- *Before the age of 2 years*: The child's temperament was ranked as primarily active (61%), happy (82%), sociable (57%), alert (60%), affectionate (60%), curious (57%), and playful (66%).
- *Between the age of 2 and 5 years*: Comparing parent report for before the age of 2 years to 2–5 years indicated the following. The child's temperament was ranked with increased activity (61% before the age of 2 years to 74% for the age of 2–5 years).

Happiness remained the same (82%–81%) although sociability increased (57%–64%) and alertness declined (60%–53%). Being affectionate slightly increased (60%–66%) similar to curiosity (57%–62%) and playfulness (66%–67%). Temperament remained relatively stable (excluding activity), suggesting that these children were not behaviorally problematic and that problems tended to escalate with attention deficits becoming more glaring as school becomes more demanding and taxing. This would explain the increased level of activity, which could be related more to anxiety. It would also explain why more children were evaluated in the 1st through the 5th grades when school involves reading and writing and independent work.

Developmental Milestones

Seventy-two percent of the parents reported later development of physical skills (sitting, crawling, and reaching), while walking was within normal developmental limits (50% before 1 year and 44% by 1–1½ years). Talking was also within normal limits (32% before 1 year and 38% by 1–1½ years), whereas toilet training was somewhat later (28% at 2 years and 33% by 2–2½ years), which again is similar to what we know about this population and the problem of bedwetting (although bedwetting was only reported in 6% of the population). Problems with toilet training were indicated as more often moderately problematic (91%).

From age 2 to 5 years, the child's motor development was primarily seen as average (64%, 20% as advanced) and language was similar (54% as average and 31% as advanced), indicating that development is more than age appropriate for these early years. Social development was indicated as average in comparison to other children (70%) and 14% as advanced. Finally, mental development was indicated as average (55%) primarily or advanced (24%).

Current Health

At the time the children were evaluated, they reported having headaches (18%), stomachaches (17%), and muscle aches (10%). Illnesses reported by parents were more often ear infections (36%) and chicken pox (31%). There was a report of tonsillitis (9%) as well as asthma and pneumonia at 7%, representing the medical issues most often seen. The surgery most often that the child had was tonsillectomies at 13%. Children were under doctor care for allergies (10%–11%).

Sleep

Difficulty getting to sleep was reported in 12% of the children and sleeping too much at 31%.

Health of Parents

There were questions about the parent's health. The two symptoms rated more often for the mother was low back pain (18%) and problems with digestion (10%) compared to fathers who indicated hypertension (10%) and low back pain (12%). Alcohol problems were indicated as 17% for the fathers and 12% for drugs when the question was asked if anyone had alcohol or drug problems (mothers did not report substance abuse at 4% and 3%). The highest medical problem for the siblings had to do with lungs or breathing at 5%.

Peer Relationships

Children who were seen as being sociable between the ages of 2 and 5 years, at the time of evaluation, were being reported as having few close friends (29%) or no close friends (60%). Peer problems that were significant included being teased (22%), being rejected (18%), and having peers who had better grades (12%). The child's self-esteem was rated as mixed (60%) with only 24% indicating positive self-esteem.

Relationship with Parents and Household Management

The relationship with the parents was seen as both positive and negative (41%) parents were yelling (22%) and withdrawing privileges (28%). The highest reason for arguments in the home was about homework (18%) and chores (16%). Relationships with the siblings were seen primarily as both positive and negative (51%). Thirty percent were rated as either very positive or positive. Parents rated themselves as average in terms of strictness (75%). Responsibilities most often assigned to the child were setting the table for meals (16%), helping to clean up afterward (19%), and more often cleaning up their room (31%). Fifty percent of both parents used recognition and praise as the primary reinforcement.

Arguments were primarily over homework (18%) and chores (16%). Family relationships were seen as supportive (39%), warm, and close (41%).

Religion was important (49%) and somewhat important (34%).

Strong emphasis was placed upon achievement, which either strongly emphasized (29%) or emphasized (63%) achievement.

Sports Activities

Sports were apparently important; 41% of the children actively participated in games and 28% had a strong drive to win. Only 14% of the children did not participate in sports. Forty-one percent were in organized sports, 27% in neighborhood games, and 18% in individual sports.

School Experience

Children in the sample began kindergarten at the typical age of 5 years (70%) and did not tend to have any problems (53%) although 20% were afraid of school and 10% complained of being ill to avoid going to school. However, parents reported that 68% enjoyed school and 64% got along well with their teacher. Distractible behavior was attributed to 28% and activity to 27%. Performance in kindergarten was mostly average (62%).

Children generally began first grade at the age of 6 years (64%), and 70% did not have any problems when first starting. However, by the end of first grade, 50% enjoyed school and 20% felt neutral with 14% disliking school although 55% got along well with their teachers and 26 got along fairly well. Twenty percent of the children were reported as having to be disciplined frequently, 30% as distracted, and 23% as active. Grades were good for 24%, average for 32%, and poor for 15%, with only 14% getting excellent grades.

At the time of our testing, parents rated their child's strengths in school subjects as highest in math, science, and social studies with the weakest area as reading (26%). One of the highest skill strengths was pleasing the teacher and behaving correctly. Skill weaknesses reported more often were symptoms of paying attention in class, getting assignments done on time, and being careful and checking work.

Forty percent of the children completed homework assignments on a regular basis compared to 18% who rarely completed homework. Extra tutoring help was required (30%). The most problematic behaviors in the classroom reported by parents were talking out of turn (20%), being distractible (29%), and overly active (19%). Problems with attention and concentration in the classroom were primarily indicated as not getting assignments done (18%), materials disorganized or messy (16%), and forgetting teacher instruction (19%).

RESULTS OF THE CHILD NEUROPSYCHOLOGICAL HISTORY

The Child Neuropsychological History is a checklist that the parents completed provided demographic information about the parents as well as their child and the child's symptomatology. This measure has been in use since 2006 and replaced the Developmental History Form. Ninety-eight parents completed this form about their child providing historical and family information as well as their current and past symptoms. Symptoms were reported as historical, new or both new and historical. There was more of an indication of historical than new problems consistent with the lifelong diagnosis of ADD. Primary behavior problems present for the last 6 months or more with the highest percentages are described in the following:

- 74% had a hard time concentrating for long periods.
- 65% were highly distractible.
- 54% were often rude or interrupted other people.
- 50% were reported to be very fidgety.
- 49% frequently lost things needed for school.
- 43% could not remain seated.
- 43% frequently made noise while playing.
- 42% rarely followed instructions of others.

Developmental Milestones

For most of the population, development of gross motor skills, language, and self-help was within early to average limits. Eighty-seven percent of the children crawled, and 87% walked alone within early to average limits. Ninety percent of the children followed simple language commands, and 85% used single-word sentences within early to average limits. Seventy-eight percent toilet training was within early to average limits, and toilet training was easy for 66%.

Pregnancy and Birth

Pregnancy revealed the trend of slightly greater use of caffeine (52%) and tobacco was down (for the years 2004–2008) to 18%.

Children were born prematurely (63%) similar to that seen on the developmental checklist for the years 1989–2004. Fetal distress was present 13% of the time, and the remainder of possible issues (such as breathing and cord wrapped) fell below 10%.

Medical History

Medical history revealed that 46% had allergies, 21% brain infection or disease and fevers, 15% colds, 22% epilepsy, and 14% meningitis. All other conditions such as heart problems, oxygen deprivation, pneumonia, and poisoning were below 10%.

Twenty-seven percent of the children wore glasses. Twenty-seven percent had some type of therapeutic intervention (29% psychological and 26% speech).

Family Medical History

Family medical history was significant of attention 6% of the time, compared to learning disability at 24% and psychological problems and reading or spelling difficulties at 35%. This suggests that the more problematic outcome from attention problems is not attention but instead difficulties with reading or psychological upset.

Family Income

Family income was over $50,000 and above for 70% of the population.

School History

School history reflected that 47% were provided with special education services. Forty-three percent indicated problems within other children in class, and 16% had been retained or repeated a grade. Twenty percent had satisfactory grades, and 27% had grades of C and above.

Social Functioning

Socially, 33% had problems making friends, and 17% had difficulty getting along with their teacher. Twenty-two percent tended to get sick in the morning before school started.

RESULTS OF THE SLEEP EVALUATION QUESTIONNAIRE

The Sleep Evaluation Questionnaire was administered to only a small number of 20 parents and has been in use since 2008.

Parents reported that 41% of the children had bedtime resistance, 29% had difficulty falling asleep, 31% awakened during the night, 18% had difficulty falling back to sleep after awakening during the night, and 56% were difficult to awaken in the morning.

The most notable symptom were that 44% of the population were reported to have episodes of stopped breathing and 22% were reported to have restless sleep. Seventeen percent were reported to experience sweating when sleeping, daytime sleepiness, and nightmares.

Children did not have difficulty remaining in their room to sleep. Parents indicated that 89% slept in their own room, 83% in their own bed, and 78% woke up in their own room and in their own bed.

DESCRIPTION OF THE ADOLESCENT POPULATION

Descriptions of the adolescent and family background were recorded on two checklists, either one was administered. The Developmental History Checklist was the measure used until 2006. In 2006, the Child Neuropsychological History was used to record basic data on the child. The Sleep Evaluation Questionnaire was another measure in use from 2008 onward.

RESULTS OF THE DEVELOPMENTAL HISTORY CHECKLIST

The Developmental History Checklist was completed by 181 parents. Questions noted in the following address reasons for the evaluation, severity of the problem, school and academic issues, pregnancy and birth, health history, family relationships, emotions, and overall behavior. Percentages were computed for the individual questions from this measure, resulting in the following findings. This is the same checklist used for the children allowing comparisons to be made between what the parents of children reported versus parents of adolescents.

The parent is able to check off several reasons that led to them coming to our clinic for help or as their reason for referral.

Reason for Evaluation

Reasons for seeking evaluation for the adolescents were primarily related to their refusal to go to school and continued academic problems as well as additional emotional issues not seen in the child sample. The changes suggest that time spent trying to cope with either identified or unidentified ADD symptoms was having a more serious effect.

Parents of adolescents indicating refusal to go to school as a reason for referral were at 30% (compared to only 2% for the children). Academic problems were at 29% (which is decreased from 46% indicated for the children). Depression accounted for 14% of the population (compared to only 4% reported for the child sample). Suicidal actions accounted for 21% of the population (compared to only 2% for the child sample). Problems with thinking clearly were at 24% (compared to 14% for the child sample). Behavior problems in school were decreased to 4% (compared to 35% for the child sample).

Ninety-two percent of the parents indicated the referral problem as moderate to severe compared to 82% for the child population. This suggests that parents of adolescents waited longer for things to get better and came in when they did not and when it was clear that things were not working. Sixty-nine percent indicated the problem had been present for several years (compared to 49% for the children) pointing to the likelihood that there was again a hope that things would get better. Adolescents referred for evaluation and treatment were more of a last-ditch effort to try to address the issues and problems that accompany the long-term presence of ADD. This suggests the long-term presence of this disorder and reinforces the thinking that things do not get better and in fact worsen with time.

Attention Problems

The presence of attention problems was primarily seen as affecting academic performance (similar to the child population) and secondarily affecting relationships with family members as well as the adolescent's emotional health and behavior. To a lesser degree was the impact upon peer relationships (again similar to the child population). Only 27% had been treated before (likely with medication) with only partial success. A total of 19% had been treated without success and only 5% reported success. However, evaluation or reevaluation would probably not have been indicated if treatment had been successful. Generally, diagnosis had occurred without testing (or testing included an intellectual and achievement assessment and no attention measures) and was based upon self-report measures completed by the parent and teacher as was the gold standard at the time. On the child sample, only 19% had been treated previously with only partial success and only 7% without success.

Emotional Issues

In the adolescent population, other emotional problems were indicated such as depression (26%), anxiety (23%), suicidal actions (43%), and arguments with parents (61%). This suggests that the adolescents were clearly more emotional, and the problem had morphed from attention into something far bigger, which is what we typically see clinically. Following the track of increased anxiety, increased attention problems, and increased anxiety and depression that follows in a cyclical manner, emotions were clearly escalating.

Behavioral Issues

Behavior problems in school were indicated for 40% of the population. By the time of adolescence, depression had increased from 10% to 26%, anxiety from 19% to 23%, suicidal actions from 0% to 43%, and arguments with parents from 32% to 61%. Behavior problems in the home reported at 45% for the children were 0% for the adolescents. While the adolescents were not regarded as a behavior problem per se, they were seen as more argumentative and more emotional.

School History

The majority of adolescents were in full-time regular education classes, 71% similar to the children (with 14% on summer vacation). Parents tend to get their children evaluated during the summer after a bad year or in their determination to have a better year. Evaluation during the year occurs when things are escalating or in response to report card periods or school conferences. A greater proportion of adolescents were in the 7th and 8th grades (79%); most were attending public school (83%).

School began at the age of 5 years for kindergarten for 70% of the children. Sixty-six percent were reported to have enjoyed kindergarten, while 23% were neutral (similar to the children). Academic performance was seen by the parents as average to advanced for 81%.

By first grade, only 59% were reported as enjoying school. Twenty-six percent were indicated as being distracted by first grade although 68% retained average and overall good grades.

This declined slightly to 60% from the first grade onward for those who had average and good grades. Adolescents were seen as performing better in art followed by science and music. Weaknesses were noted for math, followed by English and reading.

Forty-nine percent were rarely completing homework assignments (compared to 18% for the children), suggesting less parental control over homework completion. Thirty-three percent were getting help or extra help from a tutor (children reported tutorial help 46% of the time).

Behavior problems requiring reprimand such as sitting somewhere else (near the teacher or in an isolated area) or being sent to the principal's office were present for 48% of the population.

Problems of attention and concentration occurring in the classroom (daydreaming, forgetting teacher instructions, disorganized or messy material, and not getting assignments done) were indicated for 71% of the population. Behavioral issues of acting without deliberation, difficulty sitting still, or being quiet were noted for 28% of the adolescents. Thirty-three percent were distractible (similar to the children).

The primary teacher concern indicated to the parents was failing to finish assignments at 18% (compared to 12% of children).

Education and Socio-Economic Background

The majority lived in a home (87%). Similar to the child population, 71% were either the youngest or oldest, suggesting a trend that either parents are more aware of the problems of their oldest and youngest child and/or perhaps this is a genetic trend. Sixty-five percent of the fathers or male caretakers had some college, a college degree, or extended degree. Sixty percent of the mother or female caretakers had some college, a college degree, or extended degree. Only 1% of the mothers were not employed outside of the home compared to 20% of the mothers from the child sample. Mothers tend to go to work around the time of adolescence of their children if initially stayed at home. Eighty-four percent identified themselves as middle class and 7% as upper class. Parents were primarily between the age of 20 and 39 (91% for fathers and 90% for mothers).

Pregnancy and Birth

Only 64% indicated a normal birth without any kind of a problem. Sixteen percent reported long labor, and 12% had complications with delivery (similar to the child population). Normal birth without any after birth problems was present in 73% of the population. Fifty-three percent reported infection (compared to 2% for the children), and 28% had jaundice (compared to 8% for the children), suggesting that the adolescents were a more vulnerable population, which would be consistent with why treatment with medication did not work, and the children were a more naive population in terms of not being diagnosed priorly.

Parents reported smoking cigarettes (52%) and 25% at less than one pack per day. Two percent reported use of illegal drugs, and 15% reported taking prescription drugs.

Temperament Characteristics

Parents reported temperament descriptors for children before the age of 2 years and between 2 and 5 years.

Before Age 2 Years

Parents indicated that their child was happy (81%), playful (66%), sociable (55%), alert (55%), active (53%), curious (49%), and calm (38%). Thirty-five percent were seen as affectionate (decreased from the children at 60%). All descriptions were similar to the children other than affectionate, again suggesting that perhaps the adolescents were a more vulnerable population and representing the nonresponders to medication.

Age 2–5 Years

Temperament reported from before the age of 2 years is compared to parental report on the age of 2–5 years. A decline was seen for happiness to 77% for age 2–5 years (from 81% before the age of 2 years), playfulness to 58% (from 66%), calmness to 26% (from 38%), and alertness to 48% (from 55%). Temperament remained similar or the same for socialness at 54% (from 55%). Activity was slightly increased at 58% (from 53% and compared to 74% of the children) and curiosity at 53% (from 49%).

Developmental Milestones

Seventy-two percent developed later than most children for physical skills (similar to the children) establishing this group as less coordinated, a phenomenon seen clinically. Talking and walking occurred by 1½ years for 71% and 94% of the population. Sixty-six percent were toilet trained between 2 and 3 years similar to the child sample. Ninety-eight percent were average to advanced for motor development (motor development is different than the coordination of physical skills). Language development was reported as average or advanced for 88%. Social development was indicated as average or advanced for 81% and 84% for mental development. Birth issues and vulnerability did not significantly affect basic development.

Current Health Symptoms

The primary health issue was ear infections were at 27% (children were 36%). A normal increase for height and weight was at 21% (compared to children at 32%). There was more complaint of headaches at 26% (compared to 18% of the children).

Sleep

Difficulty getting to sleep was reported for 18% (compared to 12% of the children), and 9% of the adolescents were seen as not getting enough sleep (compared to 5% of the children). Five percent of the adolescents were reported to be falling asleep in school (compared to 1% for the children). Twelve percent refused to get up in the morning (compared to 6% of the children). Almost complete reduction of enuresis (bedwetting) and encopresis (soiling) was noted at 93% compared to 72% for the children.

Family Relationships

Relationships with parents had declined. Only 16% of the parents indicated a very positive relationship with their child compared to 32% for the children. Seeing the relationship as both positive and negative was at 60% compared to 41% for the children indicating the difference in the relationships between adolescents and parents (which may be more typical of adolescence and not necessarily ADD). Forty-nine percent of the parents used withdrawal of privileges or grounding for discipline similar to the children.

Relationships with siblings declined in adolescence; 67% of the parents rated these relationships as both positive and negative (compared to the children at 51% for reported positive and negative relationships with siblings). Sibling relationships that were rated as positive and very positive were only 20% for the adolescents compared to 30% for the children.

Overall family relationships revealed deterioration; 23% of the parents indicated frequent arguments (14% indicated for children), 37% reported relationships as supportive, and 29% as warm and close (compared to 41% indicated for the children). Achievement was emphasized in the home at 95%.

Household Chores

Chores and responsibilities had changed with age. Thirteen percent were doing yard work (compared to 6% for children) and 15% taking out the garbage (compared to 10% of the children), which is also more adolescent specific. Only 23% of the adolescents cleaned their room compared to 31% of the children. Either the parents gave up on the room being significant to them and/or the room became less important as the adolescent was capable of performing other chores. Generally, it is easier to close the door than argue.

Thirty-nine percent of the adolescents received an allowance if the chores were done, and 19% received an allowance regardless of completed chores.

Arguments were primarily over homework (18%) and school (10%). Bedtime was less of an argument than the children at 5% versus 14% for the children.

Social and Peer Relationships

There were more friendships reported for the adolescents; 46% had several or many close friends (compared to 10% indicated for the children). The presence of having few or no close friends in adolescence was declined at 54% compared to 89% for the children, suggesting improved social relationships in adolescence.

Being teased by peers was reported 14% of the time (compared to 22% for the children). However, 11% had friends who engaged in delinquent behavior (compared to 3% for the children). Twenty-two percent had peers with better grades (compared to 12% of the children) showing the trend of improved social relationships, but decreased grades with respect to friends and more risk of associating with those in trouble with the law.

Self-Esteem

As expected, self-esteem showed a decline in adolescence; 17% indicated that their adolescent child had very positive and positive self-esteem (compared to 31% for the children), 52% indicated mixed/positive and negative self-esteem (compared to 60% for the children), and 30% were negative and very negative (compared to 9% for the children). Declining self-esteem is not surprising given what we know in terms of increased school difficulties and the attention problem becoming more apparent and less hidden.

Sports

Participation in games offers another method to increase self-esteem when school is going poorly. Forty percent reported active participation, and 28% had a strong drive to win, very similar to the report for the children. Eighty-two percent participated in some type of sports by the time of adolescence, which is similar to the children, suggesting this as an outlet to cope with the school difficulties. Sports are often the only area the child or adolescent feels on an equal playing field.

Current Emotional Descriptors

Adolescents were described as more moody (12% vs. 8% for the children), not as happy (9% vs. 13% for the children), and more unhappy (8% vs. 3% for the children). Parental description of the adolescent at the time of the referral was considerably more negative than when the same child was described by their parent for the age range of 2–5 years. Happiness was at 9% (compared to 77%) calm at 2% (compared to 26%) and active temperament at 11% (compared to 58%).

RESULTS OF THE PERSONAL HISTORY CHECKLIST FOR ADOLESCENTS

The Personal History Checklist for Adolescents was completed by 109 adolescents who responded to questions about their history, general background, and the background of their family. Some items had more than one response that could be indicated. This measure was in use until 2004.

Reason for Evaluation

Adolescents reported that their reason for seeking an evaluation was more often at the request of their parent (58%), and only 8% reported coming in as a result of their own decision. Other reasons included physician (12%) or school referral (11%). The primary problem indicated was that of school grades (34%) although 15% reported problems with school behavior. Eleven percent reported problems thinking clearly, 9% reported depression and arguments with parents, and 5% reported anxiety. Sixty-four percent indicated that their problem was moderate to severe, and 60% indicated that the problem had been ongoing for several years. This suggests that when adolescents finally agreed to evaluation, it was because things were clearly escalating for them in their life. Up to this point in time, their methods used to get by had been successful. Primarily, the consequences were the impact to their performance at school (40%) and their relationship with their parents (24%) similar to that reported by the parents.

Either adolescents were dealing with problems that have exacerbated (often symptoms were present in elementary years although not identified as problematic) or treatment for attention problems had not been successful or were no longer successful. In my experience, treatment that relies solely upon medication loses its effect after the initial honeymoon period. Either the medication is not sufficient to change the already embedded patterns of avoidance of homework, poor study habits, and reading difficulties and/or increased medication results in unwanted side effects. More often, the failure of medication to fix overtly seen attention problems would seem to suggest that the problem is far greater than attention symptoms and more a lifestyle of avoidance and procrastination spurred by a dislike of school, low frustration tolerance (due to prior failure), and escalating anxiety. The primary problem of reading comprehension is what seems to change the tide between those who like and dislike school.

In this sample, 54% of the adolescents reported not being treated before; 4% were treated with success, 20% with only partial success, 10% were treated without success, and 5% did not want to cooperate when initially diagnosed. Thirty-three percent were currently taking medication for ADHD, and 30% had taken medication in the past. Adolescents' reported reasons for consenting to the testing were arguments with parents (23%), problems thinking clearly (19%), and anxiety (12%).

The oldest and youngest children were identified more than the middle child for attention problems, whether as a result of being the first born with higher expectations or the youngest with higher expectations and more parental time to devote to their issues. This is the same trend seen on the parent self-report measures. Forty-three percent were the oldest child, and 28% were the youngest child.

School and Work History

Sixty-nine percent were in full-time regular classes with only 9% receiving either part- or full-time special education help or support. Seventeen percent were in the 8th grade, and 67% in high school (9th to 12th grade). Seventy-five percent were attending public school and 19% private or parochial school. Forty-one percent were employed part time, and 42% were not employed or looking for a job. The majority of the adolescents had not worked full time (91%) or part time at (60%).

School was not initially indicated as problematic, which is different from the child population; 81% reported no problems for kindergarten. By the first through 8th grade, however, only 53% were reporting no problems, and 10% were in a special class part time for learning issues. Average grades for this time period were indicated by 38%; only 22% indicated good grades, and 25% had poor grades, which is consistent with the report of poor grades being a primary reason for evaluation.

High school revealed increased problems. Twelve percent were anxious about starting high school, 19% were afraid they would not do well academically, and 17% were fearful of not doing well socially. Only 11% report good grades, and only 15% of the adolescents reported getting along well with their teachers, suggesting they liked school and their teachers.

Much of the time, the problem was more that of feeling neutral and not connected to school. Only 40% reported getting along well with all but a few teachers (likely the ones they were not getting their assignments done for). This is consistent with only 15% indicating that they actually enjoyed school.

Behavioral problems do erupt in high school; generally as a result of skipping school, 25% indicated having to be disciplined frequently or were suspended.

Thirty-two percent were involved in team sports and 25% in no activities while in high school. Math was indicated as both a strength and weakness; 19% indicated it as one of the stronger subjects and 18% as one of the weakest subjects. English was indicated as the strongest subject for 12% and 19% as one of the weakest subjects. Science was indicated as a stronger subject by 10% and a weaker subject by 19%.

Described Skill Strengths and Weaknesses

Only 2% indicated concentration as a strength and only 4% test taking. Only 9% indicated reading speed or comprehension as a strength. Only 5% indicated working hard and not giving up.

Weaknesses reported more often were that of handwriting, vocabulary and expression, spelling, and reading speed.

Few of the adolescents saw themselves as a good student; 19% classified themselves as good to excellent students although only 6% saw themselves as a poor student. Perhaps they did not think about themselves as a student at all and were simply trying to get through school.

Eighty-six percent of the adolescents planned to graduate from high school. Following high school, 45% planned to attain additional training by attending college, vocational school, or business school.

Socio-Economic Status

Eighty-nine percent lived in a house. Ninety-one percent reported being middle or upper class.

Fifty percent to fifty-four percent were a first marriage for each parent and 18%–24% a second marriage for each parent. Parents were in their 20s and 30s at the time of birth for 84%–88% of the population.

Education of Parents

Adolescents report their parents to be educated; 58% of the fathers had attended some college, graduated from college, and/or had an extended degree (master's or doctorate). Sixty-four percent of the mothers had attended some college and/or graduated from college and/or an extended degree.

Learning problems in school for both parents were indicated at 23% (there was little differentiation between mothers and fathers at 12% and 11%, respectively).

Birth Conditions

Conditions of birth were indicated as normal without any problems (51%), while 35% reported either premature birth, long labor, or complications with delivery. Illnesses indicated more often were ear infections (14%), chicken pox (22%), and tonsillitis, asthma, allergies, and pneumonia (23%), and 16% had tonsillectomies as a child. At the time of evaluation, 13% were being treated for asthma or allergies, and 22% were treated in the past for asthma and allergies.

Sleep

The presence of sleep problems were indicated by the adolescents, 30% reported trouble getting to sleep and waking up a lot at night, and 18% reported not getting enough sleep. Only 20% reported no sleep problem at all. Other symptoms were not feeling rested (13%), restlessness (7%), and waking up too early in the morning (8%).

What we see in the clinic more often in the adolescents is not getting enough sleep for various reasons including staying up late to get homework done that takes them twice as long (due to poor reading comprehension and study habits). As they continue to get poor sleep and sleep deprivation sets in, the problem only becomes worse. Adolescents seem to have significant time management issues and a pervasive lack of balance between friend and social obligations and school and family obligations.

If they try to maintain a part-time job once they are driving, this seems to only heighten the problematic picture. Then there is the need to belong to social clubs and activities to promote getting into college, factors today that have become more predominant recently to a greater degree than this sample between 1989 and 2009.

Peer Relationships

During elementary school years, 38% indicated few or no close friends during elementary school years, and 40% indicated getting into trouble frequently or all of the time.

Socially things were better, however, still problematic; 59% either were not currently dating or had never dated. Twenty-two percent reported few or no close friends indicating that social issues beginning at the age of 5 –12 years have remained problematic through time.

Family Relationships

Eighteen percent reported not getting along with their siblings, and 11% had parents who were divorced. Family relationships were indicated as supportive, warm, and close (72%). Parents were described as being average to permissive (68%) and 20% as strict or very strict.

Adolescents reported more arguments with their parents over homework, followed by chores, and school in general. Discipline was primarily withdrawal of privileges and yelling at 46%. Lectures and grounding were at 36%.

Relationships with parents were seen as positive or very positive 36% of the time and both positive and negative 46% of the time. Relationships with siblings were seen as both positive and negative 35% of the time.

Family relationships were described by 60% as being mostly supportive, warm, and close. Forty-two percent felt they were important in the family. Eleven percent reported physical abuse; 14% reported emotional, physical, and sexual abuse; and 7% reported feeling neglected.

Alcohol and drug use was reported for 11%, and 6% had legal problems. Twenty-one percent indicated that they used to smoke and were not smoking presently, while 13% were continuing to smoke. Eighteen percent reported occasional drinking. Past drug use was 8%, and current occasional use was 6%. More often, the drug was marijuana (17%). Police involvement was 38% for various issues from curfew violation to drinking, drug use, assault, and theft.

Parental Substance Abuse

Twenty-two percent of the mothers were indicated to have alcohol problems compared to 14% of the fathers. Fifteen percent of the mothers and 6% of the fathers were indicated to have had drug problems.

Hobbies and Recreation

Adolescents responded to the question of what they do for fun; 23% indicated they play video or computer games or work on the computer. Eleven percent reported listening to music, and 10% talk on the phone. Only 7% indicated reading.

Home Responsibilities

The adolescents described their home responsibilities and chores; 25% indicated cleaning up their room, 14% indicated homework, 12% helped to clean up after meals, 11% did yard work, and 10% did babysitting and taking out garbage.

Current Emotional Descriptors

Adolescents described themselves currently as happy and content, nervous, fearful, and moody. Only 7% described themselves as intelligent, pointing to the far and long-reaching consequences of a continual struggle with attention symptoms.

Temperament characteristics described through life ranged from shy to content to fearful and moody. Only 13% saw themselves as happy.

RESULTS OF THE CHILD NEUROPSYCHOLOGICAL HISTORY

This is completed by the parents of the adolescents beginning in 2006 providing demographic information about themselves as well as their child. Fifty-one parents completed this form about their children, providing historical and family information as well as their current and past symptoms. Behaviors seen more often in the last 6 months were the following:

- 76% had a hard time concentrating for long periods.
- 57% reported being highly distractible.
- 55% frequently lost things needed for school.
- 54% rarely followed others' instructions.
- 43% reported being very fidgety.
- 40% did not listen to other people.

Pregnancy and Birth

Parents described their pregnancy accompanied by the following: 33% reported using caffeine, 50% reported premature birth and 26% late, and 19% indicated birth by Caesarian section.

Birth was reported as generally intact for 89%; 91% indicated first Apgar scores of 8 and 9 and second Apgar between 9 and 10.

Developmental Milestones

A developmental history was reported; 81% indicated average attainment for gross motor (although 85% reported late walking), 75% indicated late attainment of language for following simple commands, 71% indicated average attainment for using single-word sentences, 83% indicated average attainment for self-help skills, and 67% reported easy toilet training.

Health History

Information reported on prior diseases and diagnosed disorders indicated the presence of allergies (55%) and excessive colds (23%). Forty-one percent indicated use of glasses, 39% had psychological therapy, and 31% had reading or spelling difficulties, suggesting more additional issues than the child population.

Household Income

Family income was indicated to be over $50,000 in 72% of the population.

School History

Parents reported that 48% had special education services, 31% problems with other children in class, 37% difficulty making friends, and 39% had grades of C through F.

Unlike the child population, parents of adolescents reported higher percentages of new symptoms, suggesting that they were seeking evaluation due to problems arising that had not been present before. The most problematic behavior seen in the last 6 months was maintaining concentration.

DESCRIPTION OF THE ADULT POPULATION

Adults completed the Personal History Checklist from 1989 to 2006 when replaced by the Adult Neuropsychological History.

RESULTS OF THE PERSONAL HISTORY CHECKLIST FOR ADULTS

Adults completed the *Personal History Checklist for Adults*. There were 985 adults who completed this measure asking general questions about their reason for seeking evaluation, medical history, socio-economic status (living conditions as a child and adult), education (experiences in school for different grades), job history, current medical information, sleep, and substance abuse.

Reason for Referral

The primary reason for referral indicated for almost one-half of the population was problems thinking clearly. One-third reported depression as the primary reason for referring themselves for evaluation at our clinic. In response to a question about the problems they were having, approximately one-third were equally divided in reporting symptoms of depression (29%), anxiety (31%), and problems thinking clearly (35%).

Socio-Economic Status

One-half of the population came from the suburbs, and 80% were upper class.

Health History

Health was not indicated as highly problematic. Almost two-thirds reported normal birth. Ten percent indicated a long labor and 9% complications with delivery. Developmental milestones were reported as early for over one-half of the population, and 84% were within normal limits or above. Childhood illness was more often that of chicken pox (43%) followed by measles and mumps (26% and 20%).

One-third (35%) of the adults were being treated for low back pain possibly related to the type of work they did. Slightly less than one-fourth (21%) had problems with their digestive system, and 14% had problems breathing.

Slightly less than one-third (30%) were not smoking but used to smoke, 28% were smoking, and 17% one pack or more each day. Forty-one percent had been smoking from 5 to more than 20 years indicating this as a historical issue.

Almost two-thirds (61%) reported drinking alcohol occasionally and 11% regularly to daily. For those who indicated that they were drinking, 35% reported three or more drinks. So while the problem of alcohol was not seen overall as a major issue, those who did drink may have had a significant problem. Alcohol was also tolerated more in prior years than it is today. Almost one-third (35%) had used illegal drugs in the past.

Sleep

Sleep was indicated as a problem on a number of different levels: sleep onset, waking up at night, sleep maintenance, not getting enough sleep, and not feeling rested. Seventy percent reported sleep problems of trouble getting to sleep, waking up at night, not getting enough sleep, waking up too early in the morning, and sleeping enough but not feeling rested.

School History

Average grades were reported by the adults for elementary and junior high although one-third felt neutral (36%) and one-third disliked school (33%). Eighty percent reported grades of average and above. However, almost one-half (47%) did have special classes for a learning disability, and almost one-half (45%) repeated a grade.

One-half (52%) of the adult population rarely got into trouble, although one-third (35%) frequently got into trouble. Ninety percent got along well with teachers or all but a few of their teachers. Problems indicated in eighth grade or junior high were that of anxiety and fear of not fitting in, making social issues of greater concern than academic. One-quarter (27%) worried about fitting in; almost one-quarter (23%) was anxious about starting high school and fearful of their academic performance (21%).

Average and above grades were reported for 69% of the population for high school for almost one-half of the sample. Two-thirds of the population felt neutral (38%) or did not like school (35%) leaving only 28% who reported actually enjoying school. While in high school, 88% reported getting along with their teachers or all but a few of their teachers. However, almost one-half (44%) reported being disciplined frequently, and 45% reported suspension. Most of the population graduated from high school (93%). A majority of the population (79%) had some type of educational pursuit beyond high school (junior college, college, and technical or vocational program).

Experiences as a teenager indicated that the majority of the population (71%) reported rarely getting into trouble.

Employment

Eighty-one percent of the population reported being employed, and only 8% reported being out of work for more than 1 year. Most of the population spent minimal if any time being unemployed. Forty-one percent did report being fired once from a job, 22% indicated being fired twice, and 24% indicated being fired three or more times, suggesting some issues of maintaining a job, which could be related to attention symptoms.

Daily Life

One-half of the population was married (49%) and only one time.

Money matters were more often the given reason for argument and financial problems often experienced in almost one-fourth of the population. Arguments occurred daily to weekly in 31% of the population.

Relationships within the family were described as good in 43% and fair to poor for 30%.

RESULTS OF THE ADULT NEUROPSYCHOLOGICAL HISTORY

The Adult Neuropsychological History was the self-report measure used from 2006. The Adult Neuropsychological History provided demographic information about the adult population as well as symptomatology. There were 107 adults who completed this form and responded to these questions about their functioning and past history. Symptoms were reported as historical, new or both new and historical. There was more indication of historical than new problems consistent with the lifelong diagnosis of ADD. The following are the responses to specific questions about the adult's functioning in the following areas: problem solving, language (speech and math skills), nonverbal skills, concentration and awareness, memory, motor and coordination, sensory, physical issues, emotions, and behavior.

Symptoms Reported Most Often

Adults reported significant symptoms of sadness or depression (63%), anxiety (64%), stress (75%), sleeping problems (53%), and becoming angry more easily (47%) as well as being more emotional (32%) and feeling like they do not care anymore (36%).

Health History

Birth was not indicated as problematic (80% were on time), and the time period after birth was devoid of problems indicated by 87% of the population. Maternal smoking was present 22% of the time. There was no indication of alcohol abuse (91%) or illness (95%).

Frequent ear infections were indicated in almost one-fourth of the population (24%) during childhood. Some type of head injury was noted for 12% and clumsiness and speech problems for 13%. History of physical illness during childhood was only significant for allergies (31%), chicken pox (59%), and measles (27%), suggesting that health was generally intact. The isolation of allergies is significant, which may relate to the sleep-disordered breathing issues and prior research, suggesting the relationship between attention symptoms and allergies.

Developmental milestones were within early to average limits for walking (95%), language (89%), toilet training (92%), and overall development (96%).

Current Health Symptoms

Almost one-third of the population (30%) reported a head injury, which may explain some of the memory issues noted that are not seen as consistent with a genetic attention disorder. Allergies were significantly seen and present in one-third of the population (39%) indicating this as an ongoing problem commencing in childhood, which may be related to sleep-disordered breathing issues. Arthritis was at 14%, hypertension at 12%, psychiatric problems at 10%, and thyroid disease at 12%.

Attention History

Attention problems were identified during childhood in almost one-half of the sample (43%). Hyperactivity was indicated in one-fourth of the population (25%) during childhood. Learning problems were indicated in almost one-fourth of the population (22%) during childhood.

Educational History

One-third of the population (32%) completed high school, almost one-quarter (23%) attended college, and one-third (33%) completed a bachelor's or graduate degree. Sixty-four percent pursued some type of education beyond high school. This would suggest an educated population in the community that sought evaluation for ADD as an adult. Receiving special services while in school was reported by almost one-third of the population (31%). Thirty-seven percent reported income over $50,000.

Substance Abuse History

One-third (36%) began drinking during teenage years (16–18 years) and another almost one-third began in late teens to early twenties (19–21 years). Almost one-half of the population indicated that they rarely drank or did not drink at all, while one-third (34%) indicated drinking 1–2 days per week, likely on the weekend. Problems with alcohol use and substance abuse were not reported to be highly problematic.

3 Description of Tests Administered

INPUT INTO THE BRAIN: IS THE INFORMATION GETTING INTO THE BRAIN FOR USE?

Seashore Rhythm Test

The Seashore Rhythm Test is a measure of fast-paced nonverbal basic brain input. The child or adult is asked to differentiate between 30 pairs of rhyming beats. It is utilized to provide a measure of basic brain input, as well as sustained attention capacity. This measure requires alertness to nonverbal auditory stimuli, sustained attention, and the ability to perceive and compare rhythmic sequences. Scoring is based upon a number of correct items resulting in the assigning of an NDS (Neuropsychological Deficit Score) ranked score. Ranked scores range from 0 to 3 where 0 means intact performance, 1 is mildly impaired, 2 is moderately impaired, and 3 is severely impaired (Boone and Rausch, 1989; Reitan and Wolfson, 1993). There are three trials. Errors tend to occur at the end of the trial or on the last trial when there are issues with sustained attention.

Speech–Sounds Perception Test

The Speech–Sounds Perception Test is a measure of slow-paced verbal input into the brain. This measure is also from the Halstead–Reitan Neuropsychological Test Battery. The test has a version for older children (i.e., age 9–14 years) and adults (15 years and older). This task is a measure of slow-paced, verbal stimuli and the ability to correctly distinguish the sound of nonsense syllables from a visual array of choices (Reitan and Wolfson, 1990). It consists of 60 spoken nonsense words, which are variants of the "ee" sound, and the subject responds by underlining one of the four alternatives printed for each item on the test form. This measure requires the ability to pay close and continued attention to the stimulus material. Very few errors are expected. Those with a genetic attention disorder tend to become bored on this measure, losing their focus, drawing pictures on the paper, or zoning out as a result (Fisher, 1998; Reitan and Wolfson, 1993).

INFORMATION PROCESSING: ANSWERS THE QUESTION OF WHETHER OR NOT THE INFORMATION IS GETTING PROCESSED TO GO TO OTHER AREAS OF THE BRAIN

Paced Auditory Serial Addition Test and Children's Paced Auditory Serial Addition Test

Information processing was assessed using the Paced Auditory Serial Addition Test (PASAT) and Children's Paced Auditory Serial Addition Test (CHIPASAT) (an average of the four trials of these measures was used in our research). These measures are tasks of serial addition, assessing the capacity and rate of information processing, as well as sustained and divided attention that also load on memory. There are four trials during which the subject is listening to a tape that is providing numbers in a specifically paced manner (which increases with each trial) and asked to add the previous number to the next number and to say the answer aloud. For the PASAT, all of the numbers are under 10, and the score is the number of errors or omitted items for each trial, which consists of approximately 45–50 items (Gronwall, 1977). For the CHIPASAT, all of the numbers are under 5, and the score is the number of correct items for each trial. The CHIPASAT is used in individuals age 9–15, and the PASAT is generally used in those age 16 and older (Spreen, 1998).

The test was originally designed by Gronwall and associates in 1977 for use with adults. This measure is thought to assess information processing and the tendency of ADD individuals to miss small details of information such as instructions and directions. In addition to information processing, performance can reflect sustained attention deficits and distractibility, as well as emotional issues of giving up in frustration, math phobia, and/or memory problems related to additional issues beyond that of a genetic attention disorder (Fisher, 1998). While arithmetic was not seen as having a significant impact, the lack of math fluency would result in poor scoring or an inability to complete the test. Three components are indicated: working memory, information processing capacity, and information processing speed (Shucard et al., 2004). Research has cited this measure as a measure of memory problems when there is substance abuse or a brain injury affecting memory processes (Hooker and Jones, 1987; Lundqvist, 2005; Macciocchi et al., 1996, Rapeli et al., 2011; Webbe and Ochs, 2003). This measure is sensitive to mild concussion and has been used to measure deficits in different populations such as head injury, sports concussion, and multiple sclerosis (Bate et al., 2001; Cohen et al., 2002; Webbe and Ochs, 2003). Marijuana use has an effect on PASAT performance (Lundqvist, 2005). When individuals perform poorly, it is the result of omitting items and not responding as opposed to incorrect responses (Schachinger et al., 2003). In our experience when an individual adds an incorrect number, it is typically due to either adding the answer or adding a different number significant of a possible memory problem and presenting evidence of an attention disorder beyond that of a genetic attention problem or ADHD plus.

Another measure that is used as part of the battery of tests to measure information processing but is not part of the testing presented in this book is the Wisconsin Card Sorting Test. This measure is used clinically to address the question of whether the individual figures out things by using deductive reasoning, which is a common pattern seen with ADD/ADHD and responsible for assumptions that they are right most of the time.

DISTRACTIBILITY: VULNERABILITY TO BECOMING DISTRACTED BY SOUNDS IN THE ENVIRONMENT OR INTERNAL THOUGHTS

THE STROOP COLOR–WORD TEST

The Stroop Color–Word Test is a measure of divided attention assessing distractibility and the ease with which the individual is able to shift from a habitual response to perform the interference task. It is appropriate for use of age 7 through adulthood. The individual has 45 s to read the word and 45 s to complete the interference task. Comparisons are made to their performance of word reading versus the interference task as well as obtaining a normative data T-score (where 50 is average and 10 is the standard deviation). A T-score and interference score are derived and are age adjusted (Stroop, 1935).

When used in the diagnosis of ADHD adults, this measure has been found to involve multiple stages of attentional demand necessitating the recruitment of different brain regions (Burgess et al., 2010; Hervey et al., 2004). Chang et al. (2012) used this measure to assess effects of distractibility and exercise, finding that exercise may have calmed down the anxiety present in children sufficiently to improve Stroop scores and diminish perseverative errors.

This measure was originally developed in 1935 and modified in 1976. We have found through the years that those who have a problem on this task show an interference score that is one-half to two-thirds less than the word score (Fisher, 1998). This suggests that while able to read the words, there is a significant problem in completing the interference task, demonstrating the impact of problematic divided attention.

Another measure of distractibility that is used but not part of the testing presented in this book is a measure of cancellation showing the pattern of working through distractibility over the course of four trials by cancelling out a specific stimulus or object. Scoring is by observation and clinical analysis for time, pattern of response, and omitted items.

TESTS OF SPEED: MEASUREMENT OF SLOW THINKING (COGNITIVE) SPEED AND THE IMPACT OF PROBLEMATIC VISUAL SPATIAL ANALYSIS

SYMBOL DIGIT MODALITIES TEST

Symbol Digit Modalities Test (SDMT) is a measure of whole brain functioning given the factors of speeded processing, short-term memory, scanning ability, the use of numbers and symbols, and writing the correct number to correspond to a particular key of symbols. The SDMT was originally published in 1973 and revised in 1982 and is appropriate for individuals aged 8 years and above. Scoring represents the number of correct responses under a specific time frame for written and oral conditions (i.e., SDMT-W and SDMT-O) (Smith, 1982). The individual is asked to use a key to put the correct numbers with the correct symbol, and they have 90 s to complete as many items in order as they can. Those who have problems with visuospatial analysis tend to confuse three pairs of items, which either slows down the time taken to complete the task, creates errors, or both of these events occur.

This measure is completed using a written format and then an oral format (where the person is saying their responses out loud to the examiner). Yeudall et al. (1986) found higher scores for the oral version. Unless affected by distractibility, we will typically see higher scores on the oral portion for the ADD population.

This measure operates as a screening device to measure the general integrity and functioning of the brain. A score on the SDMT that falls 1–1.5 standard deviations below the mean should be considered suggestive of cerebral dysfunction (Smith, 1991). Problematic performance has been related to brain injury (Felmingham et al., 2004) and sleep apnea (Verstraeten et al., 2004). This test has been used to differentiate multiple sclerosis subtypes and in Huntington's disease research (Huijbregts et al., 2004; Lemiere et al., 2002). This is one of the measures that has typically been a differentiating factor to look at another disorder beyond that of a genetic attention problem. It is seen as one of the more sensitive tests in neuropsychology (Strauss et al., 2006). It can also provide a measure of someone's potential that is often not seen on the other attention scores. Normative data are available from age 8 years through adulthood.

TRAIL MAKING TESTS

The Trail Making Tests are subtests from the Halstead–Reitan Neuropsychological Test Battery used for age 8 to adulthood. There are two versions, one for age 8–14 years and the other for 15 years through adulthood. The adult measure for age 15 years and up is longer than the children's version. These tasks are designed to measure cognitive flexibility as well as the ability to switch sets, with visual spatial and sequencing components. Trail Making Test Part A is a measure of sequential ability and the ability to spatially move across a page of numbers in sequential order as quickly as possible. The score is the time taken to complete the task, which is compared to specific age range normative data. Errors are corrected during the task and counted as part of the time score. Trail Making Test Part B is a measure of switching sets, requiring the individual to maintain a particular set while switching to the next set using numbers and letters in sequential order. The score is the time taken to complete the task, which is compared to specific age range normative data (Reitan, 1958).

This test is a measure of speed of visual search, attention, mental flexibility, and motor function. The test was originally part of the Army Individual Test Battery in 1944 and was added by Reitan to the Halstead battery (Reitan and Wolfson, 1985, 1992). Part B is more sensitive to damage to the brain (frontal lobe regions). Reitan and Wolfson (2004) suggest Part B as a useful indicator of neurological integrity in adults and children, a screening device to determine the need for additional neuropsychological assessment. This test is sensitive to traumatic brain injury, and completion times increase with the severity of the injury (Felmingham et al., 2004).

We have found it important to distinguish between the types of errors obtained (confusion and/or loss of place versus inability to perform the task) as opposed to the time. Part B is one of the tests used to question the presence of an additional disorder beyond that of a genetic attention problem. Individuals can take longer to perform well without mistakes (Fisher, 1998). Visual spatial issues typically occur at the end of Trail Making Part A, resulting in one error commonly occurring. Errors on the Part B portion occur when it is difficult to keep one's place and remember the letter or number as well as what comes next. Sometimes, individuals have to count through the entire alphabet (in the manner they likely learned it) to get to one letter.

SYMBOL SEARCH TEST

The Symbol Search Test is a measure of processing speed. The score is how many correct items can be completed within 120 s. Scoring is compared to normative data for specific age range and assigned a scaled score (10 is average and 3 is the standard deviation). This subtest is from the Wechsler intellectual assessments.

COLOR FORM AND PROGRESSIVE FIGURES

The Color Form and Progressive Figures are similar in concept to the Trail Making Tests. These are tests from the Reitan–Indiana Neuropsychological Test Battery and used for children aged 5–8 years. These are measures employing the use of sequencing as well as switching of sets and cognitive flexibility.

The Color Form Test requires the child to move in sequential motion from color to shape and back to color. Errors are corrected while the time continues. Time taken to complete the task is the final score. The Progressive Figures task asks the child to go from inside to outside shape (the smaller to the larger version of the shape) and to recognize the difference in the shapes. Errors are corrected while the time continues. Time taken to complete the task is the final score.

ESTIMATE OF INTELLECTUAL ABILITY AND MEASUREMENT OF DECODING ERRORS THAT LEAD TO READING COMPREHENSION DIFFICULTIES

NATIONAL ADULT READING TEST-REVISED

The purpose of National Adult Reading Test-Revised (NART-R) is to provide an estimate of intellectual abilities. This measure was used for both the adolescents and the adult population. Individuals are asked to read a list of words out loud. The NART-R is a test of premorbid (prior to the onset of other disorders) measure of intelligence and provides an estimate of the person's intellectual ability. This measure was adapted for use in the United States and was originally developed using a British sample (Blair and Spreen, 1989; Grober and Sliwinski, 1991). The value of the test lies in its high correlation between reading ability and intelligence in the normal population (Crawford et al., 1989a,b), and it is seen as a good instrument to assess premorbid intelligence. This measure also serves to demonstrate reading recognition errors that can lead to errors in reading comprehension when the word tends to be read incorrectly due to deleting sounds or just using the first few initial letters. Words are often read incorrectly when it is obvious that the person knows the word and is familiar with it.

WECHSLER TEST OF ADULT READING

Wechsler Test of Adult Reading (WTAR) is similar to the NARDT-R and was developed for use as an intellectual estimate and conormed with the Wechsler Adult Intelligence Scale (WAIS-III) and Wechsler Memory Scale (WMS-III) and covers a wide age range from 16 to 89 years (Langeluddecke and Lucas, 2004).

REFERENCES

Bate, A.J., Mathias, J.L., and Crawford, J.R., (2001) Performance on the test of everyday attention and standard tests of attention following severe traumatic brain injury, *The Clinical Neuropsychologist*, 15(3), 405–422.

Blair, J.R. and Spreen, O., (1989) Predicting premorbid IQ: A revision of the National Adult Reading Test, *The Clinical Neuropsychologist*, 3, 129–136.

Boone, K.B. and Rausch, R., (1989) Seashore Rhythm Test performance in patients with unilateral temporal lobe damage, *Journal of Clinical Psychology*, 45(4), 614–618.

Burgess, G.C., Depue, B.E., Ruzic, L., Willcutt, E.G., Du, Y.P., and Banich, M.T., (2010) Attentional control activation relates to working memory in attention-deficits/hyperactivity disorder, *Biology Psychiatry*, 67, 632–640.

Chang, Y.-K., Liu, S., Yu, H.-H., and Lee, Y.-H., (2012) Effect of acute exercise on executive function in children with attention deficit hyperactivity disorder, *Archives of Clinical Neuropsychology*, 27, 225–237.

Cohen, J.A. et al., (2002) Benefit of interferon β-1a on MSFC progression in secondary progressive MS, *Neurology*, 59, 679–687.

Crawford, J.R., Stewart, L.E., Besson, J.A.O., Parker, D.M., and DeLacey, G., (1989a) Prediction of the WAIS IQ with the National Adult Reading Test: Cross-validation and extension, *British Journal of Clinical Psychology*, 28, 267–273.

Crawford, J.R., Stewart, L.E., Cochrane, R.H.B., Parker, D.M., and Besson, J.A.O., (1989b) Construct validity of the National Adult Reading Test: A factor analytic study, *Personality and Individual Differences*, 10, 585–587.

Felmingham, K.L., Baguley, L.J., and Green, A.M., (2004) Effects of diffuse axonal injury on speed of information processing following a severe traumatic brain injury, *Neuropsychology*, 18(3), 564–571.

Fisher, B.C., (1998) *Attention Deficit Disorder Misdiagnosis; Approaching ADD from a Brain-Behavior/ Neuropsychological Perspective for Assessment and Treatment*, CRC Press, Boca Raton, FL.

Grober, E. and Sliwinski, M., (1991) Development and validation of a model for estimating premorbid intelligence in the elderly, *Journal of Clinical and Experimental Neuropsychology*, 13, 933–949.

Gronwall, D.M., (1977) Paced auditory serial-addition task: A measure of recovery from concussion, *Perceptual and Motor Skills*, April, 44(2), 367–373.

Hervey, A.S., Epstein, J.N., and Curry, J.F., (2004) Neuropsychology of adults with attention-deficit/ hyperactivity disorder: A meta-analytic review, *Neuropsychology*, 18(3), 485–503.

Hooker, W.D. and Jones, R.T., (1987) Increased susceptibility to memory intrusions and the stroop interference effect during acute marijuana intoxication, *Psychopharmacology*, 91(1), 20–24.

Hujibregts, S.C., Kalkers, N.E., de Sonnevile, L.M.J., de Groot, V., Reuling, J.E.W., and Polman, C.H., (2004) Differences in cognitive impairment of relapsing, remitting, secondary and primary progressive MS, *Neurology*, 63, 335–339.

Langeluddecke, P.M. and Lucas, S.K., (2004) Evaluation of two methods for estimating premorbid intelligence on the WAIS III in a clinical sample, *The Clinical Neuropsychologist*, 18, 423–432.

Lemiere, J., Decruyenaere, M., and Evers-Kiebooms, G., (2002) Longitudinal study evaluating neuropsychological changes in so called asymptomatic carriers of the Huntington's disease mutation after 1 year, *Acta Neurologica Scandinavica*, 106(3), 131–141.

Lundqvist, T., (2005) Cognitive consequences of cannabis, *Pharmacology, Biochemistry and Behavior*, June, 81(2), 319–330.

Macciocchi, S.N., Barth, J.T., Alves, W., Rimel, R.W., and Jane, J.A., (1996) Neuropsychological functioning and recovery after mild head injury in collegiate athletes, *Neurosurgery*, September, 39(3), 510–514.

Rapeli et al., (2011) Cognitive functioning in opioid dependent patients treated with buprenorphine, methadone and other psychoactive medication stability and correlates, *BMC Clinical Pharmacology*, 11, 13.

Reitan, R.M., (1958) Validity of the trail making test as an indicator of organic brain damage, *Journal of Perceptual Motor Skills*, 5(3), 265–272.

Reitan, R.M. and Wolfson, D., (1985) *The Halstead-Reitan Neuropsychological Test Battery: Theory and Clinical Interpretation*, Neuropsychology Press, Tucson, AZ.

Reitan, R.M. and Wolfson, D., (1990) The significance of the Speech- Sounds Perception Test for cerebral functions, *Archives of Clinical Neuropsychology*, 5(3), 265–272.

Reitan, R.M. and Wolfson, D., (1992) *Neuropsychological Evaluation of Older Children*, Neuropsychology Press, Tucson, AZ.

Reitan, R.M. and Wolfson, D., (1993) *The Halstead-Reitan Neuropsychological Test Battery: Theory and Clinical Interpretation*, 2nd edn., Neuropsychology Press, Tucson, AZ.

Reitan, R.M. and Wolfson, D., (2004) Trail making test as an initial screening procedure for neuropsychological impairment in older children, *Archives of Clinical Neuropsychology*, 19, 281–288.

Schachinger, H., Cox, D., Linder, L., Brody, S., and Keller, U., (2003) Cognitive and psychomotor function in hypoglycemia: Response error patterns and retest reliability, *Pharmacology, Biochemistry and Behavior*, 75, 915–920.

Shucard, J.L., Parrish, J., Shucard, D.W., McCabe, D.C., Benedict, R.H.D., and Ambrus, J., (2004) Working memory and processing speed deficits in systemic lupus erythematosus as measured by the Paced Addition Serial Attention Test, *Journal of the International Neuropsychological Society*, 10, 35–45.

Smith, A., (1982) *Symbol Digits Modalities Test*, Western Psychological Services, Los Angeles, CA.

Spreen, O. and Strauss, E., (1998) *A Compendium of Neuropsychological Tests*, Oxford University Press, New York.

Strauss, E., Sherman, E., and Spreen, O., (2006) *A Compendium of Neuropsychological Tests*, 3rd edn., Oxford University Press, New York.

Stroop, J.R., (1935) Studies of interference in serial verbal reactions, *Journal of Experimental Psychology*, 18, 643–661.

Verstraeten, E., Cluydts, R., Pevernagie, D., and Hoffman, G., (2004) Executive function in sleep apnea: Controlling for attentional capacity in assessing executive attention, *Sleep*, 27(4), 685–693.

Webbe, F.M. and Ochs, S.R., (2003) Recency and frequency of soccer heading interact to decrease neurocognitive performance, *Applied Neuropsychology*, 10(1), 31–41.

Yeudall, L.T., Fromm, D., Reddon, J.R., and Stefanyk, W.O., (1986) Normative data stratified by age and sex for 12 neuropsychological tests, *Journal of Clinical Psychology*, 42, 918–946.

4 Child Neuropsychological Testing for ADD/ADHD

The age range was 5–11 years. Children were administered the following test measures:

Age 5–6 years:

- Wechsler Preschool and Primary Scale of Intelligence Scale for Children (WPPSI-R or WPPSI-III)
- Symbol Search Test (WPPSI-R or WPPSI-III)
- Progressive Figures Test
- Color Form Test

Age 7 years:

- Wechsler Preschool and Primary Scale of Intelligence Scale for Children (WPPSI-R or WPPSI-III)
- Stroop Color Word Test
- Symbol Search Test (WPPSI-R or WPPSI-III or WISC-III or WISC-IV)
- Progressive Figures Test
- Color Form Test

Age 8 years:

- Wechsler Intelligence Scale for Children (WISC-III or WISC-IV)
- Symbol Digit Modalities Test (SDMT)
- Stroop Color Word Test
- Trail Making Tests Part A and B
- Symbol Search Test
- Progressive Figures Test
- Color Form Test
- Children's Paced Auditory Serial Addition Test (CHIPASAT)

Age 9–11 years:

- Wechsler Intelligence Scale for Children (WISC-III or WISC-IV)
- Symbol Digit Modalities Test (SDMT)
- Stroop Color Word Test
- Trail Making Tests Part A and B
- Seashore Rhythm Test
- Speech–Sounds Perception Test
- Symbol Search Test
- Children's Paced Auditory Serial Addition Test (CHIPASAT)

Additional measures for the attention battery include the Bender Visual Motor Gestalt Test, Wisconsin Card Sorting Test, and the Cancellation Test. These measures were more difficult to analyze statistically and were not included in the study.

SUMMARY OF PERFORMANCE FALLING WITHIN AVERAGE AND ABOVE LIMITS (ABOVE AVERAGE TO SUPERIOR) CHILDREN

SDMT
  Written: 84%
  Oral: 80%
Stroop: 76%
Trail Making Part A Time: 87%
Trail Making Part A No Errors: 78%
Trail Making Part B Time: 80%
Trail Making Part B No Errors: 63%
Color Form: 79%
Progressive Figure: 86%
Seashore Rhythm Test Intact Score: 25%
Speech–Sounds Perception Test Intact Score: 51%
Symbol Search: 77%
CHIPASAT: 37%

Trends are reported based upon percentages obtained from the data composed of z-scores, T-scores, and standard scores.

In comparing the children to themselves, the measure of whole-brain functioning (SDMT) was not highly problematic although the oral score was slightly worse than the written score and although distractibility measured on the Stroop was somewhat more problematic, which would explain the lower oral score. It would be expected that saying numbers out loud would result in higher scores than writing them down; however, this was not the case. Suggested is that distractibility was the reason.

On speeded testing, the children had more difficulty when going from one shape to another involving the discrimination of shapes on the Progressive Figures task than when they had to remember whether they were going from form to shape (or vice versa) on the Color Form task. The Trail Making Test revealed more of a problem with errors than with time. More males than females sacrificed time for errors. Children had more difficulty on a speeded processing task (Symbol Search) when unable to compensate with thinking, and speed was the primary variable.

On input tasks, they had more difficulty on the fast-paced input task (Seashore Rhythm) than the slow-paced task (Speech–Sounds). Performance of the children on the input tasks was more problematic than the adolescents, which may be the result of almost 50% of this population being diagnosed with ADHD plus an additional disorder. The children had the most difficulty on the paced addition task (CHIPASAT) assessing information processing, and it was not unusual to find children who did not have either the necessary math fluency or memory sufficient to complete this task. This measure yielded the lowest results for the children.

RESULTS OF THE SPECIFIC TEST MEASURES

WISC IQ TEST

Full Scale IQ

The Wechsler Intelligence Scale for Children was administered to children aged 8–11 years. The Full Scale IQ is the average of the Verbal and Performance IQ values, which was completed on the children. Ninety-six percent of all children were within average limits and above for overall

Full Scale IQ, which includes low average functioning. If low average functioning is not included, then 83% fell within pure average limits and above, which is consistent with the adolescent data, pointing to intellectual levels not being problematic when considering an attention disorder. Females were slightly higher at 98% and males at 95 for all children functioning within average limits and above. The percentage was 84 for pure average and above functioning for females and 82 revealing slightly lower scoring for males than females.

Children

447 children completed this measure.

- 11% were at 121 and above (superior).
- 16% were at 111–120 (high average to above average).
- 56% were at 91–110 (average).
- 13% were at 80–90 (low average).
- 5% were at 79 and below (borderline, below average to well below average).

Females

130 females completed this measure (29%).

- 10% were at 121 and above (superior).
- 16% were at 111–120 (high average to above average).
- 58% were at 91–110 (average).
- 14% were at 80–90 (low average).
- 2% were at 79 and below (borderline, below average to well below average).

Males

317 males completed this measure (71%).

- 11% were at 121 and above (superior).
- 17% were at 111–120 (high average to above average).
- 54% were at 91–110 (average).
- 13% were at 80–90 (low average).
- 5% were at 79 and below (borderline, below average to well below average).

Performance IQ

Performance IQ was within average limits and above (low to above average to superior) in 94% of the children. Six percent of the children were within borderline (below average) limits. This did not change for males versus females although females were higher; 97% females and 93% males were within average limits. If excluding the low average category for more rigorous assessment, then 82% of the children fell within average limits and above. Females would be 86% compared to 80% for the males, again reflecting females scoring higher for Performance IQ, which is opposite the pattern seen for adolescents where males performed better.

Children

449 children completed this measure.

- 10% were at 121 and above (superior).
- 17% were at 111–120 (high average to above average).
- 55% were at 91–110 (average).
- 12% were at 80–90 (low average).
- 6% were at 79 and below (borderline, below average to well below average).

Females

132 females completed this measure (29%).

- 12% were at 121 and above (superior).
- 16% were at 111–120 (high average to above average).
- 58% were at 91–110 (average).
- 11% were at 80–90 (low average).
- 3% were at 79 and below (borderline, below average to well below average).

Males

317 males completed this measure (71%).

- 9% were at 121 and above (superior).
- 17% were at 111–120 (high average to above average).
- 54% were at 91–110 (average).
- 13% were at 80–90 (low average).
- 7% were at 79 and below (borderline, below average to well below average).

Verbal IQ

Verbal IQ was within average limits and above (low to above average to superior) in 93% of the children. Six percent of the children were within borderline (below average) limits. This did not change for males versus females; 95% females and 94% males were within average limits. If excluding the low average category, then 79% of the children fell within average limits and above. Females would be 80% compared to 82% for the males, indicating slightly less of a difference than seen on the performance testing where females scored slightly higher.

Children

449 children completed this measure.

- 12% were at 121 and above (superior).
- 18% were at 111–120 (high average to above average).
- 49% were at 91–110 (average).
- 14% were at 80–90 (low average).
- 6% were at 79 and below (borderline, below average to well below average).

Females

130 females completed this measure (29%).

- 10% were at 121 and above (superior).
- 17% were at 111–120 (high average to above average).
- 53% were at 91–110 (average).
- 15% were at 80–90 (low average).
- 5% were at 79 and below (borderline, below average to well below average).

Males

319 males completed this measure (71%).

- 13% were at 121 and above (superior).
- 18% were at 111–120 (high average to above average).
- 51% were at 91–110 (average).
- 12% were at 80–90 (low average).
- 6% were at 79 and below (borderline, below average to well below average).

Performance IQ versus Verbal IQ and Gender

Well below average functioning: There was a difference between males and females for the Performance IQ well below average functioning with females functioning higher; females at 3% compared to males at 7%. There was not a difference between males and females for Verbal IQ; females at 5% compared to males at 6% for well below average intellectual levels.

Superior functioning: There was a difference between males and females for higher functioning within superior limits; females functioned higher for Performance IQ, females at 12% compared to males at 9%. The same difference was seen for the Verbal IQ at higher functioning; however, males were higher than females for scoring within superior limits, females at 10% compared to males at 13%.

WPPSI IQ Test

The Wechsler Preschool and Primary Scale of Intelligence-III was a much smaller sample. On the WPPSI-III, testing is for the age range of 5–8 years (usually the WISC-III or IV was generally administered at age 8 years with some exceptions).

Full Scale IQ

Full Scale IQ was within average limits for 97% with only three percent falling within borderline limits or below average and well below average limits. It including only average and above average to superior functioning, then 78% of the young children were at average limits and above limits. This is similar to that seen for the larger sample of children on the WISC where 96% were within low average and above limits or 83% within average and above limits.

Children

32 children completed this measure.

- 6% were at 121 and above (superior).
- 25% were at 111–120 (high average to above average).
- 47% were at 91–110 (average).
- 19% were at 80–90 (low average).
- 3% were at 79 and below (borderline, below average to well below average).

Females

11 females completed this measure (31%).

- 9% were at 121 and above (superior).
- 55% were at 111–120 (high average to above average).
- 18% were at 91–110 (average).
- 9% were at 80–90 (low average).
- 9% were at 79 and below (borderline, below average to well below average).

Males

24 males completed this measure (69%).

- 4% were at 121 and above (superior).
- 42% were at 111–120 (high average to above average).
- 29% were at 91–110 (average).
- 21% were at 80–90 (low average).
- 4% were at 79 and below (borderline, below average to well below average).

Comparing Males and Females

Females performed better if comparing functioning of pure average limits and above, which was 82% for the females compared to 75% for males. When comparing a greater range of functioning, males and females from low average and above, then males performed better than females, 91% for the females compared to 96% for the males. The reason is that 9% of the females compared to 4% of the males performed within below and well below average limits.

Performance IQ

Performance IQ was at 100% (or to be specific 101%) when including low average and above average to superior functioning. If excluding the low average range, then 83% of the children were within average limits and above. Performance scores were higher than the Verbal IQ or Full Scale IQ. None of the children fell within borderline limits or below average and well below average limits. Young children tend to perform better on nonverbal tests that become more difficult as they get older. If they are bright, problems remain hidden until tasks increase in complexity. Also demonstrated is that problems are demonstrated first on verbal tests prior to performance testing. Performance testing was slightly lower on the WISC sample that is larger and had older children where 94% of the children fell within low average limits and above (above average to superior). Percentages were equivalent when the low average range was excluded.

Children

34 children completed this measure.

- 9% were at 121 and above (superior).
- 15% were at 111–120 (high average to above average).
- 59% were at 91–110 (average).
- 18% were at 80–90 (low average).
- 0% were at 79 and below (borderline, below average to well below average).

Females

11 females completed this measure (32%).

- 18% were at 121 and above (superior).
- 18% were at 111–120 (high average to above average).
- 55% were at 91–110 (average).
- 9% were at 80–90 (low average).
- 0% were at 79 and below (borderline, below average to well below average).

Males

23 males completed this measure (68%).

- 4% were at 121 and above (superior).
- 13% were at 111–120 (high average to above average).
- 61% were at 91–110 (average).
- 22% were at 80–90 (low average).
- 0% were at 79 and below (borderline, below average to well below average).

Comparing Males and Females

Females performed better if comparing functioning of average limits and above, which was 91% for the females compared to 78% for males. When comparing a greater range of functioning males and females from low average and above, then females and males were equal at 100% because no one was within below average limits. Another way to see that females were higher is by looking at the low average range, 9% for females compared to 22% for males.

Verbal IQ

Verbal scores were lower than the Performance IQ and similar to the Full Scale IQ when including only average and above average to superior functioning; 79% of the young children were at average limits and above limits. If including low average, then 97% were within average limits; 3% of the children fell within borderline limits or below average and well below average limits. Scoring demonstrates that verbal issues were already emerging as a problem in the young children. For the larger sample of children on the WISC, 79% of the children fell within average limits and above (above average to superior).

Children

33 children completed this measure.

- 6% were at 121 and above (superior).
- 18% were at 111–120 (high average to above average).
- 55% were at 91–110 (average).
- 18% were at 80–90 (low average).
- 3% were at 79 and below (borderline, below average to well below average).

Females

11 females completed this measure (31%).

- 9% were at 121 and above (superior).
- 9% were at 111–120 (high average to above average).
- 64% were at 91–110 (average).
- 18% were at 80–90 (low average).
- 0% were at 79 and below (borderline, below average to well below average).

Males

24 males completed this measure (69%).

- 4% were at 121 and above (superior).
- 26% were at 111–120 (high average to above average).
- 48% were at 91–110 (average).
- 17% were at 80–90 (low average).
- 4% were at 79 and below (borderline, below average to well below average).

Comparing Males and Females

Females performed better if comparing functioning of pure average limits and above, 82% for the females compared to 78% for males. When comparing a greater range of functioning by including the low average scores, females were still higher, 100% for females compared to 95% for males. If comparing lower functioning, male performed slightly worse than females; 4% of the males versus 0% of the females were within borderline, below average, and well below average limits. However, if comparing high average to superior functioning, then males performed better, 18% of the females compared to 30% of the males. This would suggest that males actually had higher scores for the Verbal IQ although more males performed at well below average limits.

Performance IQ versus Verbal IQ and Gender

Well below average functioning: For the Performance IQ, no males or females performed within well below average limits. However, for low average scoring, there were more males than females, 9% for females compared to 22% for males. Females had less difficulty for the Verbal IQ when looking at well below average scoring, 0% for females compared to 4% of the males. For the Full Scale IQ, more females had well below average scoring than males, 9% for females compared to 4% for males.

Superior functioning: Performance IQ values were higher when considering superior limits; for all children, 9% performed within superior limits compared to 6% for the Verbal IQ. More females performed within superior limits for the Performance IQ than males, 18% for females compared to 4% for males. Females were also higher on the Verbal IQ, 9% of the females compared to 4% of the males performed within superior limits. On the Full Scale IQ, more females were within superior limits than males, 9% for females compared to 4% for males.

SYMBOL DIGIT MODALITIES TEST

The Symbol Digit Modalities Test (SDMT) is a measure of whole-brain functioning. The child is asked to use a key to put the correct numbers with the correct symbol, and they have 90 s to complete as many items in the correct order as they can. This measure is completed using a written format and then an oral format (where the person is saying their responses out loud to the examiner who records their response). There is the tendency to mix up specific number symbol combinations seen through time as related to the visual–spatial difficulties. The written versus oral score allows for comparison when the act of writing is no longer a factor. However, often the impact of distractibility operates as an additional variable, and children lose their place on the oral portion, which negates the gain they would have had. This measure operates as a screening device to measure the general integrity and functioning of the brain. As such, it can be a measure of someone's potential that is often not seen on the other attention scores.

Scoring on this measure is a z-score, which is similar for the Trail Making Tests, Color Form, and Progressive Figures as well as the CHIPASAT, based upon normative data for age, and the score is represented by a standard deviation. Average is defined as 0.75 below the mean to 0.75 of a standard deviation above the mean. Low average is 0.76–0.99 of a standard deviation below the mean. High average is 0.76–0.99 of a standard deviation above the mean. Below average is 1.0–1.99 standard deviations below the mean, and above average is 1.0–1.99 standard deviations above the mean. Well below average/impaired is 2.00 standard deviations and below, while well above/superior is 2.00 standard deviations and above the mean. This can change when time is the score or for the correct number of items versus error scores.

There were 386 children for the written and oral portion.

Performance on the Written Portion

- 2% performed within well below average/impaired limits.
- 9% performed within below average limits.
- 5% performed within low average limits.
- 55% performed within average limits.
- 9% performed within high average limits.
- 14% performed within above average limits.
- 6% performed within well above/superior limits.

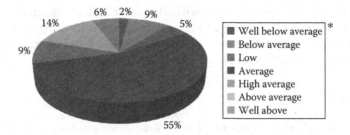

The majority of the children performed well on this measure; 84% performed within average limits and above (above average to superior) on this measure, suggesting higher abilities. Children were similar to the adolescents at 86%. Half of the children performed within average limits (55%); the adolescents were slightly higher at 60%. Children and adolescents were similar for higher functioning, above average to superior limits, at 20% for children and adolescents. Generally, this measure was not highly problematic for timed performance and tended to show the potential of children as a measure of whole-brain functioning. Often memory was seen as helping children to excel on this measure as they memorized the various combinations while having to pay specific attention to three combinations of reversed symbols.

Performance on the Oral Portion

- 2% performed within well below average/impaired limits.
- 11% performed within below average limits.
- 7% performed within low average limits.
- 50% performed within average limits.
- 8% performed within high average limits.
- 14% performed within above average limits.
- 8% performed within well above/superior limits.

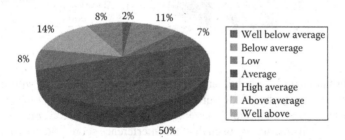

Performance on the oral portion for the children was similar to the written portion, although just slightly lower; 80% performed within average limits and above (above average to superior), which still suggests higher abilities for the children. Children did not have the increase in oral performance seen for the adolescents (at 90%), suggesting the greater impact of distractibility for children versus adolescents. Half of the child population was within average limits, 50% (similar to the adolescents at 47%). The children did not have as high functioning as that seen in the adolescents; 22% of the children compared to 36% of the adolescents were within above average to superior limits. The oral

---

* The pie graphs range from 99 to 100 to 101 due to rounding.

condition did not result in dramatically improved performance for the children as it did for the adolescents, which may be a result of increased distractibility when not writing. In addition, the child population had more individuals diagnosed as ADHD plus, which would impact performance on this measure, specifically affecting memory.

STROOP COLOR WORD TEST

The Stroop Color Word Test is a measure of divided attention assessing distractibility. We have found through the years that those who have a problem on this task reveal an interference score that is one-half to two-thirds less than the word score. The child has 45 s for the word as well as the interference portion. Comparisons are made to their performance of word reading versus the interference task as well as obtaining a normative data T-score (where 50 is average and 10 is the standard deviation). The only score that is recorded for this sample is the number of correct responses on the interference portion, which yields a T-score.

422 children completed this measure.

- 1% performed within well below average/impaired limits.
- 13% performed within below average limits.
- 10% performed within low average limits.
- 67% performed within average limits.
- 4% performed within high average limits.
- 4% performed within above average limits.
- 1% performed within well above/superior limits.

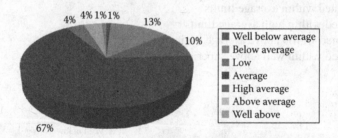

Children performed significantly higher than the adolescents; 67% were within average limits, and 5% were above average to superior compared to 4% for the adolescents for average functioning and 1% for above average and superior. The tendency was to see more average scoring while still ruling in the problem of distractibility given that this interference score tended to be half of the word score or even less than half. Children are expected to perform as well on the word score as they did on the interference score. Children performed better than the adolescents overall on this task; 76% performed within average and above limits (above average to superior) compared to 9% for the adolescents. Children may have had a higher performance due to the task being easier when there are less developed reading skills. In other words, the better the reader, the more that this measure would be distracting for them.

TRAIL MAKING TEST

The Trail Making Tests have two portions, Part A and Part B. The score is the time taken to complete the task of responding in correct sequential order for numbers and then for numbers and letters, alternating between the two. Errors are recorded, and the child is required to correct their error while the time continues to be recorded. This measure has been found to involve the use of rapid visual search and visuospatial sequencing. Part B is more sensitive to impact to the brain (executive reasoning). We have found it important to distinguish between the types of errors obtained (confusion and/or loss of place versus inability to perform the task) as opposed to the time. Children can take longer to perform well without mistakes. Mistakes can occur when the last number is missed on Part A and/or it becomes difficult to keep track of the number and letter sequence on Part B; both types of errors are seen as a result of visual–spatial issues.

Scoring is based upon errors and time taken to complete the task and compared to normative data for specific age range. The lowest speed is the most desirable.

Trail Making Part A
328 children completed the Trail Making Test Part A.

- 1% performed within well above average/superior limits.
- 31% performed within above average limits.
- 14% performed within high average limits.
- 41% performed within average limits.
- 2% performed within low average limits.
- 8% performed within below average limits.
- 2% performed within well below/impaired limits.

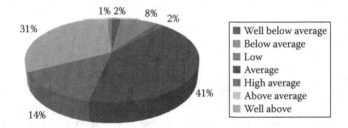

Children did not have much difficulty with measure and performed slightly better than the adolescents; 87% of the children performed within average limits and above (above average to superior) compared to 80% of the adolescents on this first portion involving the sequencing of numbers and attention to task for decreased speed and higher scoring. Less children performed within average limits and more within above average to superior when compared to the adolescents; 41% of the children were within average limits compared to 56% of the adolescents, and 32% of the children were within above average to superior limits compared to 13% of the adolescents on this task for speed. Children performed better on this task than the adolescents, and this task was not particularly problematic for them.

Trail Making Part B
315 completed the Trail Making Test Part B.

- 1% performed within well above average/superior limits.
- 21% performed within above average limits.
- 13% performed within high average limits.
- 45% performed within average limits.
- 5% performed within low average limits.
- 9% performed within below average limits.
- 6% performed within well below/impaired limits.

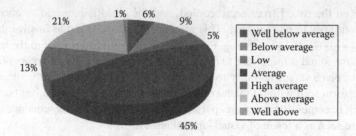

Children performed considerably better than the adolescents on the second portion of this measure, which is more demanding (requiring the use of cognitive flexibility and switching of sets); 80% of the children compared to 68% of the adolescents performed within average limits and above (above average to superior) limits on this measure for the time taken to complete the task. Children continued to perform better at higher levels of functioning; 22% of the children compared to 13% of the adolescents were within above average to superior limits. Children and adolescents were the same for average performance at 45%.

Trail Making Part A: Number of Errors Obtained

- 78% had no errors.
- 17% had one error.
- 2% had two errors.
- 2% had three errors.
- 2% had more than three errors.

The number of errors shows that only 78% performed without any errors, suggesting that although the time was not problematic, more errors were made. This holds true when compared to the adolescent population where 82% had no errors, suggesting that children sacrificed errors for time. Generally, there is one error made at the end due to visual–spatial issues, which occurred in 17% of the population (compared to 13% for adolescents) who became confused and missed the last number.

Trail Making Part B: Number of Errors Obtained

- 63% had no errors.
- 25% had one error.
- 5% had two errors.
- 6% had three errors.
- 1% had more than three errors.

Similar to Part A, children had more errors than the adolescents sacrificing errors for speed. For the children, 63% had no errors compared to 70% of the adolescents. More children than adolescents had one error; 25% of the children compared to 19% of the adolescents had one error. Errors tend to occur when there is a loss of set and forgetting where they were in the letter sequence or number sequence, which is continually alternated. Compared to 17% on Part A, there were more errors on Part B. On Part B, children having two or more errors were 12% compared to Part A, which was 6%, suggesting the increased difficulty of this task and the tendency to lose the set which is having to remember the number and position in the alphabet. Children have been observed to count out loud to recall their position, 1A, 2B, and so forth. This pattern is similar to that seen in the adolescents.

COLOR FORM TEST

The Color Form Test is a measure asking the child to move in sequential motion from color to shape or form. Errors are corrected while the time continues. Time taken to complete the task is the final score. This measure along with Progressive Figures is similar in concept to the Trail Making tasks.
   307 children completed this task.

- 1% performed within well above average/superior limits.
- 17% performed within above average limits.
- 14% performed within high average limits.
- 47% performed within average limits.
- 6% performed within low average limits.
- 8% performed within below average limits.
- 7% performed within well below/impaired limits.

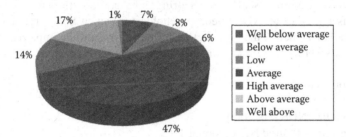

Compared to other speed measures, children had more difficulty with this task when they had to remember if they were last on form or color, 79% within average limits and above (above average to superior) on the Color Form task involving the sequencing from color to shape. Almost half were within average limits (47%) and 18% within above average to superior limits on this task for speed, suggesting that this task was not particularly problematic for the majority of children.

PROGRESSIVE FIGURES TEST

The Progressive Figures Test is another measure using sequential processing; this time, the child has to shift from the inside shape to the same outside shape. Errors are corrected while the time continues. Time taken to complete the task is the final score.
   311 children completed this task.

- 1% performed within well above average/superior limits.
- 7% performed within above average limits.
- 16% performed within high average limits.
- 62% performed within average limits.
- 5% performed within low average limits.
- 8% performed within below average limits.
- 2% performed within well below/impaired limits.

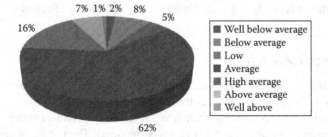

This measure was more difficult for the children seen in the slightly higher time taken to complete the task correctly; 86% performed within average limits and above (above average to superior) on the Progressive Figures task involving the sequencing and shifting from one shape to another. When compared to the Color Form task, fewer children performed within average limits (62%), although more children performed within above average to superior limits (24%). Ten percent of the children had considerable difficulty performing within below average and impaired limits.

SEASHORE RHYTHM TEST

The Seashore Rhythm Test is a measure of fast-paced nonverbal input into the brain requiring sustained attention. The child is asked to differentiate between 30 pairs of rhyming beats. It is utilized to provide a measure of basic brain input, as well as sustained attention capacity. This measure requires alertness to nonverbal auditory stimuli, sustained attention, and the ability to perceive and compare rhythmic sequences. Scoring is based upon the number of correct items resulting in the assigning of an NDS (Neuropsychological Deficit Score) ranked score. Ranked scores range from 0 to 3 where 0 means intact performance, 1 is mildly impaired, 2 is moderately impaired, and 3 is severely impaired. This test has a version for children (i.e., age 9–14 years) and adults.

231 children completed this task.

- 25% had an intact NDS score of 0.
- 32% had a mildly impaired NDS score of 1.
- 22% had a moderately impaired NDS score of 2.
- 21% had a severely impaired NDS score of 3.

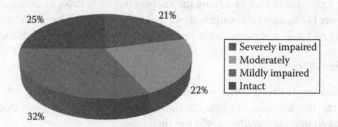

Children had a more difficult time on this task, which is fast paced and more demanding than the slow-paced measure. The child has to maintain sustained attention or it becomes quite easy to lose their place in discriminating sets of beeps; 25% of the children had intact performance, which was lower than the adolescents at 37%. Children and adolescents were similar with children actually having less difficulty when comparing those who had mildly impaired performance, 32% for children compared to 35% for adolescents. Errors tended to occur at the end of a trial or on the last trial. More children had moderate to impaired performance, which may reflect the higher presence of ADHD plus, 43% of the children compared to 28% of the adolescents. This pattern becomes clearer when examining severely impaired performance, 21% of the children compared to 11% of the adolescents.

SPEECH–SOUNDS PERCEPTION TEST

The Speech–Sounds Perception Test is a measure of slow-paced verbal input into the brain. Scoring is based upon number of errors resulting in the assigning of an NDS (Neuropsychological Deficit Score) ranked score. Ranked scores range from 0 to 3 where 0 means intact performance, 1 is mildly impaired, 2 is moderately impaired, and 3 is severely impaired. The test has a version for children (i.e., age 9–14 years) and adults. This task is a measure of slow-paced, verbal stimuli, and the ability to correctly distinguish the sound of nonsense syllables and to choose the correct syllable that they hear. Very few errors are expected. Those with a genetic attention disorder tend to become bored on this measure, losing their focus or zoning out as a result.

235 children completed this task.

- 51% had an intact NDS score of 0.
- 29% had a mildly impaired NDS score of 1.
- 14% had a moderately impaired NDS score of 2.
- 6% had a severely impaired NDS score of 3.

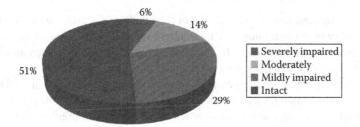

Children performed better on this measure however had a more difficult time when compared to the adolescents; 51% of the children compared to 75% of the adolescents had intact performance and no difficulty on this slow-paced task. Suggested is that the pace of the task is the reason for more problematic performance seen on the fast-paced measure (57% had intact or mildly impaired performance on the fast paced task compared to 80% on this task). Children had more mildly impaired performance than the adolescents, 29% for the children compared to 19% for the adolescents. Children also showed more moderate to severe impairment on this measure, 20% of the children compared to 7% of the adolescents.

SYMBOL SEARCH TEST

The Symbol Search Test is a measure of processing speed. The score is how many correct items can be completed within 120 s. Scoring is compared to normative data for specific age range and assigned a scaled score (10 is average and 3 is the standard deviation). This subtest is from the WISC-IV or WPPSI-III intellectual assessment.

480 children completed this task.

- 4% had a score that was well below average/impaired.
- 19% had a score in the low to below average range.
- 39% had a score within average limits.
- 27% had a score within high to above average limits.
- 11% had a score within well above average to superior limits.

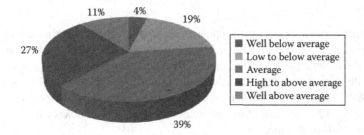

Children performed similarly to the adolescents on this measure; 77% of the children compared to 78% of the adolescents performed within average and above (above average to superior), suggesting that this measure was not as problematic. This is a measure that requires less cognitive input and is more a process of discrimination and highly speeded. Children and adolescents were similar for average performance as well as higher performance although adolescents were slightly higher; 39% of the children compared to 37% of the adolescents were within average limits, and 11% of the children compared to 14% of the adolescents were within well above average to superior.

CHILDREN'S PACED AUDITORY SERIAL ADDITION TEST

This is a measure of information processing. All of the numbers are 5 and under. The child is asked to add the last number to the next number. Children will typically struggle with this measure for two reasons, firstly a problem of math fluency (inability to add quickly enough to keep up with the tap) and secondly a memory problem whereby they do not recall the last number to add it to the next number.

This measure is thought to assess information processing and the tendency of ADD individuals to miss small details of information such as instructions and directions. In addition to information processing, performance can reflect sustained attention deficits and distractibility, as well as emotional issues of giving up in frustration, a math phobia, and/or memory problem related to additional issues beyond that of a genetic attention disorder. While arithmetic was not seen as having a significant impact, the lack of math fluency would result in poor scoring or an inability to complete the test.

The score is the number of correct items per trial. A higher score reflects more correct items obtained on each trial. The following is based upon total number of correct responses across all four trials.

299 children completed this task.

- 6% performed within well above average/superior limits.
- 6% performed within above average limits.
- 2% performed within high average limits.
- 23% performed within average limits.
- 8% performed within low average limits.
- 30% performed within below average limits.
- 25% performed within well below/impaired limits.

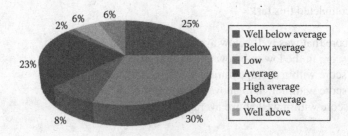

Children did not perform as well as the adolescents on this task; 37% of the children compared to 52% of the adolescents performed within average and above average limits (above average to superior) on this measure, which is one of the more difficult tasks in the attention assessment. Children had more difficulty than the adolescents when looking at average performance, 23% of the children compared to 34% of the adolescents. Adolescents remained slightly higher for the above average to superior functioning, 12% for the children compared to 15% for the adolescents.

There are four trials to this measure.

First Trial

- 4% performed within well above average/superior limits.
- 6% performed within above average limits.
- 3% performed within high average limits.
- 26% performed within average limits.
- 3% performed within low average limits.
- 30% performed within below average limits.
- 28% performed within well below/impaired limits.

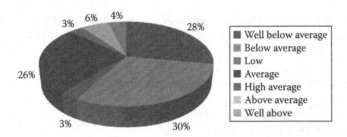

Thirty-nine percent performed within average and above (above average to superior) limits for this first trial, which is a slower pace.

Second Trial

- 5% performed within well above average/superior limits.
- 7% performed within above average limits.
- 2% performed within high average limits.
- 24% performed within average limits.
- 7% performed within low average limits.
- 27% performed within below average limits.
- 29% performed within well below/impaired limits.

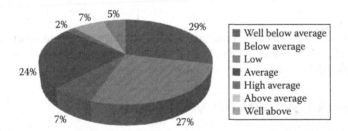

Thirty-eight percent performed within average and above (above average to superior) limits on the second trial, which is increased in pace.

Third Trial

- 7% performed within well above average/superior limits.
- 4% performed within above average limits.
- 4% performed within high average limits.
- 24% performed within average limits.
- 4% performed within low average limits.
- 32% performed within below average limits.
- 25% performed within well below/impaired limits.

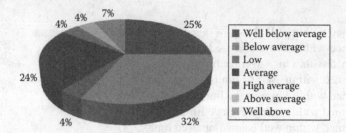

Thirty-nine percent performed within average and above (above average to superior) limits for this third trial, which has increased in pace.

Fourth Trial

- 7% performed within well above average/superior limits.
- 8% performed within above average limits.
- 5% performed within high average limits.
- 21% performed within average limits.
- 3% performed within low average limits.
- 35% performed within below average limits.
- 22% performed within well below/impaired limits.

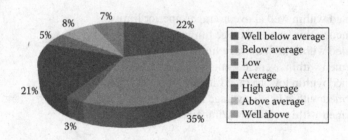

Forty-one percent performed within average and above (above average to superior) limits for this last and fourth trial, revealing improvement on the most difficult trial. The children did not struggle on this measure as much as the adults on the PASAT.

GENDER COMPARISONS: FEMALES VERSUS MALES

Symbol Digit Modalities Test

115 females (30%) and 271 males (70%)

Written Portion

Females

- 1% performed within well below average/impaired limits.
- 11% performed within below average limits.
- 4% performed within low average limits.
- 57% performed within average limits.
- 5% performed within high average limits.
- 17% performed within above average limits.
- 5% performed within well above/superior limits.

Males

- 2% performed within well below average/impaired limits.
- 9% performed within below average limits.
- 5% performed within low average limits.
- 54% performed within average limits.
- 11% performed within high average limits.
- 13% performed within above average limits.
- 6% performed within well above/superior limits.

Comparison of Males and Females

The same percentage of female and male children (84%) performed within average limits and above (above average to superior) on the written potion of this measure. Slightly more female than male children performed within above average to superior limits, 22% females compared to 19% for males. Slightly more adolescent males performed better than females, 17% for the females compared to 21% for the males. Slightly more female children were within average limits than males; 57% for females compared to 54% for males and adolescents showed greater differences at 64% for females compared to 57% for males. In comparing below average and impaired performance, female and male children were similar at 12% for females and 11% for males. For the children, females performed better on this task, which was different for the adolescents.

Oral Portion

Females

- 3% performed within well below average/impaired limits.
- 13% performed within below average limits.
- 5% performed within low average limits.
- 46% performed within average limits.
- 13% performed within high average limits.
- 11% performed within above average limits.
- 9% performed within well above/superior limits.

Males

- 2% performed within well below average/impaired limits.
- 9% performed within below average limits.
- 8% performed within low average limits.
- 52% performed within average limits.
- 5% performed within high average limits.
- 16% performed within above average limits.
- 7% performed within well above/superior limits.

Comparison of Males and Females

Males and female children performed similarly on the oral portion; 79% of the females compared to 80% of the males performed within average limits and above (above average to superior), suggesting no difference for gender on the oral portion similar to the written portion. Male children performed slightly better for above average to superior scoring, 20% of the females compared to 23% of the males. There was no gender difference for the adolescent population for above average to superior scoring, 36% females compared to 37% males. Average scores for the children revealed better performance for males than females, 46% for females compared to 52% for males. Adolescents revealed a reverse pattern although differences were slight; 48% for females compared to 46% for males. Female children performed within below average to impaired limits 16% of the time compared to 11% for males. Overall for the children, males performed slightly better on the oral portion.

When looking at more global performance, neither the children nor the adolescents revealed gender differences on the oral or written portions for scoring within average limits and above (well above average to superior) limits. Adolescents showed higher ability on this measure than the children; 85% (males and females) performed within average and above (above average to superior) limits on the written portion and the oral portion; 91% females and 90% males performed within average and above limits. The children showed gender differences for the written and oral portion when comparing performance for higher levels of functioning and less impaired functioning. The adolescents showed gender differences for only the written portion.

STROOP COLOR WORD TEST

There were 129 females (31%) and 293 males (69%).

Females

- 2% performed within impaired limits.
- 0% performed within well below average limits.
- 9% performed within below to well below average limits.
- 10% performed within low average to average limits.
- 71% performed within average to high average limits.
- 4% performed within above average limits.
- 3% performed within well above/superior limits.

Males

- 1% performed within impaired limits.
- 0% performed within well below average limits.
- 14% performed within below to well below average limits.
- 11% performed within low average to average limits.
- 70% performed within average to high average limits.
- 3% performed within above average limits.
- 1% performed within well above/superior limits.

Comparison of Males and Females

Female and male children performed equally for scoring between average and high average limits, females at 71% compared to males at 70%. For average and above (above average to superior) limits, females were at 78% compared to males at 74%. Male children had slightly more difficulty with this task when comparing functioning at below and well below average limits, males at 15% compared to females at 11%. More females performed within average to high average limits than males, 71% females compared to 70% males. Overall female children performed slightly better on this task.

The child population did not have the difficulties experienced on this measure by the adolescent population; 24% of the females were within average to high average limits compared to 25% of the males. Female adolescents were more often within average limits, while males had greater percentages above or below the average range. For the children, slightly more females were within average to well above average/superior limits, females at 78% compared to males at 74%. The adolescents struggled more on this task, with 26% females and 30% males performing within average to well above average limits. There were children who had superior scores compared to none of the adolescents.

Trail Making Part A
There were 107 females (30%) and 249 males (70%).

Females: Number of Errors Obtained
- 77% had no errors.
- 21% had one error.
- 0% had two errors.
- 1% had three errors.
- 1% had more than three errors.

Males: Number of Errors Obtained
- 77% had no errors.
- 16% had one error.
- 4% had two errors.
- 2% had three errors.
- 1% had more than three errors.

Comparison of Males and Females
Female and male children had the same percentage of no errors (77%). The adolescent population revealed slightly better performance for females than males; 85% of the females compared to 81% of the males had no errors. Adolescent males and females performed better than the children. More females than males had one error for the children, 21% for females compared to 16% for males. Adolescents, particularly females, performed better; only 12% of the females compared to 14% for the males had one error. However, for the children, more males had two or more errors, 2% of the females compared to 7% of the males. The adolescent population revealed the same pattern with slightly fewer errors for the males, 3% for the females compared to 5% for the males.

Trail Making Part B
There were 168 females (29%) and 415 males (71%).

Females: Number of Errors Obtained
- 67% had no errors.
- 22% had one error.
- 6% had two errors.
- 4% had three errors.
- 2% had more than three errors.

Males: Number of Errors Obtained
- 58% had no errors.
- 25% had one error.
- 9% had two errors.
- 6% had three errors.
- 2% had more than three errors.

Comparison of Males and Females
Part B is more difficult, requiring the shifting of sets from number to letter as opposed to just sequencing. Females performed better than males; 67% of the females compared to 58% of the males had no errors. There was more of a gender difference for the adolescents; 90% of the females

compared to 66% of the males had no errors. Females performed slightly better when considering one error, 22% of the females compared to 25% of the males. The adolescent population showed greater differences for one error, 4% for females compared to 23% for males. Two or more errors revealed the same pattern of females performing with fewer errors than males, 12% of the females compared to 17% of the males. The adolescent population revealed the same pattern with greater differences, 6% for the females compared to 11% for the males for two or more errors. Overall, across the ages, females had fewer errors on this portion.

Trail Making Part A: Overall Score

Females: Time to Complete the Task

- 0% performed within well above average/superior limits.
- 21% performed within above average limits.
- 22% performed within high average limits.
- 47% performed within average limits.
- 1% performed within low average limits.
- 8% performed within below average limits.
- 0% performed within well below/impaired limits.

Males: Time to Complete the Task

- 2% performed within well above average/superior limits.
- 35% performed within above average limits.
- 11% performed within high average limits.
- 39% performed within average limits.
- 2% performed within low average limits.
- 8% performed within below average limits.
- 3% performed within well below/impaired limits.

Comparison of Males and Females

Female children completed this task slightly faster than males; 90% of females compared to 87% of males performed within average limits and above (above average to superior) limits. In examining quality of errors, the presence of no errors was the same for females and males; however, more females had one error and more males had two or more errors. For the adolescent population, males were slightly faster, 77% for females compared to 81% for males, although males had slightly more errors.

More males than females performed within above average to superior limits, 21% females compared to 37% males. This pattern change for adolescent revealed better performance for females, 17% for females compared to 11% for males.

More female children were within average limits, 47% females compared to 39% males. In the adolescent population, more males were within average limits, 50% for females compared to 60% for males.

Slightly more male children performed within below average to impaired limits, 9% for females compared to 11% for males. In the adolescent population, females had slightly more difficulty; 17% for females compared to 13% for males performed within below average to impaired limits.

Overall male children seemed to perform better on this task for time without incurring more errors although there were slightly more males who had below average to impaired limits for a time score and definitely more males had two or more errors than females. Females performed better through time seen on the adolescent scoring, although more females performed within below average to impaired limits. Differences are greater for gender on the second portion of this measure demanding cognitive flexibility and the switching of sets.

Trail Making Part B: Overall Score

Females: Time to Complete the Task

- 1% performed within well above average/superior limits.
- 14% performed within above average limits.
- 7% performed within high average limits.
- 42% performed within average limits.
- 5% performed within low average limits.
- 7% performed within below average limits.
- 24% performed within well below/impaired limits.

Males: Time to Complete the Task

- 1% performed within well above average/superior limits.
- 19% performed within above average limits.
- 10% performed within high average limits.
- 35% performed within average limits.
- 4% performed within low average limits.
- 7% performed within below average limits.
- 23% performed within well below/impaired limits.

Comparison of Males and Females

Female and male children were similar for overall time taken to complete this task; 64% for females compared to 65% for males performed within average limits and above (above average to superior) on this more demanding measure of cognitive flexibility. However, male children had more errors than females; 67% of females had no errors compared to 58% of males on this task, suggesting that while keeping up with speed, they had more errors in their performance. In the adolescent population, there was less of a difference between males and females for time; 67% of the females compared to 69% of the males were within average and above limits, although males had far more errors.

More female than male children performed within average limits; 42% for females versus 35% for males performed within average limits. In the adolescents, males and females were similar; 46% of the females compared to 45% of the males performed within average limits.

More male than female children performed within above average to superior limits, 15% for females compared to 20% for males. Adolescents were more similar, 12% for females compared to 13% for males. Females and males were equal for below average to impaired performance for time taken to complete this task, 31% for females compared to 30% for males.

This measure was more difficult for males and females compared to the first portion (Part A). Male children performed better overall for time taken to complete the task although they had more errors. When compared to the adolescent population, males performed worse while females performed better. Males tended to sacrifice errors for speed.

COLOR FORM TEST

81 females (26%) and 226 males (74%) completed this task.

Females: Time to Complete the Task

- 1% performed within well above average/superior limits.
- 21% performed within above average limits.
- 10% performed within high average limits.
- 48% performed within average limits.

- 2% performed within low average limits.
- 5% performed within below average limits.
- 12% performed within well below/impaired limits.

Males: Time to Complete the Task

- 0% performed within well above average/superior limits.
- 16% performed within above average limits.
- 16% performed within high average limits.
- 46% performed within average limits.
- 7% performed within low average limits.
- 10% performed within below average limits.
- 5% performed within well below/impaired limits.

Comparison of Males and Females

Females were similar to males for overall performance, 80% for females compared to 78% for males for average limits and above (above average to superior) on this task requiring the sequential movement from color to shape. Almost half were within average limits, 48% for females and 46% for males. More females performed within well above average to superior limits, 22% for females compared to 16% for males.

PROGRESSIVE FIGURES TEST

94 females (29%) and 227 males (71%) completed this task:

Females: Time to Complete Task

- 2% performed within well above average/superior limits.
- 16% performed within above average limits.
- 14% performed within high average limits.
- 54% performed within average limits.
- 4% performed within low average limits.
- 10% performed within below average limits.
- 0% performed within well below/impaired limits.

Males: Time to Complete Task

- 0% performed within well above average/superior limits.
- 7% performed within above average limits.
- 16% performed within high average limits.
- 63% performed within average limits.
- 5% performed within low average limits.
- 7% performed within below average limits.
- 3% performed within well below/impaired limits.

Comparison of Males and Females

Females and males performed the same for average limits and above (above average to superior) on this measure of sequencing and requiring the shifting from one shape to another at 86%. Children performed better on this measure than the Color Form task, which would appear to be less demanding. However, this task provides an internal structure that is not present in the Color Form task, making it less vulnerable to distractibility. More females performed within higher limits (above average to superior), 18% for females compared to 7% for males.

Symbol Search

There were 139 females (29%) and 342 males (71%).

Females: Scaled Score

- 6% had a score that was well below average/impaired.
- 17% had a score in the low to below average range.
- 35% had a score within average limits.
- 29% had a score within high to above average limits.
- 13% had a score within well above average to superior limits.

Males: Scaled Score

- 3% had a score that was well below average/impaired.
- 20% had a score in the low to below average range.
- 40% had a score within average limits.
- 25% had a score within high to above average limits.
- 11% had a score within well above average to superior limits.

Comparison of Males and Females

Female and male children were similar for overall performance; 77% of the females compared to 76% of the males performed within average and above (above average to superior) limits on this task, suggesting no gender differences. This is similar to the adolescents at 77% for both females and males. At higher levels, female children were similar; 13% of the females compared to 11% of the males performed within well above average to superior limits. The adolescents showed a greater difference of females performing better than males; 21% for females compared to 10% for males performed within higher limits.

More male children performed within average limits than females, 35% for females compared to 40% for males. The adolescents showed a similar pattern of 33% for females compared to 39% for males performing within average limits.

The difference for the children is in the scoring of high average to superior limits where, similar to the adolescents, females performed better than males, 42% for females compared to 36% for males showing a higher performance for females on this measure.

CHIPASAT: Overall Score

There were 90 females (31%) and 199 males (69%). The numbers change depending upon how many children completed each trial.

Females

- 7% performed within well above average/superior limits.
- 5% performed within above average limits.
- 2% performed within high average limits.
- 13% performed within average limits.
- 13% performed within low average limits.
- 31% performed within below average limits.
- 28% performed within well below/impaired limits.

Males

- 6% performed within well above average/superior limits.
- 6% performed within above average limits.
- 2% performed within high average limits.

- 27% performed within average limits.
- 6% performed within low average limits.
- 30% performed within below average limits.
- 24% performed within well below/impaired limits.

Comparison of Males and Females

Males performed better than females for overall performance of average and above (above average to superior) limits, 27% females compared to 41% males. More males were within average limits, 13% of the females compared to 27% of the males. Females and males were the same for above average to superior limits at 12%. Males performed better on this measure.

There are four trials.

Trial 1

Females

- 7% performed within well above average/superior limits.
- 3% performed within above average limits.
- 0% performed within high average limits.
- 21% performed within average limits.
- 4% performed within low average limits.
- 31% performed within below average limits.
- 33% performed within well below/impaired limits.

Males

- 3% performed within well above average/superior limits.
- 7% performed within above average limits.
- 4% performed within high average limits.
- 29% performed within average limits.
- 3% performed within low average limits.
- 30% performed within below average limits.
- 25% performed within well below/impaired limits.

Trial 2

Females

- 5% performed within well above average/superior limits.
- 11% performed within above average limits.
- 1% performed within high average limits.
- 19% performed within average limits.
- 4% performed within low average limits.
- 28% performed within below average limits.
- 31% performed within well below/impaired limits.

Males

- 5% performed within well above average/superior limits.
- 5% performed within above average limits.
- 2% performed within high average limits.
- 26% performed within average limits.
- 8% performed within low average limits.
- 27% performed within below average limits.
- 27% performed within well below/impaired limits.

Trial 3

Females

- 6% performed within well above average/superior limits.
- 3% performed within above average limits.
- 2% performed within high average limits.
- 22% performed within average limits.
- 3% performed within low average limits.
- 38% performed within below average limits.
- 26% performed within well below/impaired limits.

Males

- 7% performed within well above average/superior limits.
- 5% performed within above average limits.
- 5% performed within high average limits.
- 25% performed within average limits.
- 4% performed within low average limits.
- 29% performed within below average limits.
- 24% performed within well below/impaired limits.

Trial 4

Females

- 8% performed within well above average/superior limits.
- 7% performed within above average limits.
- 2% performed within high average limits.
- 20% performed within average limits.
- 2% performed within low average limits.
- 39% performed within below average limits.
- 23% performed within well below/impaired limits.

Males

- 7% performed within well above average/superior limits.
- 8% performed within above average limits.
- 6% performed within high average limits.
- 21% performed within average limits.
- 3% performed within low average limits.
- 33% performed within below average limits.
- 21% performed within well below/impaired limits

SUMMATION OF THE INDIVIDUAL CHIPASAT TRIALS

Trial 1

Males performed better than females for overall scoring of average and above (above average to superior) limits, 31% females compared to 43% males. More males than females performed within average limits, 29% males compared to 21% females. Males and females were equally at above average to superior limits (10%).

Trial 2

Males performed similar to females for overall scoring of average and above (above average to superior) limits, 36% females compared to 38% males. Males performed better than females for average scoring, 26% males compared to 19% females. More females than males had above average to superior scores, 16% females compared to 10% males.

Trial 3

Males performed better than females for overall scoring of average and above (above average to superior) limits, 33% females compared to 42% males. Slightly more males than females performed within average limits, 25% males compared to 22% females. Slightly more males performed better than females within above average to superior limits, 9% for females compared to 12% for males.

Trial 4

Males performed better than females for overall scoring of average and above (above average to superior) limits, 37% females compared to 42% males. Males and females were similar within average limits, 21% males compared to 20% females. Males and females were equal for above average to superior scoring at 15%.

Overall male children tended to perform better at this task. This is the same picture seen for adolescents and adults.

SPEECH–SOUNDS PERCEPTION TEST

There were 72 females (31%) and 163 males (69%).

Females

- 49% had an intact NDS score of 0.
- 32% had a mildly impaired NDS score of 1.
- 15% had a moderately impaired NDS score of 2.
- 4% had a severely impaired NDS score of 3.

Males

- 52% had an intact NDS score of 0.
- 28% had a mildly impaired NDS score of 1.
- 13% had a moderately impaired NDS score of 2.
- 7% had a severely impaired NDS score of 3.

Comparison of Males and Females

Male children performed slightly better than females, 49% for females compared to 52% for males for intact performance on this measure of slow-paced verbal input. In the adolescent population, females had a slightly better performance than males, 77% for females compared to 74% for males. Slightly more females had mildly impaired performance, 32% for females compared to 28% for males. In the adolescent population, there was no difference between the genders; both males and females were at 19% for mildly impaired performance. Moderate to severely impaired performance revealed similar performance for females and males, 19% for females compared to 20% for males, suggesting that overall males performed better on this task.

SEASHORE RHYTHM TEST

There were 68 females (29%) and 163 males (71%).

Females

- 26% had an intact NDS score of 0.
- 38% had a mildly impaired NDS score of 1.
- 19% had a moderately impaired NDS score of 2.
- 16% had a severely impaired NDS score of 3.

Males

- 24% had an intact NDS score of 0.
- 29% had a mildly impaired NDS score of 1.
- 23% had a moderately impaired NDS score of 2.
- 23% had a severely impaired NDS score of 3.

Comparison of Males and Females

Females were similar to males for intact performance on this fast-paced input task, 26% for females compared to 24% for males. Female adolescents performed slightly worse than males on this measure; 34% of the females compared to 38% of the males had intact performance.

More female children had mildly impaired performance, 38% for females compared to 29% for males. Moderate to severely impaired performance was seen more often for males, 35% of the females compared to 46% of the males. Males seemed to have a more difficult time on this measure if comparing severity of performance similar to that seen in the adolescent population.

MALE AND FEMALE COMPARISONS FOR CHILDREN

1. Input tasks slow and fast paced: Males performed better overall. Females performed slightly worse for the slow-paced task, and males had more difficulty if comparing severity of performance on the fast-paced task.
2. Information processing: Males performed better on all of the trials. Males and females were more equivalent at higher functioning levels of above average to superior scoring.
3. Speeded tasks: There were no gender differences when comparing overall performance of average and above (above average to superior) limits. Differences occurred for errors in performance and performance at higher or lower levels. On a measure of whole-brain functioning, females performed slightly better on the written portion for higher functioning and males performed slightly better on the oral portion. Males performed better on time without incurring more errors on the sequencing task, Part A of the Trail Making Test. Males also performed better for time on the second portion that is more demanding; however, they had more errors, suggesting the sacrifice of errors for time. Females performed better than males on a task of processing speed when compared for above average to superior functioning. Females performed better than males on the two measures (sequencing and switching of sets) for younger children, likely the result of less distractibility.
4. Distractibility: Females performed slightly better than males. Males had more problematic functioning and females had slightly higher scores for average and high average limits.
5. On the WISC testing, females were slightly higher for overall global functioning within average and above limits for Full Scale IQ and Performance IQ while Verbal IQ was similar. There was a difference for well below average scoring seen for males on the performance tests compared to no difference on the verbal tests. When comparing superior functioning, females were higher for the performance tests, and males were higher for the verbal tests.
6. On the WPPSI testing for younger ages, females performed better for overall scores than males. Males had both higher and lower functioning. When comparing superior scores, females were higher for the performance and the verbal tests. If comparing high average functioning, females were higher for the performance tests, and males were higher for the verbal tests similar to the older children.

5 Adolescent Neuropsychological Testing for ADD/ADHD

The age range was 12–17 years. Adolescents were administered the following test measures:

- National Adult Reading Test Revised (NART-R)
- Wechsler Intelligence Scale for Children (WISC-III or WISC-IV)
- Symbol Digit Modalities Test (SDMT)
- Stroop Color Word Test
- Trail Making Tests Part A and B
- Seashore Rhythm Test
- Speech–Sounds Perception Test
- Symbol Search Test
- Children's Paced Auditory Serial Addition Test (CHIPASAT)
- Paced Auditory Serial Addition Test (PASAT)

Additional measures for the attention battery include the Bender Visual Motor Gestalt Test, Wisconsin Card Sorting Test, and the Cancellation Test. These measures were more difficult to analyze statistically and were not included in the study. The CHIPASAT was used for ages 8–14 years and the PASAT for ages 15–17 years.

When comparing the adolescents in their own performance, their best performance was on the measure of whole-brain functioning (SDMT). They had more difficulty on the cognitive flexibility portion (Part B) of the Trail Making Tests than the sequential portion (Part A). They had more errors on Part B than Part A as well, revealing that the task was clearly more difficult when they had to switch sets while maintaining a set. One reason for this may be distractibility. The adolescents were highly distracted and performed the worst on a measure of divided attention, the Stroop Color Word Test. A measure of processing speed (Symbol Search) was somewhat difficult compared to the other tests. On measures of input, they had more difficulty on the fast-paced task (Seashore Rhythm) demanding sustained attention than they did on the slow-paced task (speech). Finally, the measure of information processing (PASAT and CHIPASAT), a paced addition task, was the second more difficult task following the measure of distractibility.

SUMMARY OF PERFORMANCE FALLING WITHIN AVERAGE AND ABOVE LIMITS (ABOVE AVERAGE TO SUPERIOR)

SDMT
Written: 86%
Oral: 90%
Stroop: 9%

Trail Making Part A Time: 80%
Trail Making Part A No Errors: 82%
Trail Making Part B Time: 68%
Trail Making Part B No Errors: 70%
Seashore Rhythm Test Intact Score: 37%
Speech–Sounds Perception Test Intact Score: 75%
Symbol Search: 78%
CHIPASAT: 52%
PASAT: 55%

The adolescents did not perform as well when compared to the child data on the task of distractibility. There was slightly increased time on tasks of sequencing and cognitive flexibility although this was related to fewer errors. There was a decline in the overall IQ, the result of decreased Verbal IQ suggesting diminished learning. Tasks of input for fast- and slow-paced, verbal and nonverbal stimuli were improved as well as the task of information processing, the paced addition task, when compared to the children.

The adolescents did not perform as well as the adults on a measure of reading recognition used as an intellectual estimate. Their performance on the reading recognition test was worse than the IQ scores obtained on intellectual assessment pointing to the problem of reading.

Although each situation is individualized and each score comparatively assessed to the person's potential, as a whole, the data suggest that scores, while problematic, are not severely problematic in the adolescents, which would explain the delayed time of diagnosis and evaluation. Suggested is that attention symptoms for this population may not be the primary problem. Instead, the primary problem may be the emotional reactions seen in the self-report measures, the heightened depression, and the anxiety as well as the avoidance and procrastination.

Use of the term average and above means average and above average to superior limits. Trends are reported based upon percentages obtained from the data composed of z-scores, T-scores, and standard scores.

RESULTS OF THE SPECIFIC TEST MEASURES

NART-R

There were 133 adolescents who completed this measure of reading recognition. This measure is used as an estimate of intelligence. Fifty-nine percent of the adolescents performed within average and above (above average to superior) limits. In comparison, 96% of the adults however performed within average and above average to superior limits. The difficulty adolescents had with this measure is seen as a result of their lack of familiarity with the written word related to their dislike of reading. There were many unknown words that were pronounced incorrectly as well as words that are commonly known and read incorrectly. The tendency to read words incorrectly results in poor decoding skills, more arduous reading, and diminished reading comprehension (lack of recall for a passage that took too long to read):

- 21% performed within high average limits and above on this measure (110 and above).
- 38% performed within average limits (91–109).
- 25% performed within low to below average limits (76–90).
- 12% performed within below and well below average limits (51–75).
- 3% performed within impaired limits (50 and below).

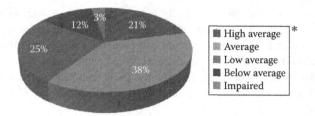

The NART-R is more a measure of problematic reading than a good intellectual estimate in the adolescent population, which was not the situation for adults. This can be seen by comparing the NART-R scores to the Full Scale IQ that was within average limits or above (above average to superior) for 72% of the population. This suggests a higher IQ than estimated by this reading recognition test and the problem of the correct pronunciation of words.

WISC IQ Test

Full Scale IQ

The Wechsler Intelligence Scale for Children was administered. The Full Scale IQ is the average of the Verbal and Performance IQ values.

Almost three-quarters of the population had intellectual scoring (Full Scale IQ) that was within average limits or above (above average limits to superior), which is what we experience clinically. This points to the fact that attention is not a problem of intelligence but instead a problem of specific attention variables. This is the reason why we stopped administering the intelligence test as part of the diagnosis of an attention disorder and used an abbreviated form or estimated IQ instead beginning in 2006.

The Verbal IQ is slightly lower than the Performance IQ. This is typical of what is often seen in the clinic. One reason for the lowered Verbal IQ is the vocabulary subtest requiring word definitions. Often ADD children described the words and personalized the definitions (their experiences with the word) or what it does rather than what it is. Low vocabulary may be the result of not reading much or inattention to the details necessary to provide an accurate definition:

- Seventy-two percent of the population had a Full Scale IQ within average limits or above (above average to superior). There is a decline when compared to the children at 83%. Full Scale IQ remained stable for males and females; 73% of the males and 72% of the females had overall Full Scale IQ within average limits or above. There is a decline when compared to the children at 82% for males and 84% for females.
- Seventy-seven percent of the population had Performance IQ values within average limits or above (above average to superior). There is a decline compared to the children at 82%. Males were slightly higher at 77% compared to 73% for females. There is a decline compared to the children at 80% for males and 86% for females. The reverse occurred in the adolescents where the males performed better than the females.
- Seventy-one percent of the population had a Verbal IQ that was within average limits and above (above average to superior). This is a decline from the 79% seen in the child population. Males were slightly higher at 71% compared to 67% for females. This is a decline from 82% for males and 80% for females in the child population that performed within average limits and above.

---

* The pie graphs range from 99 to 100 to 101 due to rounding.

This means that females had more difficulty with verbal tasks as well as performance tasks. The suggestion is that females were struggling more to be identified as needing an evaluation than males. The overall drop in IQ for the adolescents suggests their increased difficulty, which would have fueled the request for evaluation or reevaluation. When compared to the children as well as the adults, the adolescents are lower in IQ values. Finally, those who functioned within superior limits did not change much across gender (males or females) or for the difference in IQ values (Full Scale, Performance, and Verbal).

Another perspective is to include the *low average scores*, which is still seen as average although the lower end of average. This would place 93% of the adolescent population within average limits and above, which is similar to the values obtained for the children (96%), illustrating that intelligence is not the problem; attention is the symptom and the problem. Females were slightly lower at 89% and males at 94%. For Performance IQ values are similar, 94% within average limits, females are lower at 89% and males at 95%. Verbal IQ reveals less of a difference at 93%; females and males were equivalent, 92% for females and 93% for males for intelligence within the lower end of average limits or above to superior limits.

Full Scale IQ

Total of 185 adolescents completed this test:

- 6% were at 121 and above (superior).
- 12% were at 111–120 (high average to above average).
- 54% were at 91–110 (average).
- 21% were at 80–90 (low average).
- 7% were at 79 and below (borderline, below average to well below average).

Females
56 females (30%).

- 15% performed within high average limits and above on this measure (111 and above) (6% were within superior limits).
- 57% performed within average limits (91–110).
- 17% performed within low to below average limits (80–90).
- 11% performed within borderline, below average, and well below average limits (79 and below).

Males
129 males (70%).

- 20% performed within high average limits and above on this measure (111 and above) (6% were within superior limits).
- 53% performed within average limits (91–110).
- 21% performed within low to below average limits (80–90).
- 6% performed within borderline, below average, and well below average limits (79 and below).

Performance IQ

Total of 186 adolescents completed this test.

- 20% performed within high average limits and above on this measure (111 and above) (6% were within superior limits).
- 57% performed within average limits (91–110).

- 17% performed within low to below average limits (80–90).
- 6% performed within borderline, below average, and well below average limits (79 and below).

Females

56 females (30%).

- 20% performed within high average limits and above on this measure (111 and above) (7% were within superior limits).
- 53% performed within average limits (91–110).
- 16% performed within low to below average limits (80–90).
- 11% performed within borderline, below average, and well below average limits (79 and below).

Males

130 males (70%).

- 20% performed within high average limits and above on this measure (111 and above) (5% were within superior limits).
- 57% performed within average limits (91–110).
- 18% performed within low to below average limits (80–90).
- 5% performed within borderline, below average, and well below average limits (79 and below).

Verbal IQ

A total of 186 adolescents completed this test:

- 19% performed within high average limits and above on this measure (111 and above) (7% were within superior limits).
- 52% performed within average limits (91–110).
- 22% performed within low to below average limits (80–90).
- 7% performed within borderline, below average, and well below average limits (79 and below).

Females

56 females (30%)

- 21% performed within high average limits and above on this measure (111 and above) (5% were within superior limits).
- 46% performed within average limits (91–110).
- 25% performed within low to below average limits (80–90).
- 8% performed within borderline, below average, and well below average limits (79 and below).

Males

130 males (70%).

- 20% performed within high average limits and above on this measure (111 and above) (8% were within superior limits).
- 51% performed within average limits (91–110).

- 22% performed within low to below average limits (80–90).
- 6% performed within borderline, below average, and well below average limits (79 and below).

SYMBOL DIGIT MODALITIES TEST

The Symbol Digit Modalities Test (SDMT) is a measure of whole-brain functioning. The individual is asked to use a key to put the correct numbers with the correct symbol, and they have 90 s to complete as many items in correct order as they can. This measure is completed using a written format and then an oral format (where the person is saying their responses out loud to the examiner).

There is the tendency to mix up specific number symbol combinations seen through time as related to the visual–spatial difficulties. The written versus oral score allows for comparison when the act of writing is no longer a factor. However, often the impact of distractibility operates as an additional variable, and individuals lose their place on the oral portion, which negates the gain they would have had. This measure operates as a screening device to measure the general integrity and functioning of the brain. As such, it can be a measure of someone's potential that is often not seen on the other attention scores.

Scoring on this measure is a z-score, which is similar for the Trail Making Tests as well as the CHIPASAT and PASAT, based upon normative data for age, and the score is represented by a standard deviation. Average is defined as 0.75 below the mean to 0.75 of a standard deviation above the mean. Low average is 0.76–0.99 of a standard deviation below the mean. High average is 0.76–0.99 of a standard deviation above the mean. Below average is 1.0–1.99 standard deviations below the mean, and above average is 1.0–1.99 standard deviations above the mean. Well below average/impaired is 2.00 standard deviations and below, while well above/superior is 2.00 standard deviations and above the mean. This can change when time is the score or for the number of correct items versus error scores.

There were 367 adolescents for the written and oral portion.

Performance on the Written Portion
- 3% performed within well below average/impaired limits.
- 7% performed within below average limits.
- 4% performed within low average limits.
- 60% performed within average limits.
- 6% performed within high average limits.
- 16% performed within above average limits.
- 4% performed within well above/superior limit.

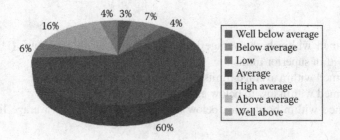

On this measure of whole-brain functioning, values are similar to that seen in the children. Whereas IQ values declined, this measure did not when comparing the children to the adolescents. The suggestion is that ability or potential is not declining with lifetime attention issues; instead, it is learning that is in decline.

For the adolescents, 86% performed within average limits and above (above average to superior) on this measure, suggesting higher abilities (this is similar to the children at 84%). Sixty percent was within average limits (similar to the children at 55%) and 20% within well above average to superior limits (children were the same at 20%). Performance was similar to that seen for the children as noted above. Generally, this measure is not highly problematic for timed performance and tends to show the potential of the individual as a measure of whole-brain functioning. Often memory was seen as helping individuals to excel on this measure as they memorized the various combinations while having to pay specific attention to three combinations of reversed symbols.

Performance on the Oral Portion

- 2% performed within well below average/impaired limits.
- 5% performed within below average limits.
- 3% performed within low average limits.
- 47% performed within average limits.
- 7% performed within high average limits.
- 19% performed within above average limits.
- 17% performed within well above/superior limits.

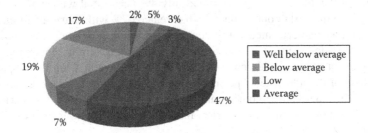

For the adolescents on the oral portion, 90% performed within average limits and above (above average to superior), suggesting higher abilities. This represents an increase from the children who were at 80%. Forty-seven percent of the adolescents performed within average limits, which is similar to the children at 50%. Thirty-six percent of the adolescents performed within above average to superior limits compared to 22% for the children, representing a substantial increase. Generally, this measure was not highly problematic for timed performance. The oral score was improved for the adolescents where it did not improve to the same degree for the children, suggesting that the adolescents benefited more from being able to provide oral responses. It would have been predicted that the adolescents would have performed worse on this measure due to the distractibility that was increased on the Stroop task of divided attention. The only explanation would be the use of memory to perform higher on the second trial of this measure as the oral condition.

STROOP COLOR WORD TEST

The Stroop Color Word Test is a measure of divided attention assessing distractibility. The adolescents has 45 s to read the word and 45 s for the interference task. Comparisons are made to their performance of word reading versus the interference task as well as obtaining a normative data T-score (where 50 is average and 10 is the standard deviation). We have found through the years that those who have a problem with this task tend to show an interference score that is one-half to two-thirds less than the word score. The only score that is recorded is the number of correct responses on the interference portion. Three hundred and fifty-six adolescents completed this task:

- 3% performed within impaired limits.
- 26% performed within well below average limits.
- 6% performed within below average limits.

- 57% performed within low average limits.
- 4% performed within average limits.
- 4% performed within high average limits.
- 1% performed within above average limits.
- 0% performed within well above/superior limits.

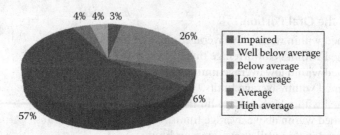

Performance for the adolescents reveals that only 4% performed within average limits. This highly declined from the child population, which revealed 67% within average limits. Fifty-seven percent of the adolescents performed within low average limits compared to 10% of the children. Four percent of the adolescents performed within high average limits compared to 4% of the children. One percent of the adolescents were within above average limits compared to 4% of the children. None of the adolescents performed within well above average/superior limits. The adolescent population performed considerably worse than the children; 9% performed within average and above (above average to superior) limits, which is far lower than the 76% indicated for the children.

TRAIL MAKING TESTS PARTS A AND B

The Trail Making Tests have two portions, Part A and Part B. The score is the time taken to complete the task of responding in correct sequential order for numbers and then for numbers and letters, alternating between the two. Errors are recorded, and the person is required to correct their error while the time continues to be recorded. This measure has been found to involve the use of rapid visual search and visuospatial sequencing. Part B assesses cognitive flexibility (ability to switch sets while maintaining a set) and is more sensitive to damage to the brain (frontal lobe regions). We have found it important to distinguish between the types of errors obtained (confusion and/or loss of place versus inability to perform the task) as opposed to the time. Individuals can take longer to perform well without mistakes. Mistakes can occur when the last number is missed on Part A and/or it becomes difficult to keep track of the number and letter sequence on Part B; both types of errors are seen as a result of visual–spatial issues. Scoring is based upon errors and time taken to complete the task and compared to normative data for specific age range. The lowest speed is the most desirable. There were 376 adolescents who completed Part A and 375 adolescents who completed Part B.

Trail Making Part A

- 3% performed within well above average/superior limits.
- 10% performed within above average limits.
- 11% performed within high average limits.
- 56% performed within average limits.
- 5% performed within low average limits.
- 9% performed within below average limits.
- 6% performed within well below/impaired limits.

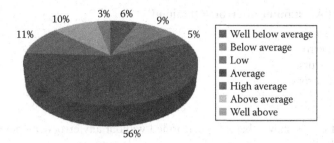

Eighty percent performed within average limits and above (above average to superior) on this first portion involving the sequencing of numbers and attention to task for decreased speed and higher scoring. This is a slight decline from 87% of the children. Fifty-six percent were within average limits, which is higher than the 41% of the children. Thirteen percent was within above average to superior limits, which is lower than the 32% seen for the children. Adolescents revealed a slight decline on their overall performance when compared to the children as a result of more adolescents performing within average limits and less within above average to superior limits. This reveals more of a qualitative decline, a decline seen in not having as high a performance when compared to the children on this task of sequencing speed. The adolescents had less errors than the children (time and errors for percentage differences between the two groups is similar), suggesting they took more time to have less errors.

Trail Making Part B
- 1% performed within well above average/superior limits.
- 12% performed within above average limits.
- 10% performed within high average limits.
- 45% performed within average limits.
- 5% performed within low average limits.
- 12% performed within below average limits.
- 14% performed within well below/impaired limits.

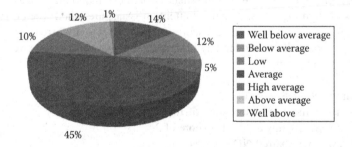

Sixty-eight percent of the adolescents performed within average limits and above (above average to superior) on this second portion involving the use of cognitive flexibility and the switching of sets from number to letter while keeping the correct sequential order. This is considerably lower than performance for the children where 80% performed within average and above limits. Thirteen percent of the adolescents were within above average to superior limits, which declined from 22% of the children. Forty-five percent of the adolescents were within average limits (children were the same). Overall this measure was more problematic for the adolescents compared to the children, and more of the children performed within higher limits. However, a slightly greater percentage of adolescents did not have any errors than the children, suggesting that the adolescents took more time to do a better job without errors, similar to the pattern seen for Part A.

Trail Making Part A: Number of Errors Obtained

- 82% had no errors.
- 13% had one error.
- 3% had two errors.
- 1% had three errors.
- 1% had more than three errors.

The number of errors shows that 82% performed without any errors compared to 78% for the children. Generally, there is one error made at the end due to visual–spatial issues, which occurred in only 13% of the population (who did not realize where the last number is) compared to 17% of the children. Errors are slightly decreased for the adolescents, which may account for the longer time to complete the task.

Trail Making Part B: Number of Errors Obtained

- 70% had no errors.
- 19% had one error.
- 8% had two errors.
- 1% had three errors.
- 2% had more than three errors.

Similar to Part A, a greater percentage (70%) of the adolescents had no errors compared to 63% of the children. Nineteen percent of the adolescents had at least one error, which tends to occur in loss of set and forgetting where they were in usually the letter sequence before the number sequence compared to 25% of the children. For the adolescents, there were slightly more errors on Part B than on Part A, which is the same pattern seen in the children.

SEASHORE RHYTHM TEST

The Seashore Rhythm Test is a measure of fast-paced nonverbal input into the brain, requiring sustained attention. Scoring is based upon the number of correct items resulting in the assigning of an NDS (Neuropsychological Deficit Score) ranked score. The individual is asked to differentiate between 30 pairs of rhyming beats. Sustained attention issues are noted when errors occur at the end of a trial; there are three trials. Ranked scores range from 0 to 3 where 0 means intact performance, 1 is mildly impaired, 2 is moderately impaired, and 3 is severely impaired. Three hundred and sixty-two adolescents completed this task:

- 37% had an intact NDS score of 0.
- 35% had a mildly impaired NDS score of 1.
- 17% had a moderately impaired NDS score of 2.
- 11% had a severely impaired NDS score of 3.

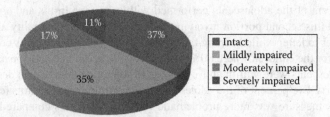

Overall the adolescents performed better on this task than the children. Thirty-seven percent of the adolescents had intact performance compared to 25% for the children. Thirty-five percent of the adolescents had a mild score, generally seen as sustained attention issues and errors, which tended to occur at the end of a trial or on the last trial, compared to 32% of the children. Seventeen percent of the adolescents had a moderately impaired score compared to 22% of the children. Eleven percent of the adolescents had a severely impaired score compared to 21% of the children. This measure tends to be more problematic than the Speech–Sounds given its faster pace. The adolescents performed better than the children overall and did not have as many moderate or severely impaired scores.

SPEECH–SOUNDS PERCEPTION TEST

The Speech–Sounds Perception Test is a measure of slow-paced verbal input into the brain and the ability to correctly distinguish the sound of nonsense syllables and to choose the correct syllable that they hear. Very few errors are expected. Scoring is similar to the Seashore Rhythm based upon the number of errors resulting in the assigning of an NDS (Neuropsychological Deficit Score) ranked score. Ranked scores range from 0 to 3 where 0 means intact performance, 1 is mildly impaired, 2 is moderately impaired, and 3 is severely impaired. Those with a genetic attention disorder tend to become bored on this measure, losing their focus or zoning out as a result. Three hundred and sixty-five adolescents completed this task:

- 75% had an intact NDS score of 0.
- 19% had a mildly impaired NDS score of 1.
- 5% had a moderately impaired NDS score of 2.
- 2% had a severely impaired NDS score of 3.

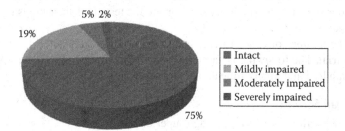

Seventy-five percent of the adolescents had no difficulty with this measure, which is much higher than the children at 51%. Ninety-four percent of the adolescents had mild or no problems compared to 57% of the children. Seven percent fell within moderate to severely impaired limits compared to 20% of the children. Adolescents clearly had no difficulty and far less difficulty than the children on this task. Some of the differences between the children and adolescents on these tasks of input may be related to more of the child population being diagnosed with ADHD plus an additional disorder.

SYMBOL SEARCH TEST

The Symbol Search Test is a measure of processing speed. The score is how many correct items can be completed within 120 s. Scoring is compared to normative data for specific age range and assigned a scaled score (10 is average and 3 is the standard deviation). This subtest is from the WISC-IV or the WAIS-III if 16 years and up. Two hundred and twenty-eight adolescents completed this measure:

- 3% had a score that was well below average/impaired.
- 19% has a score in the low to below average range.
- 37% had a score within average limits.
- 27% had a score within high to above average limits.
- 14% had a score within well above average to superior limits.

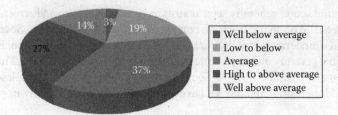

Seventy-eight percent of the adolescents had scoring within average and above (above average to superior) similar to that seen for the children at 77%, suggesting that this measure was not particularly problematic. This is a measure requiring less cognitive input and is more a process of discrimination and is highly speeded. Thirty-seven percent of the adolescents were within average limits compared to 39% of the children. Fourteen percent of the adolescents were within well above average to superior limits compared to 11% for the children, suggesting more average functioning for both groups.

CHIPASAT

This is a measure of information processing. All of the numbers are 5 and under. The adolescent is asked to add the last number to the next number. There will typically be a struggle with this measure for two reasons, firstly a problem of math fluency (inability to add quickly enough to keep up with the tap) and secondly a memory problem whereby they do not recall the last number to add it to the next number. While arithmetic was not seen as having a significant impact, the lack of math fluency would result in poor scoring or an inability to complete the test. This measure is used for ages 8–14 years. At age 15 years, the PASAT was used.

The score is the number of correct items per trial. A higher score reflects more correct items obtained on each trial. The following is based upon the total number of correct responses across all four trials. One hundred and ninety-nine adolescents completed this measure.

CHIPASAT: Overall Scoring
- 4% performed within well above average/superior limits.
- 11% performed within above average limits.
- 3% performed within high average limits.
- 34% performed within average limits.
- 7% performed within low average limits.
- 29% performed within below average limits.
- 13% performed within well below/impaired limits.

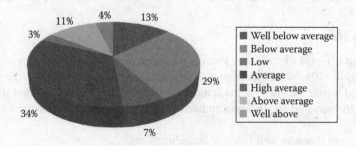

Fifty-two percent of the adolescents performed within average and above (above average limits to superior) limits on this measure, which is one of the more difficult tasks in the attention assessment.

This is significantly higher than the children at 37%. Thirty-four percent of the adolescents performed within average limits, which is higher than scoring for the children at 23%. Fifteen percent of the adolescents performed within above average to superior, which is only slightly higher than the children at 12%. The adolescents performed better than the children, which may be the result of the lower percentage of ADHD plus an additional disorder.

Data for the Four Trials

First Trial

- 4% performed within well above average/superior limits.
- 12% performed within above average limits.
- 2% performed within high average limits.
- 35% performed within average limits.
- 5% performed within low average limits.
- 22% performed within below average limits.
- 19% performed within well below/impaired limits.

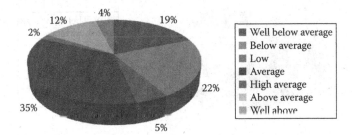

Fifty-three percent of the adolescents performed within average and above (above average to superior) for this first trial, which is a slower pace. This is higher than the children at 39%. Thirty-five percent of the adolescents were within average limits compared to 26% of the children. Sixteen percent of the adolescents were within above average to superior limits compared to 10% of the children. The adolescents performed significantly better than the children.

Second Trial

- 4% performed within well above average/superior limits.
- 9% performed within above average limits.
- 3% performed within high average limits.
- 28% performed within average limits.
- 9% performed within low average limits.
- 23% performed within below average limits.
- 23% performed within well below/impaired limits.

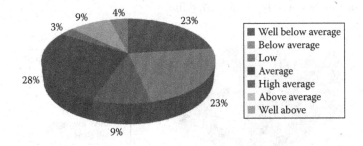

Forty-four percent of the adolescents performed within average and above (above average to superior) on the second trial, which is increased in pace. This is slightly higher than the children at 38%. Twenty-eight percent of the adolescents were within average limits compared to 24% of the children. Thirteen percent of the adolescents were within above average and superior limits compared to 12% of the children. With the increased pace, scores for the adolescents are declining and are more consistent with the children.

Third Trial

- 5% performed within well above average/superior limits.
- 11% performed within above average limits.
- 3% performed within high average limits.
- 31% performed within average limits.
- 5% performed within low average limits.
- 29% performed within below average limits.
- 17% performed within well below/impaired limits.

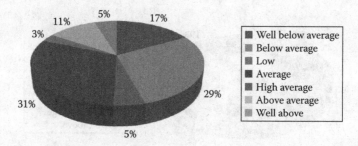

Fifty percent of the adolescents performed within average and above (above average to superior limits) for this third trial, which is more increased in pace. Scores appear to be improving, suggesting a method to cope with the pace. Sometimes adolescents tried to do every other number instead. Adolescents performed better than the children at 39%. Thirty-one percent of the adolescents were within average limits compared to 24% of the children. Sixteen percent of the adolescents were within above average to superior limits compared to 11% of the children. Adolescents seemed to figure out a method to improve their performance and were consistently performing better than the child population, representing improvement on this task.

Fourth Trial

- 6% performed within well above average/superior limits.
- 8% performed within above average limits.
- 6% performed within high average limits.
- 37% performed within average limits.
- 8% performed within low average limits.
- 28% performed within below average limits.
- 8% performed within well below/impaired limits.

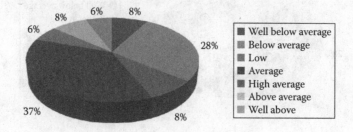

Fifty-seven percent of the adolescents performed within average and above (above average to superior limits) for this last and fourth trial, revealing improvement on the most difficult trial. Compared to the child population at 41%, adolescents performed better. Thirty-seven percent of the adolescents performed within average limits compared to 21% of the children. Fourteen percent of the adolescents were within above average to superior limits compared to 15% of the children. The children performed equivalent when considering above average to superior limits; otherwise, overall their performance was worse. The suggestion is the impact of memory issues and math fluency for the children as a result of almost half of the population being diagnosed with ADHD plus an additional disorder.

This measure does present as the most difficult task of this assessment, which is seen in the percentages remaining around 50% when the other measures ranged from 68% to 90% (other than distractibility) performing within average and above (above average to superior) limits.

PASAT

There were a total of 145 adolescents who completed the PASAT. This is a measure of information processing, a paced addition task that is used for 15 years and upward. All of the numbers are 10 and under and assess the ability to take in information, perform a simple calculation, and take in more information. The person is asked to add the last number to the next number and so on for approximately 44–45 items per trial.

Individuals will typically struggle with this measure for two reasons, firstly a problem of math fluency (inability to add quickly enough to keep up with the tape) and secondly a memory problem, not recalling the last number to add it to the next number. In addition to information processing, performance can reflect sustained attention deficits and distractibility, as well as emotional issues of giving up in frustration, a math phobia, and/or memory problem related to additional issues beyond that of a genetic attention disorder. While arithmetic was not seen as having a significant impact, the lack of math fluency would result in poor scoring or an inability to complete the test.

The PASAT is vulnerable to memory issues resulting from concussion, marijuana use, and poor sleep. Scores have improved on this measure when marijuana use is discontinued for 1 month or sleep is improved for 1 month. The score is the number of errors per trial. A higher score reflects less errors obtained on each trial. The following is based upon the total number of errors across all four trials.

PASAT Total Trials
- 0% performed within well above average/superior limits.
- 4% performed within above average limits.
- 5% performed within high average limits.
- 46% performed within average limits.
- 14% performed within low average limits.
- 24% performed within below average limits.
- 7% performed within well below/impaired limits.

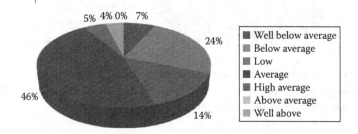

Fifty-five percent of the adolescents performed within average limits and above (above average to superior) similar to the results of the CHIPASAT. Adolescents performed similarly to the adults at 58%. Forty-six percent of the adolescents performed within average limits compared to 49% of the adults. Only 4% was within above average limits compared to 5% of the adults. None of the adolescents or adults performed within superior limits. Results suggest greater difficulty with this measure.

There are four trials and the following are the data for each trial:

First Trial

- 7% performed within well above average/superior limits.
- 25% performed within above average limits.
- 7% performed within high average limits.
- 37% performed within average limits.
- 3% performed within low average limits.
- 14% performed within below average limits.
- 7% performed within well below/impaired limits.

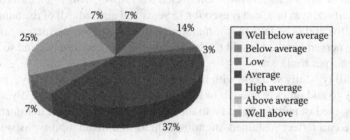

Seventy-six percent performed within average and above (above average to superior), which is significantly higher than the adults at 64%. Thirty-seven percent were within average limits (similar to adults at 39%) and 32% within above average to superior limits (higher than adults at 18%).

Second Trial

- 1% performed within well above average/superior limits.
- 8% performed within above average limits.
- 3% performed within high average limits.
- 43% performed within average limits.
- 9% performed within low average limits.
- 26% performed within below average limits.
- 10% performed within well below/impaired limits.

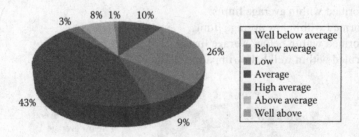

Fifty-five percent performed within average limits and above (above average to superior) on this task similar to the adults. Forty-three percent were within average limits (adults were 42%), while 9% was above average to superior limits (adults were 8%).

Third Trial

- 1% performed within well above average/superior limits.
- 3% performed within above average limits.
- 3% performed within high average limits.
- 39% performed within average limits.
- 5% performed within low average limits.
- 30% performed within below average limits.
- 20% performed within well below/impaired limits.

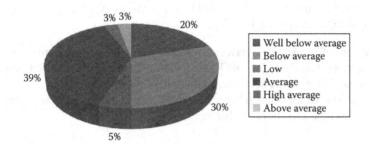

Forty-six percent performed within average and above limits (above average to superior), which was below the adults at 51%. Thirty-nine percent were within average limits similar to the adults at 40%, and only 4% (adults at 8%) was above average to superior, indicating the decline occurring as the pace of the task increased.

Fourth Trial

- 0% performed within well above average/superior limits.
- 4% performed within above average limits.
- 1% performed within high average limits.
- 32% performed within average limits.
- 11% performed within low average limits.
- 32% performed within below average limits.
- 19% performed within well below/impaired limits.

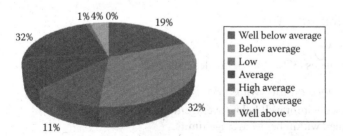

On this last trial, the adolescents did not perform as well as the adults. Thirty-seven percent performed within average and above limits (above average to superior), which is lower than the adults at 49%. Thirty-two percent was within average limits, which is again lower than the adults at 38%, and 4% was within above average (lower than adults at 8%) and no one performed within superior limits. As this task increased in pace, there was a corresponding decline in performance.

GENDER COMPARISONS: FEMALES VERSUS MALES

NART-R

There were 110 females (34%) and 218 males (66%).

Females

- 27% performed within high average limits and above on this measure (110 and above).
- 38% performed within average limits (91–109).
- 19% performed within low and well below average limits (76–90).
- 14% performed within below average and impaired limits (51–75).
- 3% performed within severely impaired limits (50 and below).

Sixty-five percent of the females performed within average or above limits (above average to superior). This is lower than the Full Scale IQ for females whereby 72% revealed average and above (above average to superior) scores but closer to the Verbal IQ where 67% performed within average and above limits. Performance is much lower than the 97% seen for the adult female population who performed within average and above on this measure.

Males

- 18% performed within high average limits and above on this measure (110 and above).
- 39% performed within average limits (91–109).
- 28% performed within low and well below average limits (76–90).
- 11% performed within below and impaired limits (51–75).
- 3% performed within severely impaired limits (50 and below).

Comparison of Males and Females

Males performed worse than females, suggesting the presence of reading difficulties or reading avoidance. Sixty-five percent of the females had average and above (above average to superior) IQ estimates on this measure compared to 57% of the males. Performance of the males on this reading recognition test is lower than the intellectual assessment showing 73% performing within average and above limits for their Full Scale IQ or Verbal IQ at 71%. Males performed worse than females on this measure; 28% of the males had low and below average IQ estimates compared to 19% of the females. The adult male population performed higher than the adolescent males on this measure with 97% revealing average and above scoring on this measure.

SYMBOL DIGIT MODALITIES TEST

Written Portion

There were 118 females (32%) and 249 males (68%).

Females: Performance on the Written Portion

- 3% performed within well below average/impaired limits.
- 9% performed within below average limits.
- 3% performed within low average limits.
- 64% performed within average limits.
- 4% performed within high average limits.
- 13% performed within above average limits.
- 4% performed within well above/superior limits.

Males: Performance on the Written Portion

- 3% performed within well below average/impaired limits.
- 6% performed within below average limits.

- 4% performed within low average limits.
- 57% performed within average limits.
- 7% performed within high average limits.
- 17% performed within above average limits.
- 4% performed within well above/superior limits.

Comparison of Males and Females

The same percentage of females and males (85%) performed within average limits and above (above average to superior) on the written potion of this measure. The child population revealed the same pattern at 84%. The difference occurs for higher functioning. Seventeen percent of the female adolescents versus 21% for males performed within above average to superior limits, suggesting slightly higher performance for males. The reverse was seen for the children; females were slightly higher at 22%, while males were at 19%.

Females were higher than males for average scoring. For the adolescents, 64% for females versus 57% for males were within average limits. The same pattern was seen in the children with slight differences, suggesting that more females perform within average limits (57% for females and 54% for males) and with age, males perform within higher limits. Adolescents revealed improved functioning on the oral portion and did not show the differences seen on the written portion.

Oral Portion

There were 117 females (32%) and 250 males (68).

Females: Performance on the Oral Portion

- 2% performed within well below average/impaired limits.
- 5% performed within below average limits.
- 3% performed within low average limits.
- 48% performed within average limits.
- 7% performed within high average limits.
- 15% performed within above average limits.
- 21% performed within well above/superior limits.

Males: Performance on the Oral Portion

- 2% performed within well below average/impaired limits.
- 5% performed within below average limits.
- 3% performed within low average limits.
- 46% performed within average limits.
- 7% performed within high average limits.
- 21% performed within above average limits.
- 16% performed within well above/superior limits.

Comparison of Males and Females

Ninety-one percent of the females versus 90% of the males performed within average limits and above (above average to superior) on the oral portion of this measure, suggesting no difference for gender similar to the written portion for overall performance. Adolescents improved when compared to the children who had more difficulty with this portion (79% for female children and 80% for male children scored within average and above limits). Males and females remained equivalent at higher scores as well; 36% of the females versus 37% of the males performed within above average to superior limits. Adolescents showed higher abilities than the children (20% for females and 23% for males). Adolescents were similar for males and females for average scoring; 48% of female adolescents had average scoring compared to 46% for males. For the children, females were slightly lower at 46% compared to the males at 52%. The children revealed differences for gender that was not seen for the adolescents.

Stroop Color Word Test

There were 111 females (31%) and 245 males (69%).

Females

- 0% performed within impaired limits.
- 3% performed within well below average limits.
- 22% performed within below to well below average limits.
- 49% performed within low average to average limits.
- 24% performed within average to high average limits.
- 2% performed within above average limits.
- 0% performed within well above/superior limits.

Males

- 0% performed within impaired limits.
- 3% performed within well below average limits.
- 26% performed within below to well below average limits.
- 40% performed within low average to average limits.
- 25% performed within average to high average limits.
- 5% performed within above average limits.
- 0% performed within well above/superior limits.

Comparison of Males and Females

Females performed slightly worse than males; 26% of the females compared to 30% of the males performed within average and above (above average to superior) limits. Males had slightly lower scores than females; 29% of the males compared to 25% of the females had scores within below average and well below average limits. Females had average scores more often; 73% of the females ranged from low average to high average limits compared to 65% of the males. Females were more often within average limits, while the males had greater percentages above or below the average range.

Trail Making Tests Parts A and B

Trail Making Part A: Number of Errors Obtained

There were 124 females (33%) and 252 males (67%).

Females

- 85% had no errors.
- 12% had one error.
- 3% had two errors.
- 0% had three errors.
- 0% had more than three errors.

Males

- 81% had no errors.
- 14% had one error.
- 3% had two errors.
- 2% had three errors.
- 0% had more than three errors.

Comparison of Males and Females

Females were slightly higher than males in obtaining no errors, 85% for females versus 81% for males. The children did not perform as well as the adolescents, 77% for females and males.

Females and males were more similar when there was one error, 12% for females versus 14% for males. The children showed greater differences for one error, 21% for females versus 16% for males.

Trail Making Part B: Number of Errors Obtained
There were 124 females (33%) and 249 males (67%).

Females
- 90% had no errors.
- 4% had one error.
- 2% had two errors.
- 1% had three errors.
- 3% had more than three errors.

Males
- 66% had no errors.
- 23% had one error.
- 9% had two errors.
- 1% had three errors.
- 1% had more than three errors.

Comparison of Males and Females

Part B is more difficult, requiring the shifting of sets from number to letter as opposed to just sequencing. Females performed significantly better than males for errors; 90% of the females versus 66% of the males had no errors. The same pattern was seen for having one error, 4% for females versus 23% for males. Making two or more errors again revealed females having less difficulty, 6% for females versus 11% for males. On this measure, there was a large gender difference revealing the superiority of females over males for the number of errors. The children revealed a similar pattern of females performing better: 67% for females versus 58% for males for no errors, 22% for females versus 25% of the males for one error, and 12% for females compared to 17% for males for two or more errors.

Trail Making Part A: Overall Score—Time to Complete the Task
Females
- 6% performed within well above average/superior limits.
- 11% performed within above average limits.
- 10% performed within high average limits.
- 50% performed within average limits.
- 5% performed within low average limits.
- 7% performed within below average limits.
- 10% performed within well below/impaired limits.

Males
- 2% performed within well above average/superior limits.
- 9% performed within above average limits.
- 10% performed within high average limits.
- 60% performed within average limits.
- 5% performed within low average limits.
- 9% performed within below average limits.
- 4% performed within well below/impaired limits.

Comparison of Males and Females

Males performed slightly better for speed and time than females; 77% for females versus 81% for males performed within average limits and above (above average to superior) on Part A involving the sequencing of numbers and attention to task with the goal of decreased speed for higher scoring. Males had slightly more errors, suggesting the compromise of quality for quantity. More males had average performance, 50% for females versus 60% for males for the time taken to complete this task. Females attained higher scores; 17% for females versus 11% for males performed within above average to superior limits. More males performed within average limits, while more females performed within above average and superior limits while simultaneously having less errors, demonstrating overall superiority on this measure.

For the child population, females were slightly higher than males for overall scoring within average and above limits, 90% for females versus 87% for males. Females were higher for average scoring, 47% females versus 39% males, which is due to more males performing within above average to superior limits, 21% females versus 37% males. There were slightly more males within below average to impaired limits, 9% females compared to 13% males. Females performed better over time, while males performed worse.

Trail Making Part B: Overall Score—Time to Complete the Task

Females
- 2% performed within well above average/superior limits.
- 10% performed within above average limits.
- 9% performed within high average limits.
- 46% performed within average limits.
- 9% performed within low average limits.
- 13% performed within below average limits.
- 10% performed within well below/impaired limits.

Males
- 0% performed within well above average/superior limits.
- 13% performed within above average limits.
- 11% performed within high average limits.
- 45% performed within average limits.
- 4% performed within low average limits.
- 12% performed within below average limits.
- 15% performed within well below/impaired limits.

Comparison of Males and Females

Sixty-seven percent of the females versus 69% of the males performed within average limits and above (above average to superior) on this more demanding measure of cognitive flexibility. Males had far more errors than females (66% for males compared to 90% for females for no errors) suggested the sacrifice of errors for time. The children showed the same pattern for time (64% for females and 65% for males), and males had more errors (percentage for no errors was 67% for females compared to 58% for males).

Female and male adolescents were similar for average scoring, 46% for females compared to 45% for males, and for scoring within above average to superior limits, 12% for females versus 13% for males. Males had no performance within well above average to superior limits.

For the child population, males performed slightly better, 15% for females compared to 20% for males for performance within well above average to superior limits. Similar to Trail Making Part A, males performed worse over time, while females performed better. Males sacrificed accuracy for speed.

Symbol Search

There were 71 females (31%) and 157 males (69%).

Females: Scaled Score
- 1% had a score that was well below average/impaired.
- 21% has a score in the low to below average range.
- 33% had a score within average limits.
- 23% had a score within high to above average limits.
- 21% had a score within well above average to superior limits.

Males: Scaled Score
- 4% had a score that was well below average/impaired.
- 18% has a score in the low to below average range.
- 39% had a score within average limits.
- 28% had a score within high to above average limits.
- 10% had a score within well above average to superior limits.

Comparison of Males and Females

Females and males were the same, 77% for average and above (above average to superior limits) on this task, suggesting no gender differences. The children showed no gender differences either, 77% for females compared to 76% for males. More females performed within well above average to superior limits, 21% of the female adolescents compared to 10% of the males. This was not seen in the children, 13% for females compared to 11% for males.

More males were within average limits, 33% of the adolescent females compared to 39% of the males. Children revealed the same pattern; 35% for females versus 40% for males attained average scoring. More adolescent males performed within high to above average scoring, 23% for females versus 28% for males (child percentages were 29 for females versus 25 for males, revealing a reverse trend).

Adolescent females performed better with higher percentages within above average to superior limits and improved in their performance over time.

CHIPASAT

There were 51 females (35%) and 94 males (65).

Females: Overall Score for Four Trials
- 2% performed within well above average/superior limits.
- 13% performed within above average limits.
- 0% performed within high average limits.
- 34% performed within average limits.
- 10% performed within low average limits.
- 32% performed within below average limits.
- 10% performed within well below/impaired limits.

Males: Overall Score
- 5% performed within well above average/superior limits.
- 9% performed within above average limits.
- 4% performed within high average limits.
- 34% performed within average limits.
- 5% performed within low average limits.
- 28% performed within below average limits.
- 15% performed within well below/impaired limits.

Comparison of Males and Females

Females did not perform as well as males when looking at performance within average and above (above average to superior) limits, 49% of females compared to 52% of males. Females performed equally to males for higher functioning, within above average to superior limits, 15% of the females compared to 14% of the males. Males and females were equivalent for average functioning; 34% of both females and males performed within average limits. Males performed better than females in adolescence similar to the child population. Females certainly improved their performance through time when comparing the child and adolescent scores. There is improvement in adolescence when compared to the child population for average and above (above average to superior) limits where males were higher, 27% for females and 41% for males. When comparing higher functioning for the children within above average to superior limits, females and males performed the same at 12%. Adolescent males overall had a slightly better performance on this paced addition task of information processing than females. There is improvement on this measure when comparing the adolescent to the child population, and females performed better in adolescents.

CHIPASAT BY TRIAL

Trial 1

Females

- 3% performed within well above average/superior limits.
- 14% performed within above average limits.
- 2% performed within high average limits.
- 35% performed within average limits.
- 6% performed within low average limits.
- 17% performed within below average limits.
- 22% performed within well below/impaired limits.

Males

- 4% performed within well above average/superior limits.
- 12% performed within above average limits.
- 3% performed within high average limits.
- 35% performed within average limits.
- 5% performed within low average limits.
- 23% performed within below average limits.
- 18% performed within well below/impaired limits.

Trial 2

Females

- 2% performed within well above average/superior limits.
- 8% performed within above average limits.
- 3% performed within high average limits.
- 37% performed within average limits.
- 3% performed within low average limits.
- 27% performed within below average limits.
- 21% performed within well below/impaired limits.

Males

- 6% performed within well above average/superior limits.
- 10% performed within above average limits.

- 4% performed within high average limits.
- 24% performed within average limits.
- 12% performed within low average limits.
- 20% performed within below average limits.
- 25% performed within well below/impaired limits.

Trial 3

Females

- 3% performed within well above average/superior limits.
- 16% performed within above average limits.
- 3% performed within high average limits.
- 26% performed within average limits.
- 2% performed within low average limits.
- 37% performed within below average limits.
- 13% performed within well below/impaired limits.

Males

- 7% performed within well above average/superior limits.
- 9% performed within above average limits.
- 3% performed within high average limits.
- 32% performed within average limits.
- 7% performed within low average limits.
- 25% performed within below average limits.
- 18% performed within well below/impaired limits.

Trial 4

Females

- 5% performed within well above average/superior limits.
- 8% performed within above average limits.
- 6% performed within high average limits.
- 42% performed within average limits.
- 10% performed within low average limits.
- 26% performed within below average limits.
- 3% performed within well below/impaired limits.

Males

- 7% performed within well above average/superior limits.
- 8% performed within above average limits.
- 6% performed within high average limits.
- 35% performed within average limits.
- 7% performed within low average limits.
- 29% performed within below average limits.
- 9% performed within well below/impaired limits.

Summation of the Individual CHIPASAT Trials

Trial 1

Comparing average and above (above average to superior) functioning, males and females were the same at 54%. Males and females were the same for average functioning at 35%. Above average to superior limits was also similar at 16% for males and 17% for females.

Trial 2

Comparing average and above (above average to superior) functioning, females were higher than males, 50% for females compared to 44% for males. Females performed better at 37% for average scoring versus males at 24%. However, more males scored higher, 16% within above average to superior range compared to 10% for females.

Trial 3

Comparing average and above (above average to superior) functioning, males were slightly higher than females, 48% for females compared to 51% for males. More males performed within average limits at 32% versus females at 26%. Females were slightly higher for above average to superior functioning at 19% compared to males at 16%.

Trial 4

Comparing average and above (above average to superior) functioning, females were higher than males, 61% for females compared to 56% for males. More females performed within average limits at 42% compared to 35% for males. Slightly more males performed within above average to superior limits at 15% versus 13% for females. On the most difficult trial, females performed slightly better.

PASAT

There were 51 females (35%) and 94 males (65%).

Females: Overall Score

- 0% performed within well above average/superior limits.
- 6% performed within above average limits.
- 6% performed within high average limits.
- 49% performed within average limits.
- 10% performed within low average limits.
- 23% performed within below average limits.
- 6% performed within well below/impaired limits.

Males: Overall Score

- 1% performed within well above average/superior limits.
- 3% performed within above average limits.
- 5% performed within high average limits.
- 44% performed within average limits.
- 15% performed within low average limits.
- 25% performed within below average limits.
- 7% performed within well below/impaired limits.

Comparison of Males and Females

Forty-nine percent of females and 44% for males performed within average limits. Sixty-one percent of females compared to 53% of males performed within average and above limits (above average to superior), suggesting better performance for the females. Six percent of the females performed within above average limits compared to 3% for the males. None of the females performed within well above average/superior limits, while 1% of the males performed within well above average/superior limits. Females generally performed better on this measure, which requires use of numbers and math fluency and is consistent with improved performance on this type of task through time. This is different from the CHIPASAT, which revealed better performance for males.

PASAT by Trials

Trial 1

Females
- 4% performed within well above average/superior limits.
- 30% performed within above average limits.
- 9% performed within high average limits.
- 41% performed within average limits.
- 2% performed within low average limits.
- 7% performed within below average limits.
- 7% performed within well below/impaired limits.

Males
- 9% performed within well above average/superior limits.
- 23% performed within above average limits.
- 6% performed within high average limits.
- 34% performed within average limits.
- 1% performed within low average limits.
- 19% performed within below average limits.
- 7% performed within well below/impaired limits.

Trial 2

Females
- 0% performed within well above average/superior limits.
- 13% performed within above average limits.
- 4% performed within high average limits.
- 37% performed within average limits.
- 13% performed within low average limits.
- 24% performed within below average limits.
- 9% performed within well below/impaired limits.

Males
- 1% performed within well above average/superior limits.
- 5% performed within above average limits.
- 3% performed within high average limits.
- 46% performed within average limits.
- 7% performed within low average limits.
- 28% performed within below average limits.
- 9% performed within well below/impaired limits.

Trial 3

Females
- 2% performed within well above average/superior limits.
- 6% performed within above average limits.
- 2% performed within high average limits.
- 37% performed within average limits.
- 2% performed within low average limits.
- 31% performed within below average limits.
- 20% performed within well below/impaired limits.

Males
- 1% performed within well above average/superior limits.
- 1% performed within above average limits.
- 3% performed within high average limits.
- 41% performed within average limits.
- 6% performed within low average limits.
- 28% performed within below average limits.
- 19% performed within well below/impaired limits.

Trial 4
Females
- 0% performed within well above average/superior limits.
- 4% performed within above average limits.
- 4% performed within high average limits.
- 31% performed within average limits.
- 15% performed within low average limits.
- 27% performed within below average limits.
- 19% performed within well below/impaired limits.

Males
- 0% performed within well above average/superior limits.
- 4% performed within above average limits.
- 0% performed within high average limits.
- 34% performed within average limits.
- 9% performed within low average limits.
- 35% performed within below average limits.
- 18% performed within well below/impaired limits.

Summation of the Individual PASAT Trials

Trial 1

Females performed better than males, 84% for females compared to 72% for males for average and above scoring (above average to superior). Females had more average scoring at 41% versus 34% for the males. Females generally performed better on the first trial given that they had a slightly higher percentage for above average to superior scoring as well, 34% versus 32% for males.

Trial 2

Females and males performed the same, 54% for females compared to 55% for males for average and above scoring (above average to superior). Males performed better at 46% for average scoring versus females at 37%. However, more females scored higher, 13% within above average to superior range compared to 6% for males.

Trial 3

Females and males performed the same, 47% for females compared to 46% for males for average and above scoring (above average to superior). Slightly more males performed within average limits at 41% versus females at 37%. Females were higher for above average to superior functioning at 8% compared to males at 2%.

Trial 4

Females and males were the same for overall performance, 39% for females compared to 38% for males for average and above scoring (above average to superior). Slightly more males performed within average limits at 34% compared to 31% for females. Males and females were equivalent at 4% for performance within above average to superior limits on the most difficult trial with the fastest pace.

SPEECH–SOUNDS PERCEPTION TEST

There were 118 females (32%) and 247 males (68%).

Females

- 77% had an intact NDS score of 0.
- 19% had a mildly impaired NDS score of 1.
- 3% had a moderately impaired NDS score of 2.
- 2% had a severely impaired NDS score of 3.

Males

- 74% had an intact NDS score of 0.
- 19% had a mildly impaired NDS score of 1.
- 6% had a moderately impaired NDS score of 2.
- 2% had a severely impaired NDS score of 3.

Comparison of Males and Females

Females were slightly higher at 77% compared to 74% males for intact performance. There is improvement through time for both males and females with males showing slightly higher performance when compared to the child population (49% females compared to 52% males). Mildly impaired performance was equal at 19% for females and 19% for males showing improvement through time when compared to the child data of 32% females and 28% males and females performing slightly worse. Females performed slightly better than males when looking at greater severity levels. Five percent for females compared to 8% for males revealed moderately to severely impaired performance (ranked scores of 2 and 3). Adolescents show substantial improvement over the child data on this slow-paced input task although there is the suggestion of males having slightly greater difficulty on this task. Females show improvement over time. Children showed more impaired functioning; 19% females and 20% males had more moderately and severely impaired performance.

SEASHORE RHYTHM TEST

There were 118 females (33%) and 244 males (67%).

Females

- 34% had an intact NDS score of 0.
- 44% had a mildly impaired NDS score of 1.
- 13% had a moderately impaired NDS score of 2.
- 9% had a severely impaired NDS score of 3.

Males

- 38% had an intact NDS score of 0.
- 31% had a mildly impaired NDS score of 1.
- 19% had a moderately impaired NDS score of 2.
- 12% had a severely impaired NDS score of 3.

Comparison of Males and Females

Females were slightly less than males for intact performance, 34% females compared to 38% males. Lower numbers of children had intact performance, which did not reveal much difference between males and females, 26% females compared to 24% males.

Females also showed more mildly impaired performance, 44% for females versus 31% for males, suggesting that males performed better on this task. The same pattern was seen for the children of 38% females compared to 29% males for mildly impaired performance.

However, greater impairment (yielding 2 and 3 ranked scores) for moderately to severely impaired performance was less for females, 22% for females compared to 31% for males, suggesting that the performance of females was not as problematic as males for severity. This is the same pattern seen for the children who had higher severity scores; 35% females and 46% males had performance that was moderately to severely impaired.

MALE AND FEMALE COMPARISONS FOR ADOLESCENTS

1. *Input tasks slow and fast paced*: Males performed somewhat worse than females for overall performance for the slow-paced task as well as more moderate to severely impaired scores. Adolescents performed better than the children for the slow-paced task. While more males had intact performance, more males also had greater moderate to severely impaired scores for the fast-paced measure of sustained attention.
2. *Information processing*: Females performed better on the PASAT, while performance on the CHIPASAT was more variable and revealed more equivalent functioning and less gender differences. Females improved their performance through time on this information processing task.
3. *Speeded tasks*: On a processing speed task, females performed better and improved in their performance over time. On measures of sequencing and cognitive flexibility, males performed worse over time, while females performed better. Males had more errors particularly on the more difficult task of cognitive flexibility, revealing the sacrifice of errors for speed. On a measure of whole-brain functioning, more females performed within average limits and more males within above average or higher limits for the written portion. Males and females improved slightly for the oral portion, and there were no gender differences.
4. *Distractibility*: Females performed slightly worse and were more often within average limits, while males had higher percentages above or below the average range.
5. Males performed worse than females on measure of reading recognition as an IQ estimate.
6. Males had a higher Performance and Verbal IQ on the intellectual testing.

6 Adult Neuropsychological Testing for ADD/ADHD

The age range was 15–80 years. Adults were administered the following test measures:

- National Adult Reading Test Revised (NART-R)
- Symbol Digit Modalities Test (SDMT)
- Stroop Color Word Test
- Trail Making Tests Part A and B
- Seashore Rhythm Test
- Speech–Sounds Perception Test
- Symbol Search Test
- Paced Auditory Serial Addition Test (PASAT)

Additional measures for the attention battery include the Bender Visual Motor Gestalt Test, Wisconsin Card Sorting Test, and the Cancellation Test. These measures were more difficult to analyze statistically and were not included in the study.

In comparing the adult performance, they had the most difficulty on the measure of divided attention, the Stroop assessing distractibility, followed by the fast-paced input task requiring sustained attention (Seashore Rhythm). The measure of information processing, a paced addition task (PASAT), was the next most problematic measure for the adults. Speed was a problem as well on tasks of whole-brain functioning (SDMT) and sequencing (Trail Making Part A) and cognitive flexibility (Trail Making Part B) performing better when speed was primary and cognitive or thinking was secondary (Symbol Search).

SUMMARY OF PERFORMANCE FALLING WITHIN AVERAGE AND ABOVE LIMITS (ABOVE AVERAGE TO SUPERIOR)

SDMT
   Written: 69%
   Oral: 69%
Stroop: 48%
Trail Making Part A Time: 72%
Trail Making Part A No Errors: 83%
Trail Making Part B Time: 63%
Trail Making Part B No Errors: 74%
Seashore Rhythm Test Intact Score: 41%
Speech–Sounds Perception Test Intact Score: 76%
Symbol Search: 84%
PASAT: 58%

The comparison of adolescents and adults on the same test measures allows assessment of the aging process of ADD symptoms through time. The adults were considerably higher than the adolescents on the reading recognition test used to estimate the intellectual level. Adults did not perform as well on a measure of whole-brain functioning, resulting in lower scores for overall performance for the written and oral portion. Adults performed better than the adolescents on the measure of distractibility although half of the population performed within below and well below average/impaired limits. Performance on a speeded sequencing task and measure of cognitive flexibility was similar to that of the adolescent population. On a task of processing speed, adults performed slightly better than the adolescents, especially on the last and most difficult trial. Adults performed better on the fast-paced input task and similar on the slow-paced task.

In comparing the adults, there was a greater struggle on the tasks of information processing, fast-paced input, distractibility, and speeded measures demanding more cognitive or thinking output.

Use of the term average and above means average and above average to superior limits. Trends are reported based upon percentages obtained from the data composed of z-scores, T-scores, and standard scores.

RESULTS OF THE SPECIFIC TEST MEASURES

NART-R

There were 1209 adults who completed this measure of reading recognition. This measure is used as an estimate of intelligence. Only 3% functioned within below average limits leaving 96% within average and above average limits:

- 68% performed within high average limits and above on this measure (110 and above).
- 28% performed within average limits (91–109).
- 3% performed within low and well below average limits (76–90).

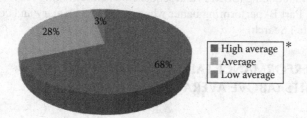

Average scoring to high average tends to be the result of using memory to develop a reading recognition vocabulary and familiarity with how the word appears. This task requires the correct pronunciation of words that the adult is asked to read out loud. Common mistakes are to read a word, colonial as colonel or recipe and receipt. The result is more difficulty decoding, the loss of the flow of reading, and ultimately what the passage actually said, appearing as a reading comprehension problem. Only 21% of the adolescents had scores within high average and above limits compared to 68% of the adults. More adolescents had average scores, 38% compared to 28% for the adults. However, adolescents had more scoring within low and below average limits, 25% compared to 3% of the adults. Adolescents also had scores below well below average limits, which the adults did not have.

SDMT

The Symbol Digit Modalities Test (SDMT) is a measure of whole-brain functioning. The individual is asked to use a key to put the correct numbers with the correct symbol, and they have 90 s to

---

* The pie graphs range from 99 to 100 to 101 due to rounding.

complete as many items in the correct order as they can. This measure is completed using a written format and then an oral format (where the person is saying their responses out loud to the examiner). There is the tendency to mix up specific number symbol combinations seen through time as related to the visual–spatial difficulties. The written versus oral score allows for comparison when the act of writing is no longer a factor. Distractibility can operate as an additional variable for the oral portion when individuals lose their place, which negates the gain they would have had. This measure operates as a screening device to measure the general integrity and functioning of the brain. As such, it can be a measure of someone's potential that is often not seen on the other attention scores.

Scoring is based upon normative data for age for the adults, and the score is represented by a standard deviation or z-score. This type of scoring is used for the Trail Making Tests and the PASAT. Average is defined as 0.75 below the mean to 0.75 of a standard deviation above the mean. Low average is 0.76–0.99 of a standard deviation below the mean. High average is 0.76–0.99 of a standard deviation above the mean. Below average is 1.0–1.99 standard deviations below the mean, and above average is 1.0–1.99 standard deviations above the mean. Well below average/impaired is 2.00 standard deviations and below, while well above/superior is 2.00 standard deviations and above the mean. When time is a factor for errors versus the score for the correct number of items, this can change.

Performance on the Written Portion

There were 1197 adults for the written portion:

- 8% performed within well below average/impaired limits.
- 17% performed within below average limits.
- 6% performed within low average limits.
- 47% performed within average limits.
- 6% performed within high average limits.
- 11% performed within above average limits.
- 5% performed within well above/superior limits.

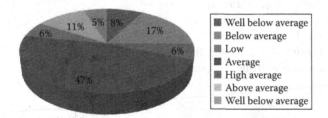

Adults performed worse than the adolescents on this measure; 69% of the adults performed within average limits and above (above average to superior) compared to the adolescents at 86%. Forty-seven percent of the adults performed within average limits compared to the adolescents at 60%. Sixteen percent of the adults performed within above average to superior compared to 20% of the adolescents.

Performance on the Oral Portion

There were 1191 adults for the oral portion:

- 7% performed within well below average/impaired limits.
- 20% performed within below average limits.
- 5% performed within low average limits.
- 46% performed within average limits.
- 4% performed within high average limits.
- 12% performed within above average limits.
- 7% performed within well above/superior limits.

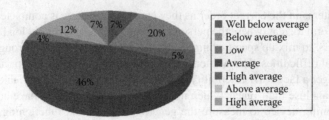

Once again, the adults showed a decline when compared to the adolescent population; 69% performed within average limits and above (above average to superior) when not having to write their responses compared to 90% of the adolescents. Nineteen percent performed within above average to superior limits, which is a slight improvement over the written score compared to the adolescents at 36%. The oral score may reflect increased distractibility when not writing. To illustrate this point, 52% of the adults performed within low average to impaired limits on the following measure of distractibility.

STROOP COLOR WORD TEST

The Stroop Color Word Test is a measure of divided attention assessing distractibility. The individual has 45 s to read the word and 45 s for the interference task. Comparisons are made to their performance of word reading versus the interference task as well as obtaining a normative data T-score (where 50 is average and 10 is the standard deviation). Individuals who have a problem on this task show an interference score that is one-half to two-thirds less than the word score. The only score that is recorded is the number of correct responses on the interference portion.

There were 1190 adults for the oral portion:

- 12% performed within well below average/impaired limits.
- 33% performed within below average limits.
- 7% performed within low average limits.
- 42% performed within average limits.
- 2% performed within high average limits.
- 3% performed within above average limits.
- 1% performed within well above/superior limits.

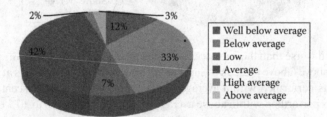

Forty-eight percent of the adults performed within average and above (above average to superior) limits, suggesting more difficulty on this measure and problems with distractibility and divided attention. Distractibility can often be impacted by other additive factors related to sleep, stress, depression, and poor diet. The performance of the adults was significantly higher than the adolescents; 9% of the adolescents performed within average and above limits (above average to superior). Seven percent of the adults were within low average limits compared to 57% of the adolescents. Not many of the adults performed higher than average; only 6% were within high average to superior limits compared to 9% for the adolescents.

TRAIL MAKING TESTS

The Trail Making Tests have two portions, Part A and Part B. The score is the time taken to complete the task of responding in correct sequential order for numbers and then for numbers and letters, alternating between the two. Errors are recorded, and the person is required to correct any errors made during the time of their performance, which continues to be recorded. This measure has been found to involve the use of rapid visual search and visuospatial sequencing. Part B is more sensitive to impact to brain processes (executive reasoning) and cognitive flexibility. We have found it important to distinguish between the types of errors obtained (confusion and/or loss of place versus inability to perform the task) as opposed to the time. Individuals can take longer to perform well without mistakes. Mistakes can occur when the last number is missed on Part A and/or it becomes difficult to keep track of the number and letter sequence on Part B; both types of errors are seen as a result of visual–spatial issues. Scoring is based upon errors and time taken to complete the task and compared to normative data for specific age range. The lowest speed is the most desirable.

Trail Making Part A: Time Score
There were 1233 adults for this portion:

- 1% performed within well above average/superior limits.
- 9% performed within above average limits.
- 9% performed within high average limits.
- 53% performed within average limits.
- 6% performed within low average limits.
- 12% performed within below average limits.
- 11% performed within well below/impaired limits.

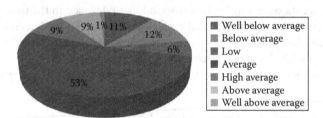

Adults were slightly lower than adolescents; 72% of the adults performed within average limits and above (above average to superior) compared to 80% for the adolescents. Adults were slightly lower than the adolescents for average scoring, 53% compared to 56% for the adolescents. Adults were slightly lower for above average to superior scoring at 10% compared to 13% for the adolescents.

Trail Making Part B: Time Score
There were 1239 adults for the oral portion:

- 0% performed within well above average/superior limits.
- 8% performed within above average limits.
- 6% performed within high average limits.
- 49% performed within average limits.
- 5% performed within low average limits.
- 15% performed within below average limits.
- 16% performed within well below/impaired limits.

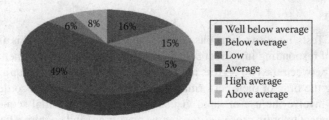

Adults were slightly below the adolescents for average and above (above average to superior) scoring, 63% for the adults compared to 68% for the adolescents on this second portion involving the use of cognitive flexibility and the switching of sets (from number to letter) while keeping the correct sequential order. Adults were slightly higher than the adolescents for average scoring, 49% compared to 45% for the adolescents. Adults were slightly lower for performance within above average to superior limits, 8% for the adults compared to 13% for the adolescents. This measure can take longer due to visual–spatial issues and needing to continually count from the beginning due to losing one's place in the alphabet. Individuals tend to keep count internally of the number and letter set (sometimes going back to the beginning each time, e.g., instead of going 4 then D, they would go A, B, C, D) while looking for the next number or letter.

Trail Making Part A: Number of Errors Obtained

- 83% had no errors.
- 11% had one error.
- 3% had two errors.
- 2% had three errors.
- 1% had more than three errors.

Adults and adolescents were similar for errors, adding relevance to the time score; 83% of the adults and 82% of the adolescents performed without any errors. Those that do make an error tend to miss the number in the corner due to visuospatial issues, which occurred with 11% of the population. Adults were slightly less for one error, 11% compared to 13% for the adolescents. Adults and adolescents were similar for two errors or more, 6% for the adults compared to 5% for the adolescents.

Trail Making Part B: Number of Errors Obtained

- 74% had no errors.
- 10% had one error.
- 4% had two errors.
- 2% had three errors.
- 10% had more than three errors.

Adults had slightly less errors than the adolescents, 74% for the adults compared to 70% for the adolescents. Adults were lower for one error and less than the adolescents, 10% compared to 19% for the adolescents. Adults however were higher for two or more errors, 16% compared to 11% for the adolescent population. This measure is more difficult and more susceptible to other conditions affecting the brain, resulting in more errors than Part A for the adults.

Seashore Rhythm Test

The Seashore Rhythm Test is a measure of fast-paced nonverbal input into the brain requiring sustained attention. The adult is asked to differentiate between 30 pairs of rhyming beats. This measure requires alertness to nonverbal auditory stimuli, sustained attention, and the ability to perceive and compare rhythmic sequences. Sustained attention issues are noted when errors occur at the end of a trial; there are three trials. Scoring is based upon the number of correct items resulting in the assigning of an NDS (Neuropsychological Deficit Score) ranked score. Ranked scores range from 0 to 3 where 0 means intact performance, 1 is mildly impaired, 2 is moderately impaired, and 3 is severely impaired.

There were 1208 adults:

- 41% had an intact NDS score of 0.
- 36% had a mildly impaired NDS score of 1.
- 18% had a moderately impaired NDS score of 2.
- 4% had a severely impaired NDS score of 3.

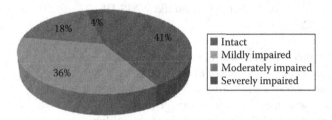

Adults had more difficulty on this measure; only 41% had no errors. Adults performed slightly better than the adolescents at 37% for no errors. Adults and adolescents were similar for a mildly impaired score (36% for the adults compared to 35% for the adolescent population) and for moderate impairment (18% of the adults compared to 17% for the adolescents). More of the adolescents had a severely impaired score, 11% compared to 4% of the adults.

SPEECH–SOUNDS PERCEPTION TEST

The Speech–Sounds Perception Test is a measure of slow-paced verbal input into the brain. Scoring is based upon number of errors resulting in the assigning of an NDS (Neuropsychological Deficit Score) ranked score. Similar to the Seashore Rhythm, ranked scores range from 0 to 3 where 0 means intact performance, 1 is mildly impaired, 2 is moderately impaired, and 3 is severely impaired. This task is a measure of slow-paced, verbal stimuli and the ability to correctly distinguish the sound of nonsense syllables and to choose the correct syllable that they hear. Very few errors are expected due to the slow pace. Those with a genetic attention disorder tend to become bored on this measure, losing their focus or zoning out as a result.

There were 1212 adults:

- 76% had an intact NDS score of 0.
- 17% had a mildly impaired NDS score of 1.
- 5% had a moderately impaired NDS score of 2.
- 2% had a severely impaired NDS score of 3.

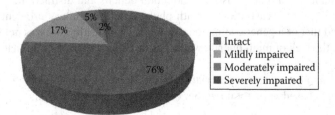

Adults were similar to the adolescents; 76% compared to 75% of the adolescents had no impairment. Seventeen percent of the adults compared to 19% of the adolescents had a mildly impaired score. Five percent of the adults and adolescents had a moderately impaired score, and 2% for the adults and adolescents had a severely impaired score. Sleep significantly impacted performance on this measure.

SYMBOL SEARCH TEST

Symbol Search Test is a measure of processing speed. The score obtained is based upon the number of correct items completed within 120 s. Scoring is compared to normative data for specific age range and assigned a scaled (standard) score (10 is average and 3 is the standard deviation). This subtest is from the WAIS-III intellectual assessment. The WAIS-IV was not used due to the difference in font that was significantly different from the WAIS-III.

There were 1212 adults:

- 4% had a score that was well below average/impaired.
- 12% had a score in the low to below average range.
- 40% had a score within average limits.
- 31% had a score within high to above average limits.
- 13% had a score within well above average to superior limits.

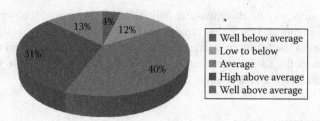

Adults performed better than the adolescents; 84% had scoring within average and well above (above average to superior) limits, suggesting that this measure was not particularly problematic, compared to 78% of the adolescents. This is a measure that requires less cognitive input and is more a process of discrimination and is highly speeded. Adults were slightly higher for average scoring; 40% adults compared to 37% adolescents performed within average limits. Adults and adolescents were similar for the highest performance within well above average to superior limits, 13% for the adults compared to 14% for the adolescents.

PASAT

This is a measure of information processing. All of the numbers are 10 and under. The person is asked to add the last number to the next number and so on for approximately 44–45 items per trial. Individuals will typically struggle with this measure for two reasons, firstly a problem of math fluency (inability to add quickly enough to keep up with the tape) and secondly a memory problem whereby they do not recall the last number to add it to the next number. In addition to information processing, performance can reflect sustained attention deficits and distractibility, as well as emotional issues of giving up in frustration, a math phobia, and/or memory problem related to additional issues beyond that of a genetic attention disorder. While arithmetic was not seen as having a significant impact, the lack of math fluency would result in poor scoring or an inability to complete the test.

The score is the number of errors per trial. A higher score reflects less errors obtained on each trial. The following is based upon total number of errors across all four trials.

There were 1108 adults:

- 0% performed within well above average/superior limits.
- 5% performed within above average limits.
- 4% performed within high average limits.
- 49% performed within average limits.
- 9% performed within low average limits.
- 22% performed within below average limits.
- 10% performed within well below/impaired limits.

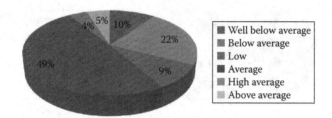

Fifty-eight percent or slightly more than half performed within average limits and above (above average to superior) on this measure, which is one of the more difficult tasks in the attention assessment. Average scoring was 49%, while below average to impaired was at 32%, suggesting the overall difficulty of this measure. Only 5% were within above average limits, and no one was within well above average to superior limits. As the trials continued, the overall score within average and above limits declined as the below average to impaired score increased. Overall scoring is similar to the adolescent population. This measure was significantly impacted by sleep.

Data for the Four Trials

First Trial

- 5% performed within well above average/superior limits.
- 13% performed within above average limits.
- 7% performed within high average limits.
- 39% performed within average limits.
- 6% performed within low average limits.
- 13% performed within below average limits.
- 18% performed within well below/impaired limits.

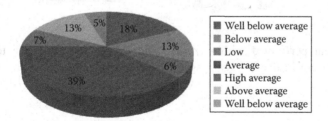

Sixty-four percent performed within average and above (above average to superior) limits. Thirty-nine percent were in the average range. Thirty-one percent were within below average to impaired limits.

Second Trial

- 1% performed within well above average/superior limits.
- 7% performed within above average limits.
- 5% performed within high average limits.
- 42% performed within average limits.
- 8% performed within low average limits.
- 23% performed within below average limits.
- 15% performed within well below/impaired limits.

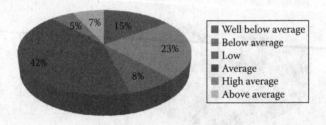

Fifty-five percent performed within average and above (above average to superior) limits. Forty-two percent were in the average range. Thirty-eight percent were within below average to impaired limits.

Third Trial

- 1% performed within well above average/superior limits.
- 7% performed within above average limits.
- 3% performed within high average limits.
- 40% performed within average limits.
- 7% performed within low average limits.
- 27% performed within below average limits.
- 15% performed within well below/impaired limits.

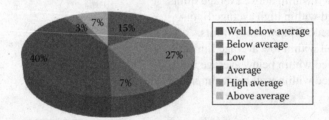

Fifty-one percent performed within average and above (above average to superior) limits. Forty percent were in the average range. Forty-two percent were within below average to impaired limits.

Fourth Trial

- 2% performed within well above average/superior limits.
- 6% performed within above average limits.
- 3% performed within high average limits.
- 38% performed within average limits.
- 10% performed within low average limits.

- 27% performed within below average limits.
- 13% performed within well below/impaired limits.

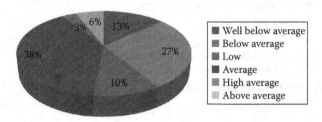

Forty-nine percent performed within average and above (above average to superior) limits. Thirty-eight percent were in the average range. Forty percent were within below average to impaired limits.

Over the course of four trials, the percent within average and above limits declined while the percentage within below average to impaired limits increased substantially.

GENDER COMPARISONS: FEMALES VERSUS MALES

NART-R

There were 435 females (36%) and 767 males (64%):

Females

- 70% performed within high average limits and above on this measure (110 and above).
- 27% performed within average limits (91–109).
- 3% performed within below and well below average limits (76–90).

Males

- 68% performed within high average limits and above on this measure (110 and above).
- 29% performed within average limits (91–109).
- 3% performed within below and well below average limits (76–90).

Comparison of Males and Females

Males and females were similar in their performance; 97% performed within average and above (above average to superior) limits. Adolescents were considerably lower with 65% for the females and 57% for the males performing within average and above limits. Three percent of the adult population was within low to well below average limits compared to 36% of the females and 42% of the males. Females showed the most improvement over time when comparing the adolescent to the adult population.

SDMT: WRITTEN PORTION

There were 435 females (36%) and 767 males (64%):

Females

- 7% performed within well below average/impaired limits.
- 16% performed within below average limits.
- 3% performed within low average limits.
- 47% performed within average limits.

- 7% performed within high average limits.
- 14% performed within above average limits.
- 6% performed within well above/superior limits.

Males

- 9% performed within well below average/impaired limits.
- 19% performed within below average limits.
- 8% performed within low average limits.
- 46% performed within average limits.
- 5% performed within high average limits.
- 10% performed within above average limits.
- 4% performed within well above/superior limits.

Comparison of Males and Females

Females performed better for overall scoring of average and above (above average to superior) limits, 74% for females compared to 65% for males. Average functioning was similar; 47% of the females compared to 46% of the males performed within average limits. However, above average to superior scoring showed better performance for females, 20% for females compared to 14% for males. Suggested is better performance for females on the written portion of this task.

SDMT: Oral Portion

There were 435 females (36%) and 767 males (64%):

Females

- 6% performed within well below average/impaired limits.
- 18% performed within below average limits.
- 6% performed within low average limits.
- 48% performed within average limits.
- 5% performed within high average limits.
- 11% performed within above average limits.
- 6% performed within well above/superior limits.

Males

- 7% performed within well below average/impaired limits.
- 21% performed within below average limits.
- 5% performed within low average limits.
- 44% performed within average limits.
- 3% performed within high average limits.
- 12% performed within above average limits.
- 7% performed within well above/superior limits.

Comparison of Males and Females

Similar to the written portion, females performed better; 70% of the females versus 66% of the males performed within average limits and above (above average to superior) on the oral portion of this measure. Forty-eight percent of the females compared to 44% of the males performed within average limits. Males were slightly higher when comparing above average to superior performance, 17% for females compared to 19% for males. Females performed better overall; however, when comparing performance at higher levels, there is less of a gender difference.

STROOP COLOR WORD

There were 435 females (36%) and 767 males (64%):

Females

- 2% performed within impaired limits.
- 11% performed within well below average limits.
- 31% performed within below average limits.
- 7% performed within low average limits.
- 43% performed within average limits.
- 2% performed within high average limits.
- 4% performed within above average limits.
- 1% performed within well above/superior limits.

Males

- 1% performed within impaired limits.
- 9% performed within well below average limits.
- 34% performed within below average limits.
- 7% performed within low average limits.
- 42% performed within average limits.
- 2% performed within high average limits.
- 3% performed within above average limits.
- 1% performed within well above/superior limits.

Comparison of Females and Males

Overall, males and females were similar in functioning; 50% of the females performed within average and above (above average to superior) compared to 48% of the males.

TRAIL MAKING TEST PARTS A AND B

Trail Making Part A: Number of Errors Obtained

There were 435 females (36%) and 767 males (64%):

Females

- 86% had no errors.
- 9% had one error.
- 2% had two errors.
- 1% had three errors.
- 1% had more than three errors.

Males

- 82% had no errors.
- 12% had one error.
- 3% had two errors.
- 2% had three errors.
- 1% had more than three errors.

Comparison of Males and Females

Males had slightly more errors than females; 86% of females compared to 82% of males had no errors on this task. Slightly more males had one error, 9% for females compared to 12% for males. Males had a slightly greater severity of errors; more males had two or more errors, 4% for the females compared to 6% for the males.

Trail Making Part B: Number of Errors Obtained

There were 435 females (36%) and 767 males (64%):

Females

- 73% had no errors.
- 12% had one error.
- 4% had two errors.
- 2% had three errors.
- 9% had more than three errors.

Males

- 74% had no errors.
- 9% had one error.
- 4% had two errors.
- 2% had three errors.
- 11% had more than three errors.

Comparison of Males and Females

Males and females were similar for having no errors, 73% of the females compared to 74% of the males. Slightly more females had one error than males, 12% for females compared to 9% for males. Males had a slightly greater severity of errors, for two or more errors were made by 15% females compared to 17% males.

Males had slightly more errors on Part A, the sequencing task, while males and females were more equivalent on Part B demanding cognitive flexibility and the switching of sets.

Trail Making Part A: Time Score

There were 435 females (36%) and 790 males (64%):

Females

- 1% performed within well above average/superior limits.
- 12% performed within above average limits.
- 10% performed within high average limits.
- 51% performed within average limits.
- 5% performed within low average limits.
- 11% performed within below average limits.
- 9% performed within well below/impaired limits.

Seventy-four percent performed within average limits and above (above average to superior) on this first portion involving the sequencing of numbers and attention to task for decreased speed and higher scoring.

Males

- 0% performed within well above average/superior limits.
- 7% performed within above average limits.
- 8% performed within high average limits.
- 53% performed within average limits.
- 7% performed within low average limits.
- 12% performed within below average limits.
- 13% performed within well below/impaired limits.

Comparison of Males and Females

Females performed better for overall time on this task for average and above (above average to superior) scoring, 74% of females compared to 68% of the males. More females performed within above average to superior limits for time, 13% of the females compared to 7% of the males. Females performed better than males on this task for speed.

Trail Making Part B: Time Score

There were 435 females (36%) and 767 males (64%):

Females

- 1% performed within well above average/superior limits.
- 9% performed within above average limits.
- 7% performed within high average limits.
- 52% performed within average limits.
- 5% performed within low average limits.
- 14% performed within below average limits.
- 12% performed within well below/impaired limits.

Males

- 0% performed within well above average/superior limits.
- 7% performed within above average limits.
- 6% performed within high average limits.
- 47% performed within average limits.
- 5% performed within low average limits.
- 16% performed within below average limits.
- 19% performed within well below/impaired limits.

Comparison of Males and Females

More females than males performed within average limits and above (above average to superior) limits on this task, 69% of the females compared to 60% of the males on this measure of cognitive flexibility. Slightly more females had above average to superior scores, 10% of the females compared to 7% of the males. Females performed better overall on this task for speed.

SYMBOL SEARCH

There were 76 females (44%) and 95 males (56%):

Females: Scaled Score
- 4% had a score that was well below average/impaired.
- 12% had a score in the low to below average range.
- 43% had a score within average limits.
- 25% had a score within high to above average limits.
- 16% had a score within well above average to superior limits.

Males: Scaled Score
- 3% had a score that was well below average/impaired.
- 13% had a score in the low to below average range.
- 38% had a score within average limits.
- 36% had a score within high to above average limits.
- 11% had a score within well above average to superior limits.

Comparison of Males and Females

Eighty-four percent of the females compared to 85% of the males performed within average and above limits (above average to superior) on this task, suggesting no gender differences. Females were lower for high average performance and higher for performance within well above average to superior limits, 25% for females compared to 36% for males for high average scoring and 16% for females compared to 11% for males for scoring within well above average to superior limits. Females were higher for average scoring; 43% of the females compared to 38% of the males were within average limits. Males and females performed similarly; however, more females performed within well above average to superior limits.

PASAT

There were 425 females (35%) and 776 males (65%):

Females: Overall Score

- 2% performed within well above average/superior limits.
- 3% performed within above average limits.
- 3% performed within high average limits.
- 41% performed within average limits.
- 11% performed within low average limits.
- 26% performed within below average limits.
- 14% performed within well below/impaired limits.

Males: Overall Score

- 0% performed within well above average/superior limits.
- 6% performed within above average limits.
- 5% performed within high average limits.
- 53% performed within average limits.
- 8% performed within low average limits.
- 20% performed within below average limits.
- 8% performed within well below/impaired limits.

Comparison of Males and Females

Forty-nine percent of the female adults performed within average limits and above (above average to superior) compared to 64% of the males, suggesting that adult males performed better on this measure, which requires use of numbers and math fluency. Females showed a decline when compared to adolescent scores of 61% females and 53% males performing within average limits and above. More males were within average limits than females, 41% females versus 53% males. Females showed a decline through time, while males improved when compared to adolescent percentages of 49% females and 44% males for average scoring. Two percent of the females performed within well above average to superior limits compared to 0% for the female adolescents. None of the adult males performed within well above average to superior limits compared to 1% for adolescent males.

Data for the Four Trials

Females: First Trial

- 3% performed within well above average/superior.
- 9% performed within above average limits.

- 7% performed within high average limits.
- 38% performed within average limits.
- 7% performed within low average limits.
- 16% performed within below average limits.
- 22% performed within well below/impaired limits.

Males: First Trial
- 5% performed within well above average/superior limits.
- 16% performed within above average limits.
- 7% performed within high average limits.
- 39% performed within average limits.
- 5% performed within low average limits.
- 12% performed within below average limits.
- 15% performed within well below/impaired limits.

Females: Second Trial
- 2% performed within well above average/superior limits.
- 4% performed within above average limits.
- 3% performed within high average limits.
- 37% performed within average limits.
- 8% performed within low average limits.
- 26% performed within below average limits.
- 20% performed within well below/impaired limits.

Males: Second Trial
- 1% performed within well above average/superior limits.
- 8% performed within above average limits.
- 5% performed within high average limits.
- 44% performed within average limits.
- 7% performed within low average limits.
- 22% performed within below average limits.
- 12% performed within well below/impaired limits.

Females: Third Trial
- 1% performed within well above average/superior limits.
- 5% performed within above average limits.
- 2% performed within high average limits.
- 31% performed within average limits.
- 7% performed within low average limits.
- 35% performed within below average limits.
- 18% performed within well below/impaired limits.

Males: Third Trial
- 1% performed within well above average/superior limits.
- 8% performed within above average limits.
- 3% performed within high average limits.
- 44% performed within average limits.
- 7% performed within low average limits.
- 23% performed within below average limits.
- 13% performed within well below/impaired limits.

Females: Fourth Trial
- 3% performed within well above average/superior limits.
- 5% performed within above average limits.
- 1% performed within high average limits.
- 34% performed within average limits.
- 10% performed within low average limits.
- 33% performed within below average limits.
- 15% performed within well below/impaired limits.

Males: Fourth Trial
- 2% performed within well above average/superior limits.
- 7% performed within above average limits.
- 4% performed within high average limits.
- 41% performed within average limits.
- 9% performed within low average limits.
- 24% performed within below average limits.
- 12% performed within well below/impaired limits.

Summation of the Individual PASAT Trials—
There Is an Increased Difficulty with Each Trial
Trial 1

Females did not perform as well as males for average and above (above average to superior) scoring, 57% of the females compared to 67% of the males. Females and males were equally within average limits, 38% of the females compared to 39% of the males. However, more males performed at the highest level within above average to superior limits, 12% of the females compared to 21% of the males. Females showed a decline through time when compared to the adolescents who performed better than males on the first trial (more average scoring at 41% versus 34% for the males and slightly higher percentage for above average to superior scoring as well, 34% versus 32% for males).

Trial 2

Females did not perform as well as males for the second trial for average and above (above average to superior) scoring, 46% versus 58% for males. More males were within average limits and at the highest level of functioning (above average to superior); 37% of the females versus 44% of the males were within average limits, while 6% females compared to 9% males performed within above average to superior limits. When compared to the adolescent data, there is a decline for females and improved functioning for males at the higher functioning levels (13% females compared to males at 6%).

Trial 3

Males performed better than females for overall performance; 39% of the females compared to 56% of the males performed within average and above limits (above average to superior). More males were within average limits and had higher functioning scores; 31% females compared to 44% males were within average limits, and 6% females compared to 9% males were at above average to superior functioning. There is a decline seen for females as the pace of the task increased. Females are declining through time, while males are improving.

This is seen when compared to the adolescents; 37% females and 41% males had average functioning; 8% females compared to 2% males had the highest functioning at above average to superior.

Trial 4

Females continued to have more difficulty; 43% of the females compared to 54% of the males performed within average and above limits (above average to superior). More males were within average limits than females; 34% females compared to 41% males were within average limits. However, higher functioning was more equal and showed improvement for the females; 8% of the females compared to 9% of the males were within above average limits. No one performed within superior limits. Males continued to improve through time and showed superiority on this measure; 34% males compared to 31% female adolescents were within average limits. Males and females improved over the adolescents on performance within above average to superior limits; male and female adolescents were at 4%.

SPEECH–SOUNDS PERCEPTION TEST

There were 432 females (36%) and 780 males (64%):

Females
- 78% had an intact NDS score of 0.
- 16% had a mildly impaired NDS score of 1.
- 4% had a moderately impaired NDS score of 2.
- 2% had a severely impaired NDS score of 3.

Males
- 75% had an intact NDS score of 0.
- 17% had a mildly impaired NDS score of 1.
- 6% had a moderately impaired NDS score of 2.
- 2% had a severely impaired NDS score of 3.

Comparison of Males and Females

Females were slightly higher at 78% compared to 75% males for intact performance. Adolescents were at 77% for females and 74% for males, revealing a similar pattern. Mildly impaired performance was equal at 16% for females and 17% for males showing improvement through time; adolescents were at 19%. Females performed slightly better with less moderate to impaired scoring, 6% for females compared to 8% for males. Adolescents were similar at 5% for females compared to 8% for males.

SEASHORE RHYTHM TEST

There were 428 females (35%) and 780 males (65%):

Females
- 41% had an intact NDS score of 0.
- 33% had a mildly impaired NDS score of 1.
- 19% had a moderately impaired NDS score of 2.
- 6% had a severely impaired NDS score of 3.

Males
- 41% had an intact NDS score of 0.
- 38% had a mildly impaired NDS score of 1.
- 17% had a moderately impaired NDS score of 2.
- 3% had a severely impaired NDS score of 3.

Comparison of Males and Females

Females and males were the same for intact performance at 41%. Performance for the adults is improved compared to adolescents of 34% for female and 38% for male for intact performance. Females performed better than males for mildly impaired performance, 33% for females compared to 38% for males. Adolescents had higher mild impairment for females and less for males; females were at 44% and males at 31%. Adult females had more severe performance with a higher percentage of moderate to severely impaired scores, females at 25% compared to males at 20%. Moderate to serve performance for adolescents was 22% for females and 31% for males which showed improved performance for males but not for females over time. Females had a more difficult time on this task when comparing moderate to severe performance, while more males had one error for mildly impaired performance.

MALE AND FEMALE COMPARISONS FOR ADULTS

1. *Input tasks slow- and fast- paced*: Females performed slightly better on the slow-paced verbal task. More females had no errors and less moderate to severely impaired scoring. Females had more difficulty on the fast-paced task demanding sustained attention. Males had more mildly impaired performance, while females had more moderate to severely impaired performance.
2. *Information processing*: Males performed higher than females on the paced addition task for overall scoring. Females revealed a decline when compared to adolescent scores. Males continued to improve through time and had higher scores on this measure through each of the individual trials.
3. *Speeded tasks*: Females performed better on the written portion of a measure of whole-brain functioning, while the oral portion was not as clear. While somewhat better overall, there was less of a gender difference when comparing above average to superior performance. Females performed better on tasks of sequencing and cognitive flexibility, taking less time with slightly fewer errors or similar amount of errors. On a task of processing speed while performing similarly for the overall scoring, females had more scores within well above average to superior limits.
4. *Distractibility*: Females and males were similar on a measure of divided attention assessing distractibility.
5. Males and females were similar on the reading recognition test. Females showed the most improvement over time when compared to the adolescent population.

7 Description of the Self-Report Measures Administered

In the following pages, you will find the statistics on the numerous checklists that were administered. There were checklists given to the adults to complete regarding their own symptoms. For children, checklists were given to parents to complete as well as to the teacher or teachers (scores were averaged when there were multiple teachers), and checklists were completed by the adolescent. For the ages of 15–17 years, the adolescents completed the same checklists used for the adults. The adult battery for testing begins at the age of 15 years.

Checklists that the parents completed are as follows:

- ADHD Rating Scale
- Child Behavior Checklist
- Children's Problems Checklist
- Children Symptom Inventory
- Child Neuropsychological History
- Developmental History Checklist
- Sleep Evaluation Questionnaire
- ADDES Home Version
- Home Situations Questionnaire

Checklists that the teacher or teachers completed are as follows:

- Academic Performance Rating Scale
- Child Attention Profile
- Social Situations Questionnaire
- ACTeRS

Checklists that the adolescent completed are as follows:

- Patient Behavior Checklist
- Physical Complaints Checklist
- Beck Depression Inventory
- Beck Anxiety Inventory
- Personal Problems Checklist for Adolescents
- Personal History Checklist for Adolescents

Checklists that the adult completed are as follows:

- CAARS
- Patient Behavior Checklist
- Physical Complaints Checklist
- Personal Problems Checklist for Adults
- Personal History Checklist for Adults

- Adult Neuropsychological Questionnaire
- Sleep Questionnaire
- Quality of Life Inventory
- Beck Depression Inventory
- Beck Anxiety Inventory

ADHD RATING SCALE

The ADHD Rating Scale is a measure completed by the parent regarding attention problems seen in their child. There are a total of 14 items that the parent can respond to as not present or seen just a little, pretty much, or very much of the time that address symptoms of inattention, hyperactivity, and impulsivity. A total of 454 parents of children and 175 parents of adolescents responded and reported on attention symptoms about their child. This measure was published in 1998 by DuPaul et al.

CHILD BEHAVIOR CHECKLIST

The Child Behavior Checklist is a self-report measure completed by the parent for the age range of 4–18 years, 1991 version. It was revised in 2001, and the current version uses the age range of 6–18. The majority of the parents used the version from 4 to 18 years (we began using the updated current version in 2007/2008). There are a total of 118 problem items designed to address behavioral and emotional problems present in children, yielding a multiaxial empirically based assessment to provide diagnosis and severity of emotional symptoms. Scoring is based upon a serevity, not present, and occurs some of the time and very often (Achenbach, 1991, 2001). There were 212 parents of adolescents who responded to this checklist. Only 17 of the parents of children responded to this measure; so these data were not used for the child population.

CHILDREN'S PROBLEM CHECKLIST

The Children's Problem Checklist is utilized to assess a variety of areas of functioning, including emotions, academics, concentration, behaviors, language, thinking, health, and habits. The questionnaire consists of 202 yes and no response items and was written by Schinka (1985a). There were a large number, 550 parents of children, who responded to this questionnaire asking them to report areas of concern regarding their child for emotions, self-issues, social interaction, school, language/thinking, concentration/organization, actions/motor skills, behavior, values, habits, and health. Parents do not rate how significant the problem is; they respond only as to whether they think that it is a concern or not. There were 186 parents of adolescents who responded to this questionnaire.

CHILD SYMPTOM INVENTORY-4: PARENT CHECKLIST (CSI-4)

The Child Symptom Inventory-4: Parent Checklist (CSI-4) is a parent-completed rating scale that allows for the screening of attention deficit/hyperactivity disorder (ADHD) and other emotional and behavioral disorders described in the American Psychiatric Association's (1994) Diagnostic and Statistical Manual for Mental Disorders. Questions are asked regarding the following types of disorders: attention deficit/hyperactivity disorder, oppositional defiant disorder, conduct disorder, anxiety, schizophrenia, major depressive disorder, dysthymic disorder, autistic disorder, Asperger's disorder, social phobia, and separation anxiety disorder. There were 107 parents of children and 32 parents of adolescents who responded to this questionnaire used between the years 2006 and 2009 and currently in use. Parents rated the symptoms as occurring never, sometimes, often, or very often.

ADULT AND CHILD NEUROPSYCHOLOGICAL HISTORY

The Adult and the Child Neuropsychological History was created in 1990 by Glen D. Greenberg (Greenberg, 1990a,b). The adult checklist is similar to the child checklist only completed by the adult patient as opposed to the parent/guardian of a child. The child checklist, which the parents completed, provided demographic information about themselves as well as their child and the child's symptomatology. This measure was in use from 2006 on and replaced the Developmental History form for children and the Adult Personal History.

There were 51 parents of adolescents and 98 parents of children who completed this form about their child, providing historical and family information as well as their current and past symptoms in the following areas: problem solving, language (speech and math skills) spatial skills, concentration and awareness, memory, motor and coordination, sensory, physical issues, emotions, and behavior. Parents were also able to mark if a symptom did not exist or if the problem was both new and old. Symptoms were reported as historical, new, or both new and historical. There were 107 adults who completed this form.

SLEEP EVALUATION QUESTIONNAIRE

The Sleep Evaluation Questionnaire (Mindell and Owens, 2003) was administered to only a small number of parents (20) and has been in use from 2008 onward. The Sleep Evaluation Questionnaire addresses historical information as well as sleep symptoms. Parents are asked to indicate current sleep symptoms covering all of the sleep disorders. There is a rating scale to determine how often the symptom is seen throughout the week. Only two parents of adolescents completed this form so that data are not reported.

DEVELOPMENTAL HISTORY CHECKLIST

The Developmental History Checklist is a general measure providing basic information that the parents provided regarding their child. There were 496 parents of children and 181 parents of adolescents who completed this measure. This measure was in use until replaced in 2006. Questions in this checklist addressed reasons for the evaluation, severity of the problem, school and academic issues, pregnancy and birth, health history, family relationships, emotions, and overall behavior. This measure was developed in 1989 by Dougherty and Schinka.

ADDES HOME AND SCHOOL RATING FORM VERSION

The ADDES Home and School Rating Form Version has two editions and both were used. The first edition was published in 1989 and the second in 1995. This is a measure of attention symptoms that subdivides when scored into two diagnostic categories: ADHD inattentive and ADHD combined subtype or hyperactive. The parent and the classroom teacher or teachers rated children on these symptoms using a scale from 0 to 4 depending upon how often the symptom is seen: weekly, daily, or hourly. Typically, symptoms were seen as significant when occurring daily or hourly.

There were 536 parents and 84 teacher ratings for the children. Two hundred and fourteen parents of adolescents completed the home version. Often testing was completed during the summer, resulting in teacher ratings not being completed all of the time.

This measure, originally created by McCarney, was designed to be a relevant measure of attention deficits in the home and school environment relying upon the reporting of the teacher, parent, or primary caregiver. There are 46 items developed according to the recommendations of diagnosticians professionally involved in measuring an attention disorder (McCarney, 1989).

HOME SITUATIONS QUESTIONNAIRE

The Home Situations Questionnaire has 16 specific situations occurring in and out of the home setting that the parent is asked to indicate if the child's behavior is problematic. Four hundred and forty-five parents of children and 170 parents of adolescents completed this measure. This measure was created by Barkley and published in 1987 (Barkley, 1987).

ACADEMIC PERFORMANCE RATING SCALE

The Academic Performance Rating Scale is a measure completed by the classroom teacher. There were 414 teachers for the children and 133 classroom teachers for the adolescents who completed this measure. Teachers rated the work completed as well as the child's attention (following directions and instruction), learning skills, academic development, work characteristics (quality versus quantity), and overall behavior in class. This is a measure that was developed by DuPaul et al. in 1990.

CHILD ATTENTION PROFILE

The Child Attention Profile is a measure completed by the classroom teacher to describe attention symptoms in the classroom. Four hundred and one classroom teachers completed this measure addressing attention symptoms seen in the child, while 136 teachers completed forms for the adolescents. There are a total of 12 symptoms of attention using a scale of not true, sometimes true, and very often true to rank the degree that the attention symptom is seen in the classroom setting. This is a form developed by Edelbrock in 1989.

SCHOOL SITUATIONS QUESTIONNAIRE

The School Situations Questionnaire is completed by teachers addressing the child's behavior in 12 specific situations occurring in the school setting as well as to and from the school setting (if riding the bus). Three hundred and eighty-six teachers completed this form for the children and 104 for the adolescents. Teachers respond to a question whether the problem exists (yes or no), and then the teacher ranks the severity of the problem. We used only the score for the problem being in existence. This is a measure designed to identify the problem settings and reflects more behavioral issues. This measure was created by Barkley and published in 1987 (Barkley, 1987).

The ACTeRS is a measure that provides descriptions of the child's behavior in the classroom falling into categories of attention, hyperactivity, social kills, and oppositional. There are versions created in 1986, 1988, and 1991; the latter two versions were used (Ullmann et al., 1991). There are a total of 24 items relevant to classroom behavior that fall into the previously described areas. The measure is completed by teachers who have observed the behavior of the child or adolescent in the classroom. Items are ranked from 1 to 5 (almost never to almost always seen). A total score is provided for each of the areas: attention, hyperactivity, social skills, and oppositional. Three hundred and sixty-seven teachers completed this form for the children, and 114 teachers responded for the adolescents.

PERSONAL PROBLEMS CHECKLIST FOR ADOLESCENTS

The Personal Problems Checklist for Adolescents is a measurement of various aspects of everyday functioning, including areas of social, emotional, academic, interpersonal skills, and health. The questionnaire was written by John Schinka and published in 1985, consisting of 240 items with yes and no responses. Adolescents indicated their concerns regarding questions about the following areas: social, appearance, vocation, family, school, money, religion, emotions, sexuality, legal, health, attention, and crisis. One hundred and seventy-nine to hundred and eighty three adolescents completed this measure.

PERSONAL HISTORY CHECKLIST FOR ADOLESCENTS

The Personal History Checklist for Adolescents, created by Schinka and published in 1989, was completed by 109 adolescents who responded to questions about their history, general background, and the background of their family. Adolescents respond to questions about the reason for coming in for evaluation, how they feel about home, school, their peers, parental relationships, medical history, sleep symptoms, their likes and dislikes, as well as symptoms regarding cognitive or thinking processes as well as emotions. This measure was in use until 2004.

PHYSICAL COMPLAINTS CHECKLIST FOR ADHD ADULTS

The Physical Complaints Checklist for ADHD Adults is a questionnaire consisting of 17 items that examines a variety of physical symptoms. On the Physical Complaints Checklist for ADHD Adults, responses to the items are ranked on a 5-point scale (i.e., less than four times a year to nearly daily) (Barkley, 1991b). One thousand one hundred twelve (1112) adults responded to this measure asking about their physical complaints. There were 121 adolescents who completed this measure.

PATIENT BEHAVIOR CHECKLIST FOR ADHD ADULTS

The Patient Behavior Checklist for ADHD Adults is a checklist consisting of 18 items that assess symptoms of hyperactivity, distractibility, and inattention. Responses to items are ranked on a 4-point scale (i.e., not at all to very much) (Barkley, 1991). A large sample, 1195 adults, completed this measure responding to questions regarding their behavior. Adolescent responders were 123.

CAARS: LONG VERSION

The CAARS: Long Version was completed by a very small sample of 22 adults who responded to this measure that was in use from 2006 to 2009. Symptoms of attention, impulsivity, and overactivity are addressed by the adult to see if present currently, and symptoms are rated as 0, 1, 2, and 3 depending upon the severity and how often the symptoms occur in daily life. This measure was designed by Conners et al. (1998) and addresses four factors: inattention/memory, hyperactivity/restless, impulsivity/emotional liability, and problematic self-concept. There are a total of 66 questions with a rating from 0 to 4 for severity.

EPWORTH SLEEPINESS SCALE OF DAYTIME SLEEPINESS

On the Epworth Sleepiness Scale of Daytime Sleepiness, there are a total of 8 items that are rated from 0 to 3 in terms of a high chance of dozing in specific situations. It is used to provide a measure of daytime sleepiness. The Epworth Sleepiness Scale asks individuals to rate the chance that they might doze off or fall asleep in eight different situations or activities that people generally engage in during daytime hours. The scale is really asking people to imagine being in a particular situation or to make a mental judgment about such a situation and to indicate if they would doze off. However, individuals tend to respond with a score of 0 when they are not in the situation, which then changes the measurement. Nonetheless, it remains a valid indicator of daytime sleepiness and is used universally. A score of 10 or above is significant of daytime sleepiness. Only 20% of the general population tend to have scores above 10. This measure was completed by 46 adults.

SLEEP DISORDERS QUESTIONNAIRE

Sleep Disorders Questionnaire provides questions for the various possible sleep disorders: sleep apnea, insomnia, sleep hygiene, narcolepsy, restless legs, periodic limb movement, nightmares, parasomnias, and bruxism. This measure was developed for use at the Sleep Disorders Clinic located at the JFK Neuroscience Center in Edison, New Jersey. There were 48 adults who responded to this measure. The use of this measure began in 2006.

PERSONAL PROBLEMS CHECKLIST FOR ADULTS

The Personal Problems Checklist for Adults is a measurement of various aspects of everyday functioning, including areas of social, emotional, academic, interpersonal skills, and health. The questionnaire was written by John Schinka and published in 1985, consisting of 208 items with yes and no responses. The checklist had 1196 adults who completed this measure asking them about their concerns in the following areas: social, appearance, vocation, family, school, finances, religion, emotions, sexuality, legal, health, attention, and crisis.

PERSONAL HISTORY CHECKLIST FOR ADULTS

The Personal History Checklist for Adults, created by Schinka and published in 1989, was completed by 985 adults who responded to questions about their history, general background, and the background of their family. Adults responded to questions about the reason for coming in for evaluation, medical history, socioeconomic status, education, job history and current medical information, sleep, and substance abuse. This measure was in use until 2006 when replaced by the Adult Neuropsychological History.

QUALITY OF LIFE INVENTORY

The Quality of Life Inventory is a measure inquiring about 16 areas asking how important they are to the individual and if they are satisfied or dissatisfied in any of these areas. There are rankings from not important to very important and from being dissatisfied to satisfied. The discrepancy between the degree of importance and degree of satisfaction or dissatisfaction provides a level of significance. The most significant would be when an area is very important and there is dissatisfaction. Significant items would be when the person indicated that the area was very important to them and that they were dissatisfied to some degree. Seventy-five adults completed this form from 2006 onward. It was developed in 1994 by Michael Frisch, PhD, as a criterion for mental health and adjustment.

BECK DEPRESSION INVENTORY-II

The Beck Depression Inventory-II is a measure of depression: a 21-item measure to address the presence and severity of depression in adults and adolescents. Each item requires the endorsement of four options: scoring from 0 to 3 with increasing scores reflecting greater severity of a symptom of depression. The individual is asked to respond to the following to describe their last 2 weeks. In this manner, this measure reports on symptoms of depression that are currently present. Developed in 1996, this is the second version. This measure was completed by 113 adults and 29 adolescents.

BECK ANXIETY INVENTORY

The Beck Anxiety Inventory is a measure that inquires about the past week and as such reports only on very current symptoms of anxiety. Symptoms relate to both the emotional and physical characteristics of anxiety although individuals may have symptoms of physical issues that are not the result of anxiety symptoms. There were 125 adults that completed this measure and 28 adolescents. This was developed in 1993.

REFERENCES

Achenbach, T.M., (1991) *Child Behavior Checklist for Ages 4–18*, University of Vermont Burlington, VT.

Achenbach, T.M., (2001) *Child Behavior Checklist for Ages 6–18*, University of Vermont Burlington, VT.

American Psychiatric Association (1994) *Diagnostic and Statistical Manual for Mental Disorders*, 4th edn., American Psychiatric Association, Washington, DC, 1994.

Barkley, R.A., (1987) *Defiant Children: A Clinician's Manual for Parent Training*, Guilford Press, New York.

Barkley, R., (1991a) *Patient Behavior Checklist for ADHD Adults*, Guilford Publications, New York, p. 43.

Barkley, R., (1991b) *Physical Complaints Checklist for ADHD Adults*, Guilford Publications, New York, p. 42.

Beck, A.T. and Steer, R.A., (1993) *Beck Anxiety Inventory*, The Psychological Corporation, San Antonio, TX.

Beck, A.T., Steer, R.A., and Brown, G.K., (1996b) *Beck Depression Inventory*, 2nd edn., The Psychological Corporation, San Antonio, TX.

Child Symptom Inventory-4: Parent Checklist, (1994) University of New York Checkmate Plus, LTD., Stony Brook, New York.

Conners, C.K., Erhardt, D., and Sparrow, E., (1998) *Conners' Adult ADHD Rating Scales*, Multi Health Systems, North Tonawanda, NY.

Dougherty, E. and Schinka, J., (1989) *The Developmental History Checklist for Children*, Psychological Assessment Resources, Odessa, FL.

DuPaul, G.J. et al., (2001) Self-report of ADHD symptoms in university students: Cross-gender and cross-national prevalence, *Journal of Learning Disabilities*, 34, 370–379.

DuPaul, G.J., Power, T.J., Anastopoulos, A.D., and Reid, R., (1998) *ADHD Rating Scale-IV, Checklists, Norms and Clinical Interpretation*, The Guilford Press, New York.

DuPaul, C.J., Rapport, M., and Perriello, L.M., (1990) *Academic Performance Rating Scale, Teacher Ratings of Academic Performance: The Development of the Academic Performance Rating Scale*, unpublished manuscript, University of Massachusetts Medical Center, Worcester, MA.

Edelbrock, C.S., (1989) *Child Attention Profile*, University of Massachusetts Medical Center, Worcester, MA.

Frisch, M.B., (1994) *Quality of Life Inventory, Manual and Treatment Guide*, National Computer Systems, Inc., Minneapolis, MN.

Greenberg, G.D., (1990a) *Adult Neuropsychological History*, International Diagnostic Systems, Inc, Worthington, OH.

Greenberg, G.D., (1990b) *Child Neuropsychological History*, International Diagnostic Systems, Inc, Worthington, OH.

McCarney, S.R., (1989, 1995) *ADDES Second Edition*, Hawthorne Educational Services, Inc, Colombia, MO.

Mindell, J. and Owens, J., (2003) *A Clinical Guide to Pediatric Sleep, Diagnosis and Management of Sleep Problems*, Lippincott, Williams & Wilkins, Philadelphia, PA.

Schinka, J.A., (1985a) *Children's Problems Checklist*, Psychological Assessment Resources, Odessa, FL.

Schinka, J.A., (1985b) *Personal Problems Checklist for Adolescents*, Psychological Assessment Resources, Odessa, FL.

Schinka, J.A., (1985c) *Personal Problems Checklist for Adults*, Psychological Assessment Resources, Odessa, FL.

Schinka, J.A., (1989a) *Personal History Checklist for Adults*, Psychological Assessment Resources, Odessa, FL.

Schinka, J.A., (1989b) *Personal History Checklist for Adolescents*, Psychological Assessment Resources, Odessa, FL.

Sleep Disorders Center, Sleep Disorders Questionnaire, The Neuroscience Institute at JFK Medical Center Edison, NJ.

Ullmann, R., Sleator, E.K., and Sprague, R.L., (1991) *ACTeRS*, MetriTech Inc, Champaign, IL.

8 Results of the Child Self-Report Measure/Checklist

The total sample size was 833 children from the age of 5 to 11 years. Of these, 71% were males and 29% females. Fifty-six percent were diagnosed with ADHD inattentive type and 44% with ADHD plus an additional disorder.

In the following pages, you will find the statistics on the numerous checklists that were administered. There were checklists given to the parents to complete about their child and to the child's teacher or teachers.

Checklists that the parents completed are as follows:

- Home Situations Questionnaire
- ADDES Home Version
- ADHD Rating Scale
- Children Symptom Inventory-4
- Children's Problems Checklist
- Child Behavior Checklist
- Children's Neuropsychological History
- Developmental History Checklist

Checklists that the teacher or teachers completed are as follows:

- Child Attention Profile
- Social Situations Questionnaire
- ACTeRS
- Academic Performance Rating Scale
- ADDES School Version

CHILD ATTENTION PROFILE

This is a measure completed by the classroom teacher to describe attention symptoms in the classroom. Four hundred one classroom teachers completed this measure addressing attention symptoms seen in the child. There are a total of 12 symptoms assessing attention using a scale of not true, sometimes true, and very often true to rank the degree that the attention symptom is seen by the teacher in the classroom setting.

Fails to finish things he/she starts: 79% somewhat or often true
    Not true = 21%
    Somewhat true = 39%
    Very true or often true = 40%

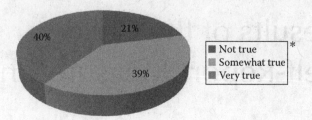

Can't concentrate, can't pay attention for long: 89%
    Not true = 11%
    Somewhat true = 32%
    Very true or often true = 57%

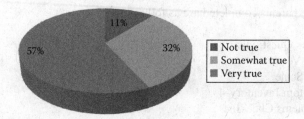

Can't sit still, restless, or hyperactive: 68%
    Not true = 32%
    Somewhat true = 31%
    Very true or often true = 37%

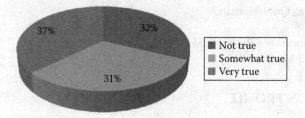

Fidgets: 75%
    Not true = 25%
    Somewhat true = 31%
    Very true or often true = 44%

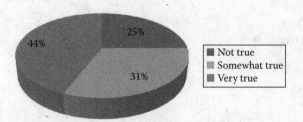

* The pie graphs range from 99 to 100 to 101 due to rounding.

Daydreams or gets lost in his/her thoughts: 82%
    Not true = 19%
    Somewhat true = 40%
    Very true or often true = 42%

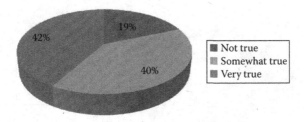

Impulsive or acts without thinking: 69%
    Not true = 31%
    Somewhat true = 30%
    Very true or often true = 39%

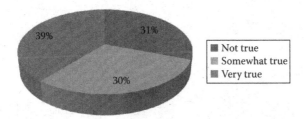

Difficulty following directions: 84%
    Not true = 16%
    Somewhat true = 42%
    Very true or often true = 42%

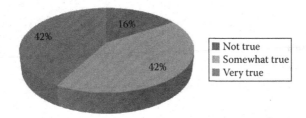

Talks out of turn: 64%
    Not true = 37%
    Somewhat true = 27%
    Very true or often true = 37%

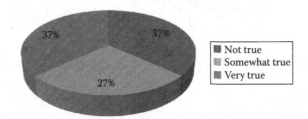

Messy work: 74%
    Not true = 26%
    Somewhat true = 40%
    Very true or often true = 34%

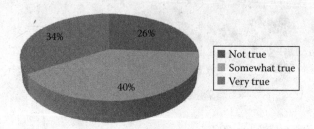

Inattentive, easily distracted: 92%
    Not true = 8%
    Somewhat true = 30%
    Very true or often true = 62%

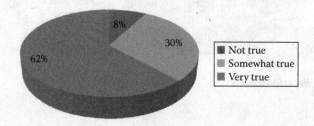

Talks too much: 66%
    Not true = 34%
    Somewhat true = 34%
    Very true or often true = 32%

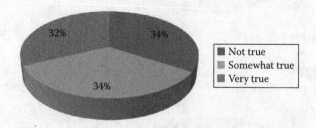

Fails to carry out assigned tasks: 79%
    Not true = 20%
    Somewhat true = 42%
    Very true or often true = 37%

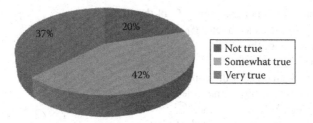

SUMMATION OF FINDINGS

Items that were marked very true and were present more than other items were that of inattention and being easily distracted. These were the only two symptoms that were reported as being seen much of the time (to an extensive degree), suggesting the diagnosis of ADHD inattentive type:

- 57% identified an inability to concentrate or sustain attention as a problem occurring much of the time.
- 62% were seen as inattentive and easily distracted with these symptoms occurring much of the time.

All of the 12 symptoms from this self-report measure occurred very often in at least one-third of the population of children from ages 5 to 11. However, there were items that were reported more often by the teacher as not being seen at all. They are the following:

- Talking out of turn (37%).
- Talking too much (34%).

Most of the symptoms are typically suggestive of inattention, other than symptoms of impulsivity or an inability to sit still, which can be seen associated with anxiety, hyperactivity, or insufficient sleep or poor sleep (growing pains, sleep-disordered breathing problem) or even injury to the brain, to name a few possibilities.

Identifying those symptoms that were indicated as present (regardless of the severity) seen either some of the time or most of the time (often true) resulted in mostly symptoms of inattention:

- Failing to finish things was seen 79% of the time.
- Failing to carry out assigned tasks was seen 79% of the time.
- Unable to concentrate or sustain attention was seen 89% of the time.
- Difficulty following directions was seen 84% of the time.
- Daydreaming or getting lost in one's thoughts was seen 82% of the time.
- Inattentive and being easily distracted was seen 92% of the time.

These symptoms are clearly suggestive of the problem being that of inattention and failure to complete tasks (seen as the combination of anxiety and avoidance of work).

SCHOOL SITUATIONS QUESTIONNAIRE

Three hundred and eighty-six teachers provided responses to this measure asking about the child's behavior in specific situations occurring in the school setting, as well as to and from the school setting (if riding the bus). This is a measure designed to identify the problem settings and reflects more behavioral issues. Teachers indicated that problem behaviors occurred in the following settings:

- While arriving at school: Seen 33% of the time.
- During individual desk work: Seen 64% of the time.
- During small group activities: Seen 63% of the time.

- During free play time in class: Seen 48% of the time.
- During lectures to the class: Seen 61% of the time.
- At recess: Seen 37% of the time.
- At lunch: Seen 33% of the time.
- In the hallways: Seen 44% of the time.
- In the bathroom: Seen 26% of the time
- On field trips: Seen 19% of the time.
- During special assemblies: Seen 35% of the time.
- On the bus: Seen 11% of the time.

SUMMATION OF FINDINGS

Frequencies indicated earlier are based upon teacher report that the problem is present in the school setting. The problem can be mild, or it can be severe (or in between the two). The measurement is based upon the child having some degree of problematic behavior significant enough to be identified.

It is apparent that arriving at school is not a primary problem. Neither is free play, recess, or lunch. Behavior is not problematic in the hallways or the bathroom, on field trips and during special assemblies, or on the bus.

This suggests the presence of more symptoms consistent with an inattentive disorder, and primary symptoms occurred when having to complete academic work. This is consistent with the idea that ADHD is more of a cognitive or thinking problem than a behavioral problem.

So where were the problems seen on this measure? They were present in class, during individual desk work, during small group activities, and during lectures:

- 64% had a problem during individual desk work.
- 63% had a problem during small group activities.
- 61% had a problem during lectures in class.

Symptoms seen less often may relate to the children diagnosed with ADHD plus who can display difficulties in unstructured settings:

- 33% had a problem when arriving at school or at lunchtime.
- 37% had a problem at recess.
- 26% had a problem in the bathroom.
- 19% had a problem on field trips.
- 11% had a problem on the bus.

Teachers did not identify any problem behaviors as occurring very often in the areas that would typically be thought of as ADHD hyperactive or the combined subtype. Symptoms that would usually be considered problematic for the hyperactive or combined subtype were not common for the previously described areas for 63%–89% of the children.

HOME SITUATIONS QUESTIONNAIRE

Four hundred and forty-five parents provided responses to this measure asking about the child's behavior in specific situations occurring in the home setting. There are 16 specific situations occurring in and out of the home setting where the parent is asked to indicate if the child's behavior is problematic. The following is the percentage of parent-indicated problem behaviors in these settings:

- Playing alone: 29%.
- Playing with other children: 48%.
- Mealtimes: 55%.

- Getting dressed/undressed: 52%.
- Washing and bathing: 39%.
- When you are on the telephone: 70%.
- Watching television: 37%.
- When visitors are in your home: 55%.
- When you are visiting someone's home: 44%.
- In public places: 58%.
- When father is home: 44%.
- When asked to do chores: 82%.
- When asked to do homework: 78%.
- At bedtime: 63%.
- While in the car: 42%.
- When with a babysitter: 35%.

SUMMATION OF FINDINGS

On this measure similar to the school situations self-report measure, the parent identifies settings where the child's behavior is seen as problematic. The severity was not used, meaning the problem identified may have existed to only a mild degree. What is being measured here is whether the problem exists at all. Therefore, it becomes more significant when the parents did not see the problem as occurring at all. Parents did not identify playing alone, washing and bathing, watching television, and being with a babysitter as a problem. Problem situations occurring half of the time were when playing with other children, getting dressed or undressed, when visitors are in the home, when visiting someone else's home, in public places, when the father is home, and while in the car. Bedtime emerged as more problematic, when asked to do chores, when asked to do homework, and while the parent is on the telephone:

- 70% indicated problems while on the telephone.
- 82% indicated problems when asking their child to complete chores.
- 78% indicated problems when asking their child to do homework.
- 63% indicated problems at bedtime.

This is consistent with the common experience of the ADD child and the known difficulty of getting their homework done or completing chores. Many interrupt parents while on the telephone to tell them something important that they do not want to forget. Having so much in their mind, it is easy to become distracted and to be unable to retain information for long, resulting in the tendency to interrupt others. Completion of homework and avoidance and procrastination of chores or work that they do not like doing are common symptoms endorsed by most mothers of diagnosed ADHD children. Bedtime resistance may often be related to sleep onset insomnia and the anxious child who reviews their day before falling asleep and/or is worried about the following day. Parents typically report bedtime resistance to be more associated with a school night.

ACTeRS

This is a measure providing descriptions of the child's behavior in the classroom falling into categories of attention, hyperactivity, social skills, and oppositional. There are a total of 24 items relevant to classroom behavior that fall into the previously described areas. The measure is completed by teachers who have observed the behavior of the child or adolescent in the classroom. Items are ranked from 1 to 5 (almost never to almost always seen). A total score is provided for each of the areas: attention, hyperactivity, social skills, and oppositional. There were 367 teachers who completed this measure.

ATTENTION

Works well independently
26% responded 1 (almost never).
29% responded 2.
25% responded 3.
12% responded 4.
8% responded 5 (almost always).

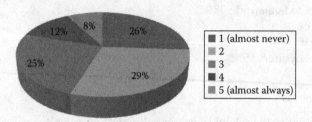

Persists with task for reasonable amount of time
21% responded 1 (almost never).
30% responded 2.
26% responded 3.
13% responded 4.
10% responded 5 (almost always).

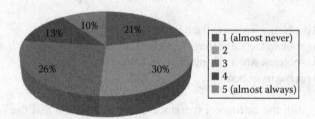

Completes assigned task satisfactorily with little additional assistance
24% responded 1 (almost never).
34% responded 2.
21% responded 3.
12% responded 4.
9% responded 5 (almost always).

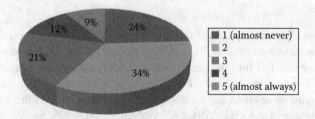

Follows simple directions accurately
    10% responded 1 (almost never).
    30% responded 2.
    29% responded 3.
    18% responded 4.
    14% responded 5 (almost always).

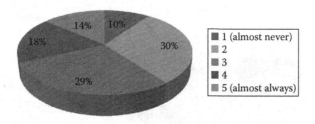

Follows a sequence of instructions
    20% responded 1 (almost never).
    34% responded 2.
    23% responded 3.
    15% responded 4.
    8% responded 5 (almost always).

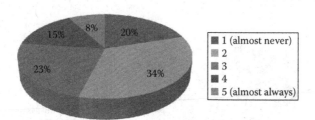

Functions well in the classroom
    13% responded 1 (almost never).
    35% responded 2.
    31% responded 3.
    12% responded 4.
    9% responded 5 (almost always).

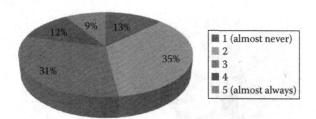

HYPERACTIVITY

Extremely overactive (out of seat, on the go)
   36% responded 1 (almost never).
   11% responded 2.
   16% responded 3.
   20% responded 4.
   17% responded 5 (almost always).

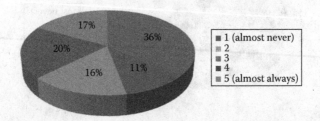

Overreacts
   33% responded 1 (almost never).
   16% responded 2.
   17% responded 3.
   21% responded 4.
   13% responded 5 (almost always).

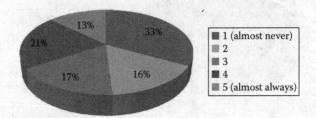

Fidgety (hands always busy)
   21% responded 1 (almost never).
   14% responded 2.
   17% responded 3.
   19% responded 4.
   29% responded 5 (almost always).

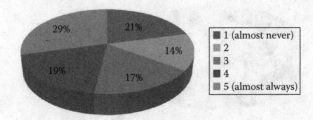

Impulsive (acts or talks without thinking)
    27% responded 1 (almost never).
    15% responded 2.
    11% responded 3.
    22% responded 4.
    25% responded 5 (almost always).

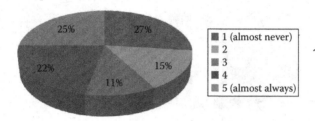

Restless (squirms in seat)
    23% responded 1 (almost never).
    15% responded 2.
    18% responded 3.
    18% responded 4.
    25% responded 5 (almost always).

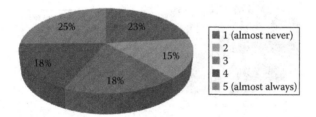

Social Skills

Behaves positively with peers/classmates
    4% responded 1 (almost never).
    17% responded 2.
    31% responded 3.
    22% responded 4.
    24% responded 5 (almost always).

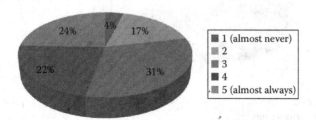

Verbal communication clear and connected
   5% responded 1 (almost never).
   17% responded 2.
   26% responded 3.
   25% responded 4.
   27% responded 5 (almost always).

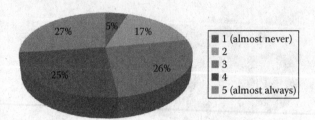

Nonverbal communication clear and connected
   5% responded 1 (almost never).
   16% responded 2.
   31% responded 3.
   30% responded 4.
   19% responded 5 (almost always).

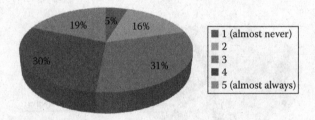

Follows group norms and social rules
   8% responded 1 (almost never).
   23% responded 2.
   22% responded 3.
   23% responded 4.
   24% responded 5 (almost always).

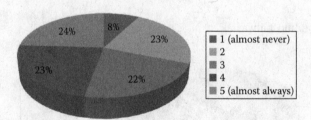

Cites general rule when criticizing
   12% responded 1 (almost never).
   13% responded 2.

27% responded 3.
27% responded 4.
22% responded 5 (almost always).

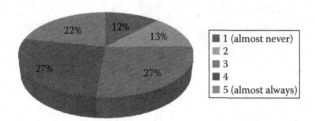

Skillful at making new friends
14% responded 1 (almost never).
19% responded 2.
33% responded 3.
21% responded 4.
13% responded 5 (almost always).

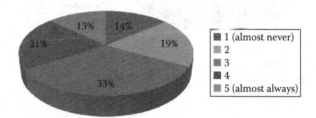

Approaches situations carefully
17% responded 1 (almost never).
23% responded 2.
30% responded 3.
17% responded 4.
13% responded 5 (almost always).

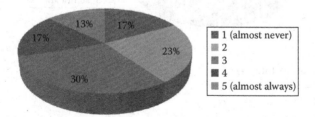

OPPOSITIONAL

Tries to get others into trouble
50% responded 1 (almost never).
16% responded 2.
15% responded 3.
14% responded 4.
4% responded 5 (almost always).

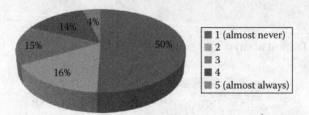

Starts fights over nothing

   63% responded 1 (almost never).

   11% responded 2.

   12% responded 3.

   11% responded 4.

   3% responded 5 (almost always).

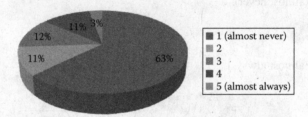

Makes malicious fun of people

   66% responded 1 (almost never).

   14% responded 2.

   11% responded 3.

   7% responded 4.

   2% responded 5 (almost always).

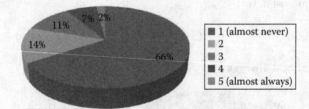

Defies authority

   54% responded 1 (almost never).

   12% responded 2.

   15% responded 3.

   15% responded 4.

   4% responded 5 (almost always).

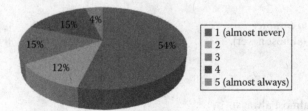

Picks on others
   57% responded 1 (almost never).
   19% responded 2.
   13% responded 3.
   8% responded 4.
   3% responded 5 (almost always).

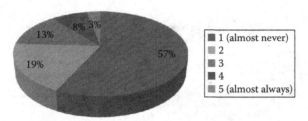

Mean and cruel to other children
   66% responded 1 (almost never).
   15% responded 2.
   9% responded 3.
   8% responded 4.
   2% responded 5 (almost always).

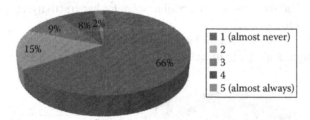

   Profile scores for each of the four categories are scored for how severe the problem is and if it is seen as representing a problem. Scoring is different for boys versus girls.

MALES COMPARED TO FEMALES

ATTENTION

Population: 25% girls and 75% boys

Girls: 65% had significant attention problems:

- 32% of the girls had the most severe possible score for attention.
- 33% had the next most severe score.
- 29% were borderline significant for attention problems.
- 6% were not significant for attention.

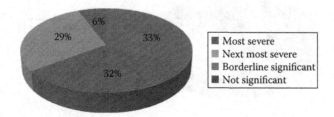

Boys: 67% had significant attention problems:

- 33% of the boys had the most severe possible score for attention.
- 34% had the next most severe score.
- 18% were borderline significant for attention problems.
- 15% were not significant for attention.

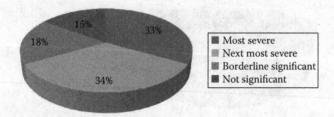

HYPERACTIVITY

Population: 28% girls and 72% boys

Girls: 47% had significant hyperactivity problems:

- 22% of the girls had the most severe possible score for hyperactivity.
- 25% had the next most severe score.
- 16% were borderline significant for hyperactivity problems.
- 38% were not significant for hyperactivity.

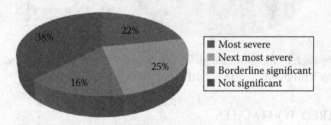

Boys: 49% had significant hyperactivity problems:

- 29% of the boys had the most severe possible score for hyperactivity.
- 20% had the next most severe score.
- 19% were borderline significant for hyperactivity problems.
- 32% were not significant for hyperactivity.

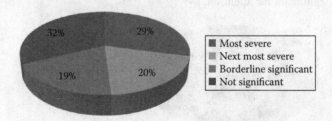

SOCIAL SKILLS

Population: 49% girls and 51% boys

Girls: 47% had significant problems with social skills:

- 19% of the girls had the most severe possible score for social skills.
- 28% had the next most severe score.
- 32% were borderline significant for social skills problems.
- 21% were not significant for social skills.

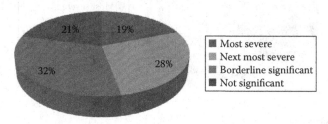

Boys: 43% had significant with social skills:

- 16% of the boys had the most severe possible score for social skills.
- 27% had the next most severe score.
- 27% were borderline significant for social skills problems.
- 30% were not significant for social skills.

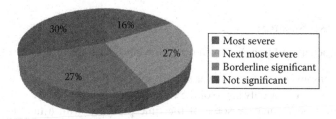

OPPOSITIONAL

Population: 28% girls and 72% boys

Girls: 34% had significant oppositional problems:

- 16% of the girls had the most severe possible score for oppositional behavior.
- 18% had the next most severe score.
- 29% were borderline significant for oppositional behavior.
- 37% were not significant for oppositional behavior.

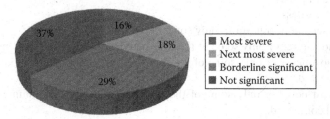

Boys: 28% had significant oppositional problems:

- 11% of the boys had the most severe possible score for oppositional behavior.
- 17% had the next most severe score.
- 29% were borderline for oppositional behavior.
- 43% were not significant for oppositional behavior.

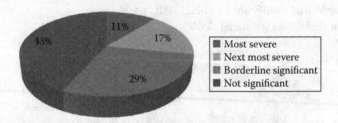

SUMMATION OF FINDINGS

- Boys and girls were similar for attention symptoms.
- Boys and girls were similar in symptoms of hyperactivity.
- Girls had slightly more social problems than boys.
- Girls had slightly more oppositional behaviors than boys.
- Attention problems were seen more often. Oppositional behavior was seen less often.
- Hyperactive behavior and problematic social skills were seen about one-half of the time.

INDIVIDUAL ITEMS AND SYMPTOMS

According to the teacher, children displayed the following symptoms:

- Attention symptoms seen almost never to only some of the time
  - 55% almost never or only some of the time worked independently.
  - 51% almost never or only some of the time persisted with a task for a reasonable amount of time.
  - 58% almost never or only some of the time completed an assigned task without assistance from the teacher.
  - 40% almost never or only some of the time followed simple directions accurately.
  - 54% almost never or only some of the time followed a sequence of instructions.
  - 48% almost never or only some of the time functioned well within the classroom.
- Hyperactive behavior seen always to most of the time
  - 37% were out of their seat and on the go.
  - 34% were overreactive.
  - 48% were fidgety.
  - 47% were impulsive.
  - 43% were restless.
- Social skills seen almost never to only some of the time
  - 21% almost never or only some of the time had positive peer interactions.
  - 22% almost never or only some of the time had verbal communication that was clear and connected.
  - 21% almost never or only some of the time had nonverbal communication that was clear and connected.

- 31% almost never or only some of the time followed group norms and social rules.
- 25% almost never or only some of the time cited a general rule when criticizing.
- 33% almost never or only some of the time were skillful at making new friends.
- 40% almost never or only some of the time approached social situations carefully.
- Oppositional behavior seen almost always to most of the time
  - 18% tried to get others into trouble.
  - 14% started fights over nothing.
  - 9% made malicious fun of others.
  - 19% defied authority.
  - 11% picked on others.
  - 10% were mean or cruel.

Inattention was the most problematic symptom seen in the problems of working independently, completing tasks, and following instruction. The question is whether the primary symptoms indicated for hyperactivity are actually overactivity or instead related to anxiety. Primary symptoms were that of being fidgety, impulsive, and restless. Hand movements and playing with objects are often descriptors of anxiety or nervousness. Anxiety is typically a reaction that manifests as impulsive behavior (not thinking, just doing) or restlessness. When we are nervous, we do not think things through. Undiagnosed restless legs certainly would have children out of their seat and moving their legs.

Socially, there was difficulty knowing how to approach social situations and skillfulness in making friends. Missing the social subtleties results in being less skillful in interpersonal interactions. Whether this is the result of information processing deficits (missing small details of information), and consequently missing the social subtleties in conversation or perhaps visual–spatial issues and not seeing the whole picture (results in saying the wrong thing at the wrong time).

Through the years, the smarter the child, the more we see this type of behavior and poor social relationships, which tends to be related to the difficulty getting along with themselves as well as the people around them. Symptoms of depression were more apparent in the adolescent population and may be revealing itself in this manner in the child population.

True oppositional behavior is not seen very often. The highest percentages were seen in trying to get others into trouble or defying authority, both of which could be related to depression and/or the compulsive need to be right about something. The need to be right about things is often seen in the ADD/ADHD population whether as a result of thinking they are right (due to missing information and taking the information they do have to form their own logical conclusions) or the actual need to be correct as a defense against feeling incorrect or wrong much of the time.

ACADEMIC PERFORMANCE RATING SCALE

This is a measure completed by the classroom teacher. There were 414 classroom teachers who completed this measure for elementary school students. Teachers rated the work completed as well as the child's attention (following directions and instruction), learning skills, academic development, work characteristics (quality versus quantity), and overall behavior in class.

Percentages of written math work completed relative to classmates: 76% are average and above
   12% responded with 0%–49%.
   12% responded with 50%–69%.
   9% responded with 70%–79%.
   19% responded with 80%–89%.
   48% responded with 90%–100%.

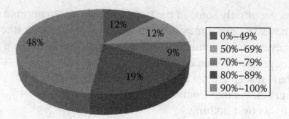

Percentage of written math work completed that was accurate: 80% are average and above
10% responded with 0%–49%.
9% responded with 50%–69%.
24% responded with 70%–79%.
31% responded with 80%–89%.
25% responded with 90%–100%.

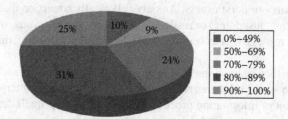

Percentage of written language arts work completed relative to classmates: 65% are average and above
18% responded with 0%–49%.
18% responded with 50%–69%.
9% responded with 70%–79%.
21% responded with 80%–89%.
35% responded with 90%–100%.

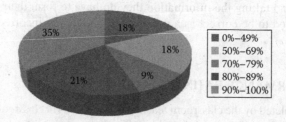

Percentage of written language arts work completed that was accurate: 69% are average and above
16% responded with 0%–49%.
16% responded with 50%–69%.
24% responded with 70%–79%.
27% responded with 80%–89%.
18% responded with 90%–100%.

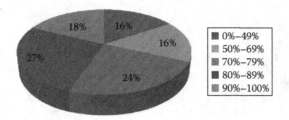

How consistent was the quality of the child's academic work over the past week? 60% are variable to consistently poor:

9% responded with consistently poor.
13% responded with more poor than successful.
38% responded with variable.
24% responded with more successful than poor.
16% responded with consistently successful.

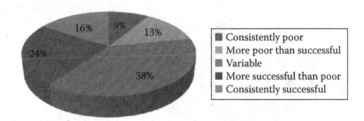

How frequent was the child able to accurately follow teacher instructions and/or class discussion during large group instruction? 66% are never to sometimes:

2% responded with never.
26% responded with rarely.
38% responded with sometimes.
26% responded with often.
8% responded with very often.

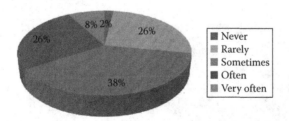

How frequent was the child able to accurately follow teacher instructions and/or class discussion during small group instruction? 55% are never to sometimes:

1% responded with never.
13% responded with rarely.
41% responded with sometimes.
34% responded with often.
11% responded with very often.

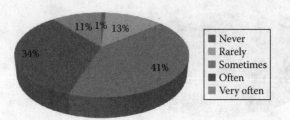

The child learns new material quickly: 69% are never to sometimes:
    9% responded with never.
    26% responded with rarely.
    34% responded with sometimes.
    19% responded with often.
    11% responded with very often.

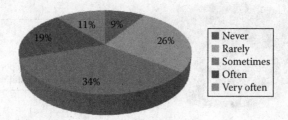

Quality or neatness of this child's handwriting: 55% are poor to fair:
    30% responded with poor.
    25% responded with fair.
    31% responded with average.
    11% responded with above average.
    4% responded with excellent.

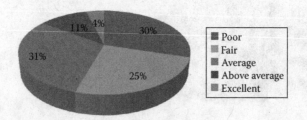

Quality of this child's reading skills: 45% are poor to fair:
    20% responded with poor.
    25% responded with fair.
    28% responded with average.
    20% responded with above average.
    8% responded with excellent.

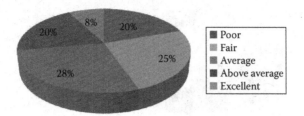

Quality of this child's speaking skills: 22% are poor to fair:
   7% responded with poor.
   15% responded with fair.
   44% responded with average.
   25% responded with above average.
   9% responded with excellent.

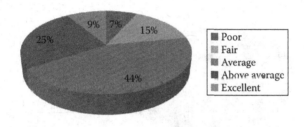

Percentage that the child completes written work in a careless, hasty fashion: 78% are sometimes to very often:
   4% responded with never.
   18% responded with rarely.
   29% responded with sometimes.
   25% responded with often.
   24% responded with very often.

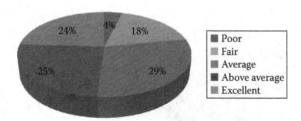

Percentage that the child takes more time to complete work than his/her classmates: 69% are sometimes to very often:
   8% responded with never.
   23% responded with rarely.
   17% responded with sometimes.
   17% responded with often.
   35% responded with very often.

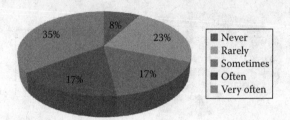

Percentage that the child is able to pay attention without you promoting him/her: 23% are often to very often:
   7% responded with never.
   37% responded with rarely.
   34% responded with sometimes.
   16% responded with often.
   7% responded with very often.

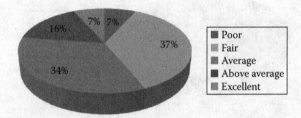

Percentage that the child requires teacher assistance to accurately complete his/her academic work: 84% are sometimes to very often:
   3% responded with never.
   14% responded with rarely.
   30% responded with sometimes.
   33% responded with often.
   21% responded with very often.

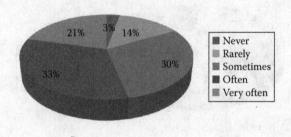

Percentage that the child begins written work prior to understanding the directions: 60% are sometimes to very often:
   13% responded with never.
   28% responded with rarely.
   33% responded with sometimes.
   22% responded with often.
   5% responded with very often.

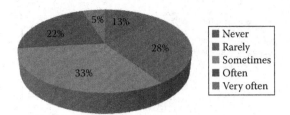

Frequency that the child has difficulty recalling material from a previous day's lesson: 69% are sometimes to very often:

    5% responded with never.

    25% responded with rarely.

    34% responded with sometimes.

    22% responded with often.

    13% responded with very often.

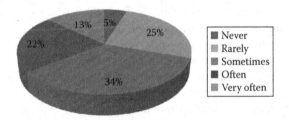

Frequency that the child appears to be staring excessively or "spaced out": 62% are sometimes to very often:

    14% responded with never.

    24% responded with rarely.

    26% responded with sometimes.

    19% responded with often.

    17% responded with very often.

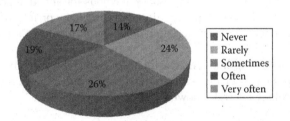

Frequency that the child appears to be withdrawn or tending to lack an emotional response in a social situation: 42% are sometimes to very often:

    27% responded with never.

    30% responded with rarely.

    24% responded with sometimes.

    10% responded with often.

    8% responded with very often.

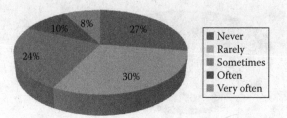

SUMMATION OF FINDINGS

This self-report measure is completed by teachers who report on the child's academic work as well as their behavior in the classroom setting. Trends observed are the following:

- 60% had variable to poor quality of academic work.
- 66% had difficulty following teacher instruction and/or class direction during large group instruction.
- 69% had difficulty learning new material.
- 78% completed work in a careless, hasty manner.
- 69% took more time to complete their work.
- 78% were unable to pay attention without teacher prompting.
- 84% required teacher assistance to accurately complete their work.
- 60% began work prior to understanding the directions.
- 69% had difficulty recalling material from the previous day's lesson.
- 62% stared excessively or appeared spaced out.

Overall results suggest difficulty following teacher instruction, learning new material, the tendency to complete work too quickly, inability to pay attention without prompting, requiring teacher assistance to complete work, and difficulty recalling information. These are common traits for ADHD inattentive type. The problem of recalling information may be the result of almost half of the population being diagnosed with ADHD plus an additional disorder that typically involves the additional symptom of memory problems.

Memory generally is not a problem for the genetic ADD. What we have found through the years is that memory is one of the primary compensation methods for attention problems, whether it is memorizing words due to phonological/word decoding problems or memorizing information to compensate for not understanding the material. In other words, memory for the genetic ADD is the solution, not the problem.

Staring episodes or appearing emotionally withdrawn could represent anxiety and distractibility and/or another problem such as seizures, which would have resulted in additional neuropsychological evaluation and neurology referral following the attention evaluation.

ADDES SCHOOL VERSION

The ADDES (from 2006 to 2009, the ADDES-second edition was used) is a measure of attention symptoms that is subdivided and is scored into two categories, ADHD inattentive and ADHD combined subtype or hyperactive. The classroom teacher rated children on these symptoms using a scale from 0 to 4 depending upon how often the symptom occurred, weekly, daily, or hourly. Typically, symptoms were seen as significant when occurring daily or hourly. There were a total of 84 teacher ratings.

DISTRACTIBILITY AND LISTENING

Is easily distracted by other activities in the classroom, other students, the teacher, etc.: 75% hourly to daily

  4% indicated does not engage in the behavior.
  6% indicated one to several times per month.
  15% indicated one to several times per week.
  33% indicated one to several times per day.
  42% indicated one to several times per hour.

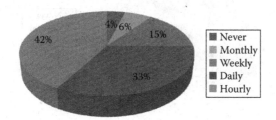

Does not listen to what other students are saying: 52% hourly to daily

  11% indicated does not engage in the behavior.
  8% indicated one to several times per month.
  29% indicated one to several times per week.
  38% indicated one to several times per day.
  14% indicated one to several times per hour.

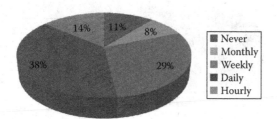

Does not hear all of what is said: 34% hourly to daily

  17% indicated does not engage in the behavior.
  15% indicated one to several times per month.
  34% indicated one to several times per week.
  27% indicated one to several times per day.
  7% indicated one to several times per hour.

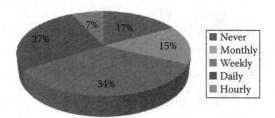

Does not direct attention or fails to maintain attention to important sounds in the immediate environment: 64% hourly to daily

   12% indicated does not engage in the behavior.
   6% indicated one to several times per month.
   18% indicated one to several times per week.
   45% indicated one to several times per day.
   19% indicated one to several times per hour.

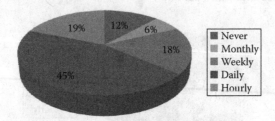

Is unsuccessful in activities requiring listening: 42% hourly to daily

   8% indicated does not engage in the behavior.
   27% indicated one to several times per month.
   23% indicated one to several times per week.
   32% indicated one to several times per day.
   10% indicated one to several times per hour.

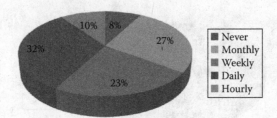

Requires eye contact in order to listen successfully: 54% hourly to daily

   8% indicated does not engage in the behavior.
   14% indicated one to several times per month.
   24% indicated one to several times per week.
   42% indicated one to several times per day.
   12% indicated one to several times per hour.

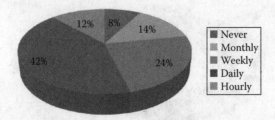

Attends more successfully when close to the source of sound: 62% hourly to daily
   6% indicated does not engage in the behavior.
   16% indicated one to several times per month.
   16% indicated one to several times per week.
   40% indicated one to several times per day.
   22% indicated one to several times per hour.

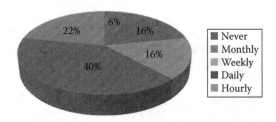

FOLLOWING DIRECTIONS

Needs oral questions and directions frequently required: 45% hourly to daily
   8% indicated does not engage in the behavior.
   12% indicated one to several times per month.
   35% indicated one to several times per week.
   25% indicated one to several times per day.
   20% indicated one to several times per hour.

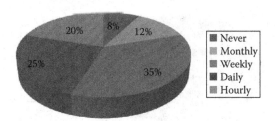

Does not listen to or follow verbal directions: 47% hourly to daily
   14% indicated does not engage in the behavior.
   13% indicated one to several times per month.
   25% indicated one to several times per week.
   34% indicated one to several times per day.
   13% indicated one to several times per hour.

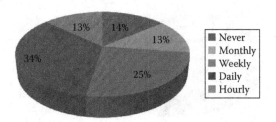

Begins assignments before receiving directions or instructions or does not follow directions or instructions: 37% hourly to daily

    16% indicated does not engage in the behavior.

    16% indicated one to several times per month.

    31% indicated one to several times per week.

    23% indicated one to several times per day.

    14% indicated one to several times per hour.

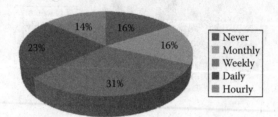

Fails to follow necessary steps in math problems: 19% hourly to daily

    23% indicated does not engage in the behavior.

    23% indicated one to several times per month.

    35% indicated one to several times per week.

    14% indicated one to several times per day.

    5% indicated one to several times per hour.

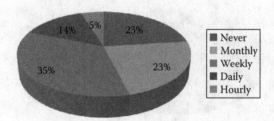

Does not read or follow written directions: 35% hourly to daily

    22% indicated does not engage in the behavior.

    15% indicated one to several times per month.

    28% indicated one to several times per week.

    23% indicated one to several times per day.

    12% indicated one to several times per hour.

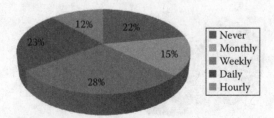

MEMORY AND CONCENTRATION

Fails to demonstrate short-term memory: 45% hourly to daily
 18% indicated does not engage in the behavior.
 10% indicated one to several times per month.
 29% indicated one to several times per week.
 35% indicated one to several times per day.
 10% indicated one to several times per hour.

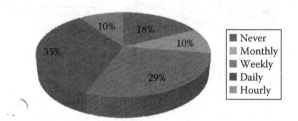

Fails to remember sequences: 34% hourly to daily
 21% indicated does not engage in the behavior.
 20% indicated one to several times per month.
 24% indicated one to several times per week.
 19% indicated one to several times per day.
 15% indicated one to several times per hour.

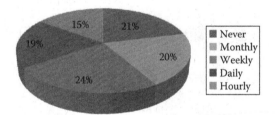

Has difficulty concentrating: 60% hourly to daily
 8% indicated does not engage in the behavior.
 11% indicated one to several times per month.
 20% indicated one to several times per week.
 39% indicated one to several times per day.
 21% indicated one to several times per hour.

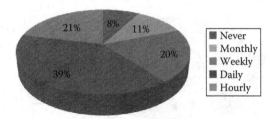

Does not perform academically at his/her ability: 41% hourly to daily
   18% indicated does not engage in the behavior.
   21% indicated one to several times per month.
   29% indicated one to several times per week.
   26% indicated one to several times per day.
   15% indicated one to several times per hour.

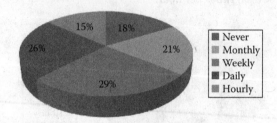

READING, READING COMPREHENSION, AND LANGUAGE

Loses place when reading: 34% hourly to daily
   25% indicated does not engage in the behavior.
   18% indicated one to several times per month.
   23% indicated one to several times per week.
   20% indicated one to several times per day.
   14% indicated one to several times per hour.

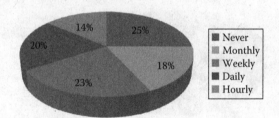

Omits, adds, substitutes, or reverses letters, words, or sounds when reading: 44% hourly to daily
   23% indicated does not engage in the behavior.
   10% indicated one to several times per month.
   24% indicated one to several times per week.
   25% indicated one to several times per day.
   19% indicated one to several times per hour.

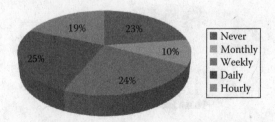

Fails to copy letters, words, sentences, and numbers from a textbook, chalkboard, etc.: 27% hourly to daily
   29% indicated does not engage in the behavior.
   24% indicated one to several times per month.
   24% indicated one to several times per week.
   13% indicated one to several times per day.
   11% indicated one to several times per hour.

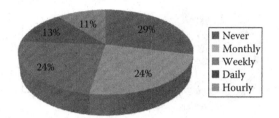

Omits, adds, or substitutes words when writing: 32% hourly to daily
   25% indicated does not engage in the behavior.
   14% indicated one to several times per month.
   29% indicated one to several times per week.
   26% indicated one to several times per day,
   6% indicated one to several times per hour.

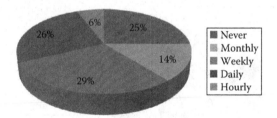

TASK COMPLETION AND DISORGANIZATION

Rushes through assignments with little or no regard for accuracy or quality of work: 57% hourly to daily
   16% indicated does not engage in the behavior.
   10% indicated one to several times per month.
   18% indicated one to several times per week.
   35% indicated one to several times per day.
   22% indicated one to several times per hour.

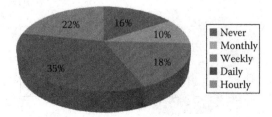

Fails to complete homework assignments and return them to school: 22% hourly to daily
   39% indicated does not engage in the behavior.
   21% indicated one to several times per month.
   17% indicated one to several times per week.
   14% indicated one to several times per day.
   8% indicated one to several times per hour.

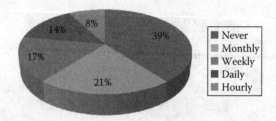

Does not perform or complete classroom assignments during class time: 38% hourly to daily
   11% indicated does not engage in the behavior.
   21% indicated one to several times per month.
   30% indicated one to several times per week.
   23% indicated one to several times per day.
   15% indicated one to several times per hour.

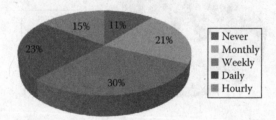

Is disorganized to point of not having necessary materials, losing materials, failing to find completed assignments, failing to follow steps of assignment in order, etc.: 26% hourly to daily
   31% indicated does not engage in the behavior.
   19% indicated one to several times per month.
   24% indicated one to several times per week.
   12% indicated one to several times per day.
   14% indicated one to several times per hour.

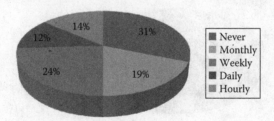

Completes assignments with little or no regard to neatness: 44% hourly to daily
    17% indicated does not engage in the behavior.
    15% indicated one to several times per month.
    24% indicated one to several times per week.
    31% indicated one to several times per day.
    13% indicated one to several times per hour.

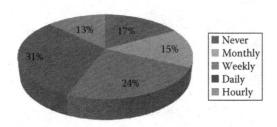

Fails to perform assignments independently: 41% hourly to daily
    15% indicated does not engage in the behavior.
    18% indicated one to several times per month.
    26% indicated one to several times per week.
    24% indicated one to several times per day.
    17% indicated one to several times per hour.

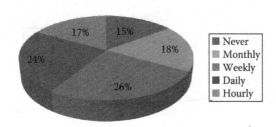

Fails to make appropriate use of study time: 33% hourly to daily
    17% indicated does not engage in the behavior.
    26% indicated one to several times per month.
    21% indicated one to several times per week.
    21% indicated one to several times per day.
    12% indicated one to several times per hour.

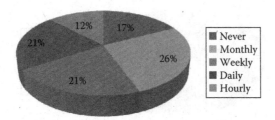

Does not prepare for school assignments: 20% hourly to daily
  37% indicated does not engage in the behavior.
  25% indicated one to several times per month.
  17% indicated one to several times per week.
  18% indicated one to several times per day.
  2% indicated one to several times per hour.

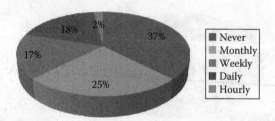

Does not remain on task: 47% hourly to daily
  19% indicated does not engage in the behavior.
  16% indicated one to several times per month.
  18% indicated one to several times per week.
  28% indicated one to several times per day.
  19% indicated one to several times per hour.

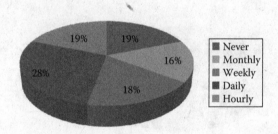

Changes from one activity to another without finishing first, without putting things away, before time to move on, etc.: 44% hourly to daily
  12% indicated does not engage in the behavior.
  19% indicated one to several times per month.
  24% indicated one to several times per week.
  31% indicated one to several times per day.
  13% indicated one to several times per hour.

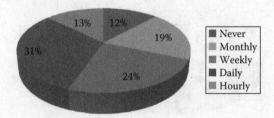

Oppositional Behavior

Does not follow school rules: 19% hourly to daily
　　30% indicated does not engage in the behavior.
　　30% indicated one to several times per month.
　　20% indicated one to several times per week.
　　13% indicated one to several times per day.
　　6% indicated one to several times per hour.

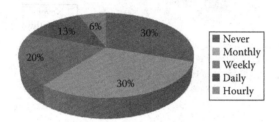

Grabs things away from others: 29% hourly to daily
　　30% indicated does not engage in the behavior.
　　22% indicated one to several times per month.
　　19% indicated one to several times per week.
　　18% indicated one to several times per day.
　　11% indicated one to several times per hour.

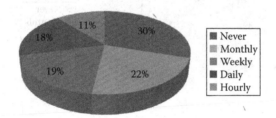

Fails to comply with teachers or other school personnel: 21% hourly to daily
　　48% indicated does not engage in the behavior.
　　13% indicated one to several times per month.
　　18% indicated one to several times per week.
　　11% indicated one to several times per day.
　　10% indicated one to several times per hour.

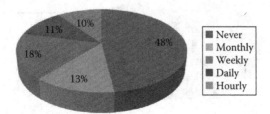

Ignores consequences of behavior: 16% hourly to daily
   54% indicated does not engage in the behavior.
   16% indicated one to several times per month.
   14% indicated one to several times per week.
   12% indicated one to several times per day.
   4% indicated one to several times per hour.

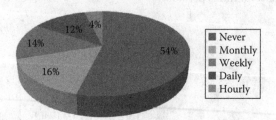

Does not follow the rule of games: 11% hourly to daily
   64% indicated does not engage in the behavior.
   14% indicated one to several times per month.
   11% indicated one to several times per week.
   8% indicated one to several times per day.
   3% indicated one to several times per hour.

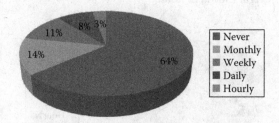

Does not wait his/her turn in activities or games: 32% hourly to daily
   25% indicated does not engage in the behavior.
   19% indicated one to several times per month.
   24% indicated one to several times per week.
   22% indicated one to several times per day.
   10% indicated one to several times per hour.

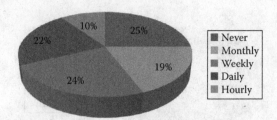

IMPULSIVE AND EMOTIONAL

Blurts out answers without being called on: 20% hourly to daily
    31% indicated does not engage in the behavior.
    28% indicated one to several times per month.
    20% indicated one to several times per week.
    12% indicated one to several times per day.
    8% indicated one to several times per hour.

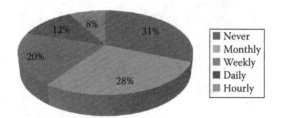

Interrupts the teacher: 51% hourly to daily
    23% indicated does not engage in the behavior.
    11% indicated one to several times per month.
    16% indicated one to several times per week.
    23% indicated one to several times per day.
    28% indicated one to several times per hour.

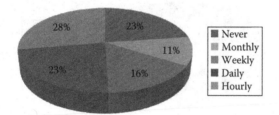

Interrupts other students: 40% hourly to daily
    28% indicated does not engage in the behavior.
    14% indicated one to several times per month.
    18% indicated one to several times per week.
    18% indicated one to several times per day.
    22% indicated one to several times per hour.

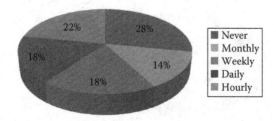

Makes unnecessary physical contact with others: 22% hourly to daily
   43% indicated does not engage in the behavior.
   16% indicated one to several times per month.
   18% indicated one to several times per week.
   14% indicated one to several times per day.
   8% indicated one to several times per hour.

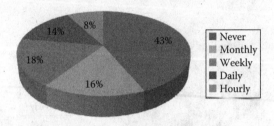

Is impulsive: 23% hourly to daily
   47% indicated does not engage in the behavior.
   16% indicated one to several times per month.
   14% indicated one to several times per week.
   13% indicated one to several times per day.
   10% indicated one to several times per hour.

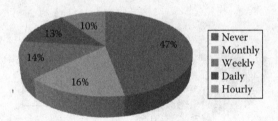

Fails to follow a routine: 9% hourly to daily
   50% indicated does not engage in the behavior.
   17% indicated one to several times per month.
   25% indicated one to several times per week.
   3% indicated one to several times per day.
   6% indicated one to several times per hour.

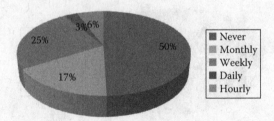

Bothers other students who are trying to work, listen, etc.: 30% hourly to daily
   30% indicated does not engage in the behavior.
   16% indicated one to several times per month.
   20% indicated one to several times per week.
   17% indicated one to several times per day.
   13% indicated one to several times per hour.

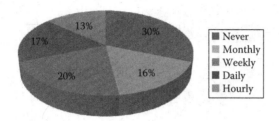

Makes unnecessary comments or noises in the classroom: 24% hourly to daily
   52% indicated does not engage in the behavior.
   11% indicated one to several times per month.
   13% indicated one to several times per week.
   14% indicated one to several times per day.
   10% indicated one to several times per hour.

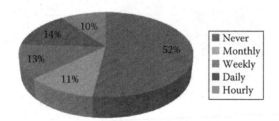

Does not adjust behavior to expectations of different situations: 22% hourly to daily
   44% indicated does not engage in the behavior.
   8% indicated one to several times per month.
   25% indicated one to several times per week.
   11% indicated one to several times per day.
   11% indicated one to several times per hour.

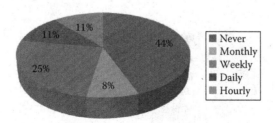

Engages in inappropriate behaviors while seated: 30% hourly to daily
   42% indicated does not engage in the behavior.
   14% indicated one to several times per month.
   14% indicated one to several times per week.
   14% indicated one to several times per day.
   17% indicated one to several times per hour.

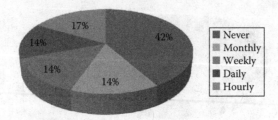

Is easily angered, annoyed, or upset: 30% hourly to daily
   36% indicated does not engage in the behavior.
   18% indicated one to several times per month.
   16% indicated one to several times per week.
   22% indicated one to several times per day.
   8% indicated one to several times per hour.

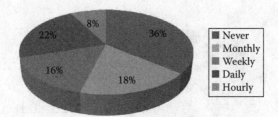

RESTLESS

Moves about while seated, fidgets, squirms, etc.: 42% hourly to daily
   20% indicated does not engage in the behavior.
   23% indicated one to several times per month.
   14% indicated one to several times per week.
   23% indicated one to several times per day.
   19% indicated one to several times per hour.

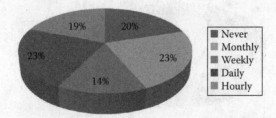

Appears restless: 33% hourly to daily
   24% indicated does not engage in the behavior.
   21% indicated one to several times per month.
   22% indicated one to several times per week.
   18% indicated one to several times per day.
   15% indicated one to several times per hour.

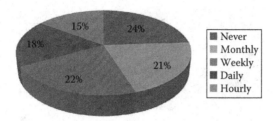

Engages in nervous habits: 25% hourly to daily
   42% indicated does not engage in the behavior.
   19% indicated one to several times per month.
   14% indicated one to several times per week.
   11% indicated one to several times per day.
   14% indicated one to several times per hour.

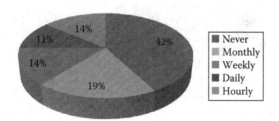

Talks to others during quiet activity periods: 24% hourly to daily
   22% indicated does not engage in the behavior.
   24% indicated one to several times per month.
   30% indicated one to several times per week.
   14% indicated one to several times per day.
   10% indicated one to several times per hour.

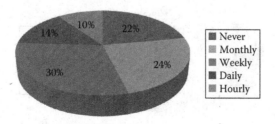

Talks beyond what is expected or at inappropriate times: 39% hourly to daily
    8% indicated does not engage in the behavior.
    31% indicated one to several times per month.
    22% indicated one to several times per week.
    14% indicated one to several times per day.
    25% indicated one to several times per hour.

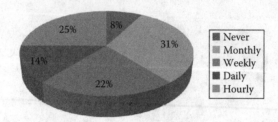

Does not wait appropriately for assistance from instructor: 33% hourly to daily
    22% indicated does not engage in the behavior.
    19% indicated one to several times per month.
    25% indicated one to several times per week.
    25% indicated one to several times per day.
    8% indicated one to several times per hour.

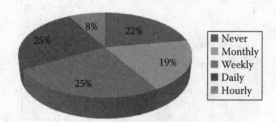

OVERLY ACTIVE

Leaves seat without permission: 31% hourly to daily
    44% indicated does not engage in the behavior.
    14% indicated one to several times per month.
    11% indicated one to several times per week.
    17% indicated one to several times per day.
    14% indicated one to several times per hour.

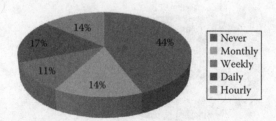

Does not work in a group situation: 47% hourly to daily
25% indicated does not engage in the behavior.
19% indicated one to several times per month.
8% indicated one to several times per week.
28% indicated one to several times per day.
19% indicated one to several times per hour.

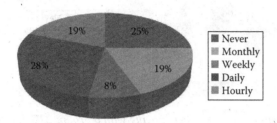

Hops, skips, and jumps when moving from one place to another instead of walking: 14% hourly to daily
42% indicated does not engage in the behavior.
28% indicated one to several times per month.
17% indicated one to several times per week.
8% indicated one to several times per day.
6% indicated one to several times per hour.

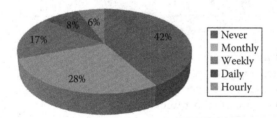

Handles objects: 39% hourly to daily
28% indicated does not engage in the behavior.
17% indicated one to several times per month.
17% indicated one to several times per week.
25% indicated one to several times per day.
14% indicated one to several times per hour.

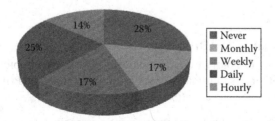

Becomes overexcited: 22% hourly to daily
   47% indicated does not engage in the behavior.
   17% indicated one to several times per month.
   14% indicated one to several times per week.
   11% indicated one to several times per day.
   11% indicated one to several times per hour.

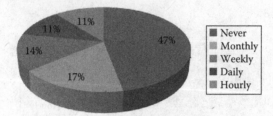

Demonstrates inappropriate behavior when moving with a group: 22% hourly to daily
   42% indicated does not engage in the behavior.
   11% indicated one to several times per month.
   25% indicated one to several times per week.
   14% indicated one to several times per day.
   8% indicated one to several times per hour.

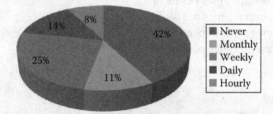

Moves about unnecessarily: 28% hourly to daily
   47% indicated does not engage in the behavior.
   11% indicated one to several times per month.
   14% indicated one to several times per week.
   11% indicated one to several times per day.
   17% indicated one to several times per hour.

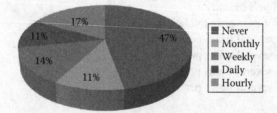

SUMMATION OF FINDINGS

Looking at Severity, What ADD/ADHD Is

Symptoms occurring daily or hourly were the following. These are symptoms that we commonly think of as associated with inattention and difficulty sustaining attention. Primary problems are that of distractibility and poor sustained attention:

- 75% are easily distracted by other activities in the classroom.
- 64% do not direct attention or fail to maintain attention to important sounds.

- 62% attend more successfully when close to the source of sound.
- 60% have difficulty concentrating.
- 57% rushed through assignments without regard to accuracy or quality of work.
- 54% requires eye contact to listen successfully.
- 51% interrupts the teacher.
- 52% do not listen to what other students are saying.
- 45% need oral questions and directions frequently repeated.

The following symptoms would be seen more often with the ADHD combined subtype or hyperactivity. That these symptoms were not seen very often suggests that ADHD is primarily a disorder of attention. The following are the percentages that these symptoms were rated by the teacher as occurring daily or hourly:

- 22% demonstrated inappropriate behavior when moving with a group.
- 22% become over excited.
- 22% do not adjust behavior to expectations of different situations.
- 22% make unnecessary physical contact with others.
- 22% fail to complete homework assignments.
- 21% fail to comply with teachers.
- 20% blurt out answers without being called on.
- 20% do not prepare for school assignments.
- 19% do not follow school rules.
- 16% ignore consequences of behavior.
- 14% hop, skip, and jump when moving.
- 11% do not follow rules of games.

What ADD/ADHD Is Not

Another way to examine the data is to look at symptoms reported as not existing at all. A very small percent (less than 10%) of the teachers reported not seeing symptoms in the areas of distractibility, not listening, needing directions repeated, attending better when closer to the source of sound, requiring eye contact to listen successfully, difficulty concentrating, and talking beyond what is expected and/or at inappropriate times. These are the traits seen *more often* in the ADD/ADHD child, which are commonly referenced as classic signs of inattention.

Most of the items are similar to that seen on the home version of this measure. Excluded were the following of verbal directions, forgetting things, changing activities, and not independently performing responsibilities.

The school version had a far smaller sample than the home version. Often parents had their children evaluated during the summer when teachers were not available to provide information on their behavior in school.

Symptoms that commonly are thought of as associated with the combined subtype and hyperactivity were not reported by the teachers, suggesting again that ADD/ADHD is a disorder of attention as opposed to behavioral disturbance. The following traits that we would commonly associate with hyperactivity were not reported by the teacher as existing at all:

- 64% did not report not following the rules of the game.
- 54% did not report ignoring consequences of their behavior.
- 52% did not report making unnecessary comments or noises in the classroom.
- 50% did not report failing to follow a routine in the classroom.
- 48% did not report failing to comply with teachers.
- 47% did not report any impulsivity.

This means that half or more of the time, none of the previously described symptoms were reported by the teacher.

The following are symptoms seen less often and reported by the teacher as either not occurring at all or only occurring monthly:

- 78% not following rules of the game
- 70% ignoring consequences of behavior
- 70% hopping, skipping, and jumping instead of walking
- 67% failing to follow a routine
- 64% becoming overly excited
- 63% making unnecessary comments or noises in class
- 63% being impulsive
- 60% failing to complete homework assignments and return them to school (this changed in adolescence)
- 62% not preparing for school assignments (this changed in adolescence)
- 61% failing to comply
- 61% engaging in nervous habits
- 60% not following school rules
- 59% blurting out answers
- 59% making unnecessary physical contact

The absence of these symptoms is due to the nature of the elementary classroom, which promotes routine. Teachers may not see children as being problematic unless they are behaviorally out of control especially when they have 25–30 children in their class. Missing assignments and failure to complete work tend to become more noticeable after the age of 12 when there is more reading and writing that has to be done commencing with the 6th grade and junior high. Our cutoff for adolescents was age 11 years. Therefore, the adolescent population reflects these symptoms more than the children.

ADDES: HOME VERSION

This is a measure to assess ADHD, symptoms of inattention, hyperactivity, and combined subtype (impulsivity), that is completed by parents. There 536 parents that completed this measure. Results include both the first and second versions of this measure. Parents rate the symptoms based upon how often it is occurring as well as if it is not occurring at all. Symptoms are assigned a score from 0 to 4 based upon how often the symptom is observed in the home setting.

DISTRACTIBILITY AND LISTENING

Is easily distracted by other things happening in the home (e.g., other kids, TV, radio, etc.): 71% occurring hourly to daily
4% does not engage in the behavior.
8% engages in the behavior one to several times per month.
17% engages in the behavior one to several times per week.
43% engages in the behavior one to several times per day.
28% engages in the behavior one to several times per hour.

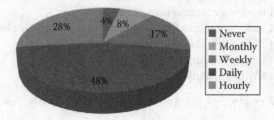

Does not listen to what others are saying: 58% occurring hourly to daily
   7% does not engage in the behavior.
   11% engages in the behavior one to several times per month.
   24% engages in the behavior one to several times per week.
   44% engages in the behavior one to several times per day.
   14% engages in the behavior one to several times per hour.

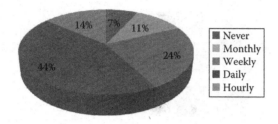

Does not direct attention or fails to maintain attention to important sounds in the immediate environment: 52% occurring hourly to daily
   15% does not engage in the behavior.
   9% engages in the behavior one to several times per month.
   22% engages in the behavior one to several times per week.
   40% engages in the behavior one to several times per day.
   12% engages in the behavior one to several times per hour.

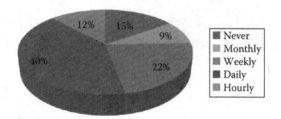

Is unsuccessful in activities requiring listening: 34% occurring hourly to daily
   15% does not engage in the behavior.
   18% engages in the behavior one to several times per month.
   33% engages in the behavior one to several times per week.
   28% engages in the behavior one to several times per day.
   6% engages in the behavior one to several times per hour.

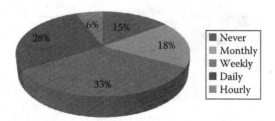

Needs oral questions and directions frequently repeated: 64% occurring hourly to daily
   8% does not engage in the behavior.
   8% engages in the behavior one to several times per month.
   19% engages in the behavior one to several times per week.
   45% engages in the behavior one to several times per day.
   19% engages in the behavior one to several times per hour.

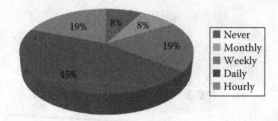

Does not listen to or follow verbal directions: 52% occurring hourly to daily
   6% does not engage in the behavior.
   12% engages in the behavior one to several times per month.
   30% engages in the behavior one to several times per week.
   41% engages in the behavior one to several times per day.
   11% engages in the behavior one to several times per hour.

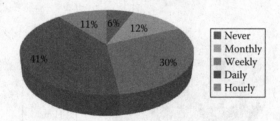

ATTENTION AND CONCENTRATION

Has difficulty concentrating: 57% occurring hourly to daily
   9% does not engage in the behavior.
   12% engages in the behavior one to several times per month.
   22% engages in the behavior one to several times per week.
   42% engages in the behavior one to several times per day.
   15% engages in the behavior one to several times per hour.

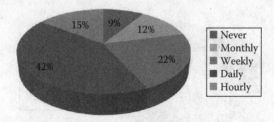

Can't concentrate, can't pay attention for long: 55% occurring hourly to daily
    11% does not engage in the behavior.
    10% engages in the behavior one to several times per month.
    24% engages in the behavior one to several times per week.
    29% engages in the behavior one to several times per day.
    26% engages in the behavior one to several times per hour.

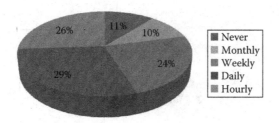

Forgets things: 50% occurring hourly to daily
    8% does not engage in the behavior.
    13% engages in the behavior one to several times per month.
    29% engages in the behavior one to several times per week.
    36% engages in the behavior one to several times per day.
    14% engages in the behavior one to several times per hour.

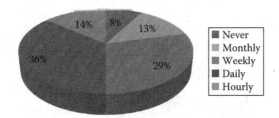

Changes from one activity to another without finishing the first, without putting things away, and before it is time to move on to the next activity: 54% occurring hourly to daily
    6% does not engage in the behavior.
    15% engages in the behavior one to several times per month.
    25% engages in the behavior one to several times per week.
    37% engages in the behavior one to several times per day.
    17% engages in the behavior one to several times per hour.

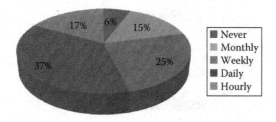

Has a short attention span: 53% occurring hourly to daily
   11% does not engage in the behavior.
   12% engages in the behavior one to several times per month.
   24% engages in the behavior one to several times per week.
   34% engages in the behavior one to several times per day.
   19% engages in the behavior one to several times per hour.

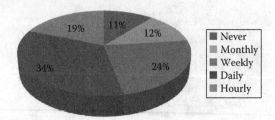

ORGANIZATION AND TASK COMPLETION

Is disorganized with possessions: 44% occurring hourly to daily
   11% does not engage in the behavior.
   14% engages in the behavior one to several times per month.
   31% engages in the behavior one to several times per week.
   29% engages in the behavior one to several times per day.
   15% engages in the behavior one to several times per hour.

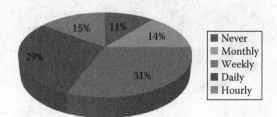

Starts but does not complete homework: 29% occurring hourly to daily
   27% does not engage in the behavior.
   16% engages in the behavior one to several times per month.
   28% engages in the behavior one to several times per week.
   18% engages in the behavior one to several times per day.
   11% engages in the behavior one to several times per hour.

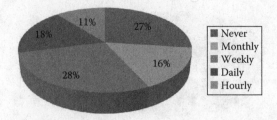

Does not independently perform chores or responsibilities: 57% occurring hourly to daily
   6% does not engage in the behavior.
   9% engages in the behavior one to several times per month.
   27% engages in the behavior one to several times per week.
   41% engages in the behavior one to several times per day.
   16% engages in the behavior one to several times per hour.

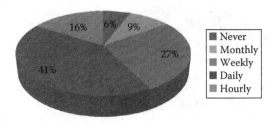

Does not remain on task to study or prepare for tests or quizzes: 34% occurring hourly to daily
   26% does not engage in the behavior.
   13% engages in the behavior one to several times per month.
   28% engages in the behavior one to several times per week.
   21% engages in the behavior one to several times per day.
   13% engages in the behavior one to several times per hour.

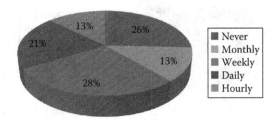

Does not organize responsibilities: 39% occurring hourly to daily
   19% does not engage in the behavior.
   15% engages in the behavior one to several times per month.
   27% engages in the behavior one to several times per week.
   28% engages in the behavior one to several times per day.
   11% engages in the behavior one to several times per hour.

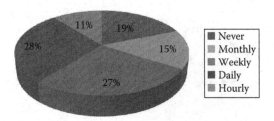

Does not prepare for school assignments: 37% occurring hourly to daily
   33% does not engage in the behavior.
   17% engages in the behavior one to several times per month.
   17% engages in the behavior one to several times per week.
   27% engages in the behavior one to several times per day.
   10% engages in the behavior one to several times per hour.

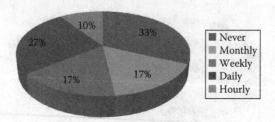

Rushes through chores or tasks with little or no regard for quality: 43% occurring hourly to daily
   11% does not engage in the behavior.
   16% engages in the behavior one to several times per month.
   29% engages in the behavior one to several times per week.
   28% engages in the behavior one to several times per day.
   15% engages in the behavior one to several times per hour.

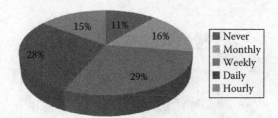

FOLLOWING DIRECTIONS

Does not read or follow written directions: 31% occurring hourly to daily
   27% does not engage in the behavior.
   17% engages in the behavior one to several times per month.
   25% engages in the behavior one to several times per week.
   20% engages in the behavior one to several times per day.
   11% engages in the behavior one to several times per hour.

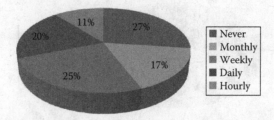

Fails to follow necessary steps in doing things: 38% occurring hourly to daily
   16% does not engage in the behavior.
   21% engages in the behavior one to several times per month.
   25% engages in the behavior one to several times per week.
   24% engages in the behavior one to several times per day.
   14% engages in the behavior one to several times per hour.

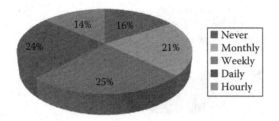

Does not follow directions from parents or other home authority figures: 19% occurring hourly to daily
   32% does not engage in the behavior.
   25% engages in the behavior one to several times per month.
   24% engages in the behavior one to several times per week.
   16% engages in the behavior one to several times per day.
   3% engages in the behavior one to several times per hour.

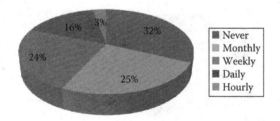

Refuses to follow requests or accept decisions made by parents: 23% occurring hourly to daily
   32% does not engage in the behavior.
   23% engages in the behavior one to several times per month.
   22% engages in the behavior one to several times per week.
   17% engages in the behavior one to several times per day.
   6% engages in the behavior one to several times per hour

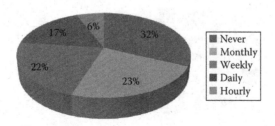

Begins things before receiving directions or instructions: 36% occurring hourly to daily
  16% does not engage in the behavior.
  22% engages in the behavior one to several times per month.
  26% engages in the behavior one to several times per week.
  24% engages in the behavior one to several times per day.
  12% engages in the behavior one to several times per hour.

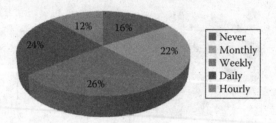

EMOTIONAL AND IMPULSIVE

Is easily frustrated: 43% occurring hourly to daily
  14% does not engage in the behavior.
  15% engages in the behavior one to several times per month.
  28% engages in the behavior one to several times per week.
  29% engages in the behavior one to several times per day.
  14% engages in the behavior one to several times per hour.

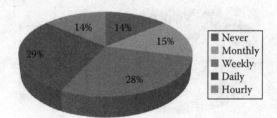

Does not wait his/her turn in activities or games: 40% occurring hourly to daily
  17% does not engage in the behavior.
  19% engages in the behavior one to several times per month.
  24% engages in the behavior one to several times per week.
  27% engages in the behavior one to several times per day.
  13% engages in the behavior one to several times per hour.

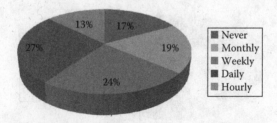

Grabs things away from others: 37% occurring hourly to daily
    25% does not engage in the behavior.
    17% engages in the behavior one to several times per month.
    21% engages in the behavior one to several times per week.
    24% engages in the behavior one to several times per day.
    13% engages in the behavior one to several times per hour.

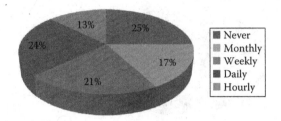

Interrupts others: 26% occurring hourly to daily
    29% does not engage in the behavior.
    24% engages in the behavior one to several times per month.
    21% engages in the behavior one to several times per week.
    18% engages in the behavior one to several times per day.
    8% engages in the behavior one to several times per hour.

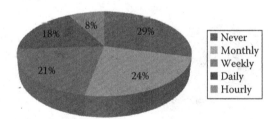

Is impulsive: 26% occurring hourly to daily
    20% does not engage in the behavior.
    24% engages in the behavior one to several times per month.
    31% engages in the behavior one to several times per week.
    17% engages in the behavior one to several times per day.
    9% engages in the behavior one to several times per hour.

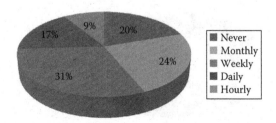

Fails to follow a routine: 45% occurring hourly to daily
   14% does not engage in the behavior.
   16% engages in the behavior one to several times per month.
   25% engages in the behavior one to several times per week.
   31% engages in the behavior one to several times per day.
   14% engages in the behavior one to several times per hour.

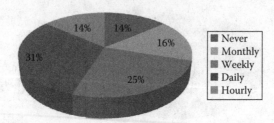

Is easily angered, annoyed, or upset: 47% occurring hourly to daily
   14% does not engage in the behavior.
   16% engages in the behavior one to several times per month.
   23% engages in the behavior one to several times per week.
   32% engages in the behavior one to several times per day.
   15% engages in the behavior one to several times per hour.

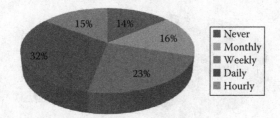

Has accidents that are the result of impulsive or careless behavior: 11% occurring hourly to daily
   37% does not engage in the behavior.
   30% engages in the behavior one to several times per month.
   22% engages in the behavior one to several times per week.
   8% engages in the behavior one to several times per day.
   3% engages in the behavior one to several times per hour.

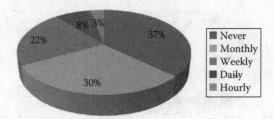

INTRUSIVE AND OPPOSITIONAL

Intrudes on others: 24% occurring hourly to daily
    23% does not engage in the behavior.
    25% engages in the behavior one to several times per month.
    28% engages in the behavior one to several times per week.
    19% engages in the behavior one to several times per day.
    5% engages in the behavior one to several times per hour.

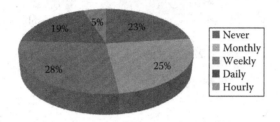

Bothers others while they are trying to work, play, etc.: 34% occurring hourly to daily
    17% does not engage in the behavior.
    23% engages in the behavior one to several times per month.
    26% engages in the behavior one to several times per week.
    25% engages in the behavior one to several times per day.
    9% engages in the behavior one to several times per hour.

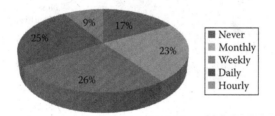

Ignores consequences of his/her behavior: 36% occurring hourly to daily
    18% does not engage in the behavior.
    21% engages in the behavior one to several times per month.
    25% engages in the behavior one to several times per week.
    23% engages in the behavior one to several times per day.
    13% engages in the behavior one to several times per hour.

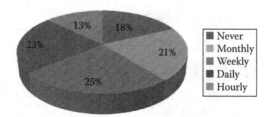

Does not follow the rules of games: 14% occurring hourly to daily
39% does not engage in the behavior.
27% engages in the behavior one to several times per month.
19% engages in the behavior one to several times per week.
12% engages in the behavior one to several times per day.
2% engages in the behavior one to several times per hour.

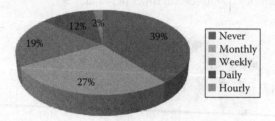

Behaves inappropriately when riding in the car: 12% occurring hourly to daily
59% does not engage in the behavior.
19% engages in the behavior one to several times per month.
11% engages in the behavior one to several times per week.
8% engages in the behavior one to several times per day.
4% engages in the behavior one to several times per hour.

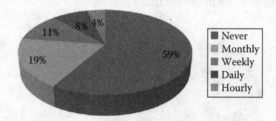

OVERACTIVE AND RESTLESS

Moves about while seated, squirms, fidgets, etc: 45% occurring hourly to daily
20% does not engage in the behavior.
15% engages in the behavior one to several times per month.
16% engages in the behavior one to several times per week.
22% engages in the behavior one to several times per day.
23% engages in the behavior one to several times per hour.

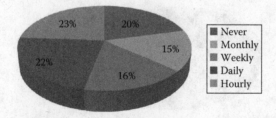

Appears restless: 41% occurring hourly to daily
　　25% does not engage in the behavior.
　　14% engages in the behavior one to several times per month.
　　20% engages in the behavior one to several times per week.
　　21% engages in the behavior one to several times per day.
　　20% engages in the behavior one to several times per hour.

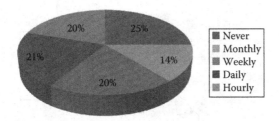

Does not remain seated: 33% occurring hourly to daily
　　30% does not engage in the behavior.
　　16% engages in the behavior one to several times per month.
　　20% engages in the behavior one to several times per week.
　　21% engages in the behavior one to several times per day.
　　12% engages in the behavior one to several times per hour.

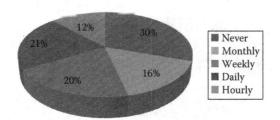

Does not adjust behavior to expectations of different situations: 27% occurring hourly to daily
　　33% does not engage in the behavior.
　　17% engages in the behavior one to several times per month.
　　23% engages in the behavior one to several times per week.
　　20% engages in the behavior one to several times per day.
　　7% engages in the behavior one to several times per hour.

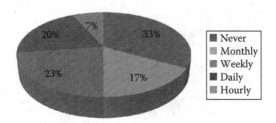

Becomes overexcited: 28% occurring hourly to daily
32% does not engage in the behavior.
20% engages in the behavior one to several times per month.
20% engages in the behavior one to several times per week.
19% engages in the behavior one to several times per day.
9% engages in the behavior one to several times per hour.

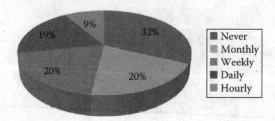

Climbs on things: 25% occurring hourly to daily
36% does not engage in the behavior.
22% engages in the behavior one to several times per month.
17% engages in the behavior one to several times per week.
16% engages in the behavior one to several times per day.
9% engages in the behavior one to several times per hour.

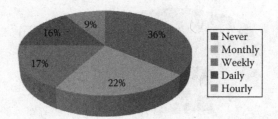

Moves about unnecessarily: 20% occurring hourly to daily
57% does not engage in the behavior.
11% engages in the behavior one to several times per month.
13% engages in the behavior one to several times per week.
13% engages in the behavior one to several times per day.
7% engages in the behavior one to several times per hour.

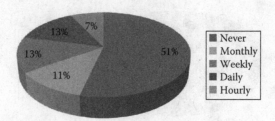

Runs in the house and does not sit appropriately on furniture: 30% occurring hourly to daily
    34% does not engage in the behavior.
    19% engages in the behavior one to several times per month.
    17% engages in the behavior one to several times per week.
    18% engages in the behavior one to several times per day.
    12% engages in the behavior one to several times per hour.

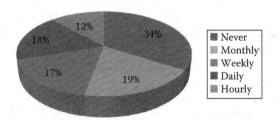

Runs in the shopping mall, pushes and makes noises in line at the movies, yells in stores, etc.: 13% occurring hourly to daily
    58% does not engage in the behavior.
    18% engages in the behavior one to several times per month.
    11% engages in the behavior one to several times per week.
    9% engages in the behavior one to several times per day.
    4% engages in the behavior one to several times per hour.

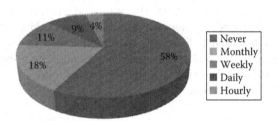

Makes excessive noise: 24% occurring hourly to daily
    45% does not engage in the behavior.
    18% engages in the behavior one to several times per month.
    13% engages in the behavior one to several times per week.
    17% engages in the behavior one to several times per day.
    7% engages in the behavior one to several times per hour.

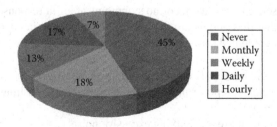

Summation of Findings

The home version of the ADDES, a measure of attention symptoms completed by the parents, confirms what has been observed in the clinic through the years: that ADHD is a thinking disorder of attention and that symptoms of restlessness are more related to anxiety while symptoms of hyperactivity are more related to sleep. The rather clear finding is that of attention symptoms not oppositional or overactivity.

What ADD/ADHD Is

A look at severity, symptoms seen more often and on a daily basis

- 71% were easily distracted.
- 64% needed oral directions repeated.
- 58% did not listen.
- 57% had difficulty concentrating.
- 57% did not independently perform chores or responsibilities.
- 55% could not sustain attention.
- 54% changed from one activity without finishing the first activity.
- 53% had a short attention span.
- 52% did not direct attention or maintain attention.
- 52% did not listen to or follow verbal direction.
- 50% forgot things.

Another way to examine the data is to look at the report of no symptoms at all.

For the attention symptoms, parents reported seeing no symptoms of distractibility less than 10% of the time. This means that 90% of the time, they saw distractibility occurring to some degree. Parents reported the absence or no symptoms in the following areas less than 10% of the time: not listening, needing directions repeated, difficulty concentrating, not following verbal directions, forgetting things, changing activities, and not independently performing responsibilities. Again, that means that these symptoms are seen to some degree 90% of the time.

Symptoms seen over 90% of the time:

- Easily distracted by other things happening in the home: 96%
- Not listening to what others are saying: 93%
- Requiring oral directions to be repeated: 91%
- Not listening to or following verbal directions: 94%
- Difficulty concentrating: 91%
- Changing from one activity to another without completion of the first activity: 94%
- Ability to independently perform chores or responsibilities in the home: 93%
- Forgets things: 92%

What ADD/ADHD Is Not

Parents reported the absence of symptoms or no symptoms at all in response to the following specific items, suggesting that these items are more rare. These are the items typically thought of as characteristic of ADHD combined subtype or overactivity:

- 57% of the parents did not report moving about unnecessarily.
- 58% of the parents did not report running in the shopping mall, pushing and making noises in line, or yelling in stores.
- 45% of the parents did not report making excessive noise.
- 59% of the parents did not report behaving inappropriately while riding in the car.

This means that approximately half or more of the time, parents saw absolutely no symptoms of moving about unnecessarily, running in the shopping mall, making excessive noise, or behaving inappropriately in the car. The remaining half of the time, parents saw these symptoms either daily, weekly, or monthly although percentages were small for daily observation of these behaviors. Moving about unnecessarily was seen 20% of the time on a daily basis. Running in the shopping mall was seen 13% of the time on a daily basis. Making excessive noise was seen 24% of the time on a daily basis and behaving inappropriately, while riding in the car was seen 12% of the time on a daily basis.

The following symptoms are reported as either not occurring at all or only monthly and therefore less significantly seen:

- 78% of the parents did not report behaving inappropriately when riding in the car.
- 76% of the parents did not report running in the shopping mall or unable to stand in line.
- 68% of the parents did not report moving about unnecessarily.
- 67% of the parents did not report having accidents resulting from impulsive or careless behavior.
- 66% of the parents did not report not following the rules of the game.

Suggested is that these behavioral issues are not seen much of the time and that the problem is in attention and anxiety, which creates procrastination in completing tasks and homework. When the previously described symptoms are seen, it is the result of additional disorders beyond that of a genetic attention disorder. Our sample of children had an almost equal number of ADHD and ADHD plus children. The child sample was the only developmental age to have such a large proportion of ADHD plus, suggesting the problem of underdiagnosis of additional disorders while overdiagnosing an attention disorder. This pattern was not seen for the adolescents or for the adults.

Emotional/behavioral symptoms seen as related to anxiety, occurring more often, daily to weekly

- 71% were easily frustrated.
- 70% became easily angered, annoyed, or upset.
- 64% found it difficult to wait for their turn.
- 61% appear restless.

ADHD RATING SCALE

This is a measure completed by the parent regarding attention problems seen in the child. A total of 454 parents responded and reported symptoms on their child. There are a total of 14 items that the parent can respond to as not present or seen just a little, pretty much, or very much of the time covering the areas of inattention, hyperactivity, and impulsivity.

Often fidgets or squirms in seat: 79%
    Not at all = 22%
    Just a little = 30%
    Pretty much = 28%
    Very much = 21%

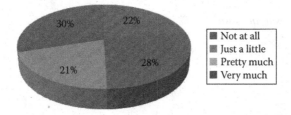

Has difficulty remaining seated: 79%
    Not at all = 22%
    Just a little = 30%
    Pretty much = 28%
    Very much = 21%

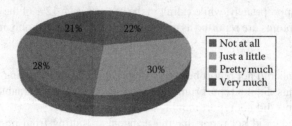

Is easily distracted: 95%
    Not at all = 5%
    Just a little = 16%
    Pretty much = 37%
    Very much = 42%

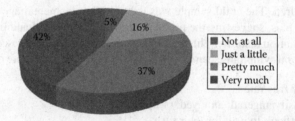

Has difficulty awaiting turn in groups: 68%
    Not at all = 32%
    Just a little = 31%
    Pretty much = 26%
    Very much = 11%

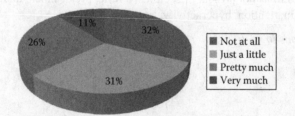

Often blurts out answers to questions: 69%
    Not at all = 31%
    Just a little = 33%
    Pretty much = 22%
    Very much = 14%

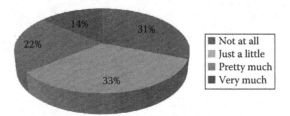

Has difficulty following instructions: 91%
    Not at all = 9%
    Just a little = 27%
    Pretty much = 37%
    Very much = 27%

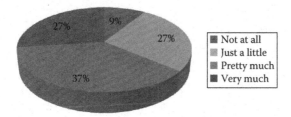

Has difficulty sustaining attention to tasks: 93%
    Not at all = 8%
    Just a little = 21%
    Pretty much – 34%
    Very much = 38%

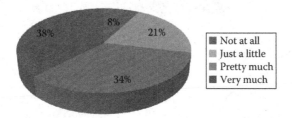

Often shifts from one uncompleted activity to another: 83%
    Not at all = 17%
    Just a little = 28%
    Pretty much = 31%
    Very much = 24%

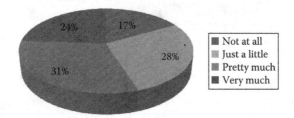

Has difficulty playing quietly: 56%
    Not at all = 44%
    Just a little = 27%
    Pretty much = 20%
    Very much = 9%

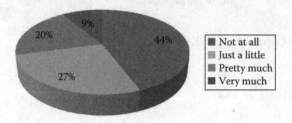

Often talks excessively: 71%
    Not at all = 30%
    Just a little = 29%
    Pretty much = 23%
    Very much = 19%

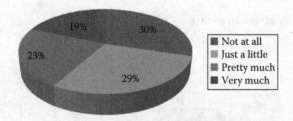

Often interrupts or intrudes on others: 83%
    Not at all = 17%
    Just a little = 30%
    Pretty much = 27%
    Very much = 26%

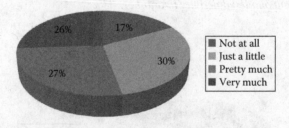

Often does not seem to listen: 93%
    Not at all = 7%
    Just a little = 24%
    Pretty much = 33%
    Very much = 36%

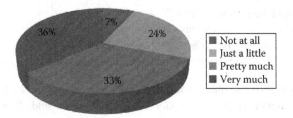

Often loses things necessary for tasks: 79%
    Not at all = 20%
    Just a little = 33%
    Pretty much = 24%
    Very much = 22%

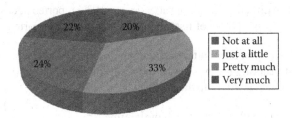

Often engages in physically dangerous activities without considering consequences: 42%
    Not at all = 58%
    Just a little = 24%
    Pretty much = 11%
    Very much = 7%

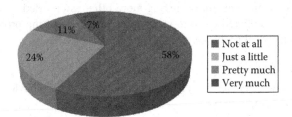

SUMMATION OF FINDINGS

Severity of Symptoms

Symptoms being seen pretty to very much of the time:

- Is easily distracted: 79%
- Has difficulty sustaining attention to tasks: 72%
- Often does not seem to listen: 69%
- Has difficulty following instructions: 64%
- Often shifts from one uncompleted activity to another: 55%
- Often interrupts or intrudes on others: 53%
- Often fidgets or squirms in seat: 49%
- Has difficulty remaining seated: 49%
- Often loses things necessary for tasks: 46%
- Often talks excessively: 42%

- Has difficulty awaiting turn in groups: 37%
- Often blurts out answers to questions: 36%
- Has difficulty playing quietly: 23%
- Often engages in physically dangerous activities without considering consequences: 18%

Primary symptoms reported by parents as occurring more often were the following: being easily distracted, difficulty following instructions, poor sustained attention, and often not seeming to listen.

Symptoms Seen More Often

The following percentages suggest that these four symptoms are more predominant and that 90% or more of the time, these symptoms were indicated as present per parental report:

- Only 5% reported no distractibility, and 95% reported distractibility.
- Only 9% reported no difficulty following directions, and 91% reported difficulty.
- Only 8% reported no difficulty sustaining attention, and 93% reported poor sustained attention.
- Only 7% reported no symptoms of listening problems, and 93 reported listening issues.

In looking at severity of symptoms, attention symptoms emerged as the most prevalent; however, there were issues of interrupting (often seen as the result of not wanting to forget what they were going to say), which can be related to distractibility:

- 79% were distracted pretty to very much of the time.
- 72% had poor sustained attention pretty to very much of the time.
- 69% often did not seem to listen pretty to very much of the time.
- 64% had difficulty following instruction pretty to very much of the time.
- 55% shifted from one uncompleted task to another pretty to very much of the time.
- 53% often interrupted or intruded upon others pretty to very much of the time.

The key is that these symptoms are occurring more often as opposed to whether *they exist or not*. Primary symptoms are related more to inattention and the thinking problems of an attention disorder and not the behavioral problems.

Symptoms Seen Less Often

Confirmation of the problem being that of attention as opposed to behavioral is provided by the absence of the following symptoms:

- 29% of the time did parents report difficulty playing quietly that occurred pretty to very much of the time.
- 37% had difficulty waiting for their turn as a symptom that occurred pretty to very much of the time.
- 18% engaged in physically dangerous activities without considering the consequences pretty to very much of the time.

This large sample of parents that completed this form indicates that attention symptoms are the primary issue with diagnosed ADD/ADHD and not behavioral problems.

CHILDREN SYMPTOM INVENTORY

The Child Symptom Inventories-4 (CSI-4) are parent-completed rating scales that allow for the screening of attention deficit/hyperactivity disorder (ADHD) and other emotional and behavioral disorders. Questions are asked to determine symptoms related to the following types of disorders: attention deficit/hyperactivity disorder, oppositional defiant disorder, conduct disorder, anxiety, schizophrenia, major depressive disorder, dysthymic disorder, autistic disorder, Asperger's disorder, social phobia, separation anxiety disorder. There were 107 parents who responded to this questionnaire used between the years 2006 and 2009, and it is currently in use. Parents rated the symptoms as occurring never, sometimes, often, or very often.

The following are the significant percentages for symptoms that parents saw as occurring often or very often:

ATTENTION–THINKING SYMPTOMS

Fails to give close attention to details or makes careless mistakes: 69% seen often and very often
    Never = 1%
    Sometimes = 30%
    Often = 44%
    Very often = 25%

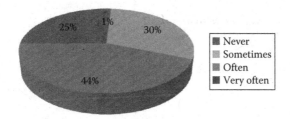

Has difficulty paying attention to tasks or activities: 61%
    Never = 1%
    Sometimes = 38%
    Often = 38%
    Very often = 23%

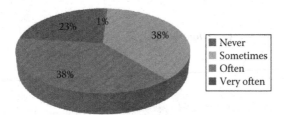

Does not seem to listen when spoken to directly: 59%
    Never = 12%
    Sometimes = 28%
    Often = 30%
    Very often = 29%

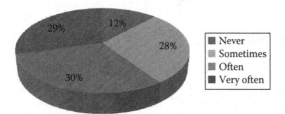

Has difficulty following through on instructions and fails to finish things: 67%
    Never = 5%
    Sometimes = 28%
    Often = 43%
    Very often = 24%

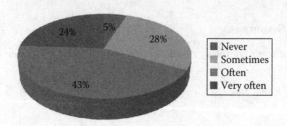

Has difficulty organizing tasks and activities: 66%
    Never = 6%
    Sometimes = 28%
    Often = 36%
    Very often = 30%

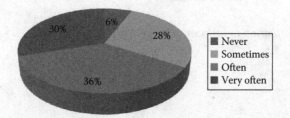

Is easily distracted by other things going on: 82%
    Never = 1%
    Sometimes = 17%
    Often = 40%
    Very often = 42%

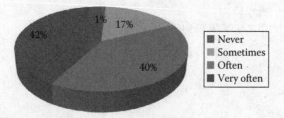

Is forgetful in daily activities: 57%
    Never = 10%
    Sometimes = 32%
    Often = 35%
    Very often = 22%

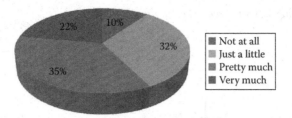

BEHAVIORAL SYMPTOMS RELATED TO ATTENTION

Avoids doing tasks that require a lot of mental effort (schoolwork, homework, etc.): 73%
    Never = 5%
    Sometimes = 22%
    Often = 39%
    Very often = 34%

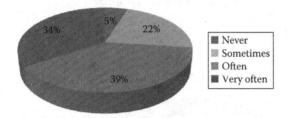

Loses things necessary for activities: 45%
    Never = 13%
    Sometimes = 42%
    Often = 28%
    Very often = 17%

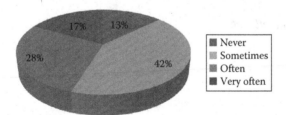

Fidgets with hands or feet or squirms in seat: 54%
    Never = 15%
    Sometimes = 34%
    Often = 23%
    Very often = 31%

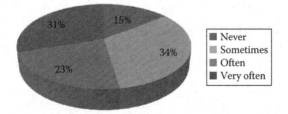

Has difficulty remaining in seat when asked to do so: 44%
> Never = 23%
> Sometimes = 34%
> Often = 25%
> Very often = 19%

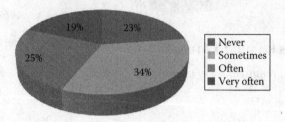

Runs about or climbs on things when asked not to do so: 31%
> Never = 33%
> Sometimes = 35%
> Often = 18%
> Very often = 13%

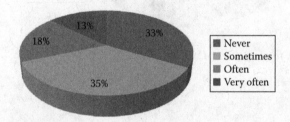

Has difficulty playing quietly: 26%
> Never = 32%
> Sometimes = 42%
> Often = 14%
> Very often = 12%

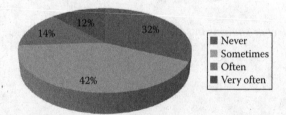

Is "on the go" or acts as if "driven by a motor": 43%
> Never = 34%
> Sometimes = 23%
> Often = 21%
> Very often = 22%

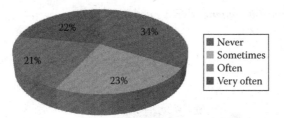

Talks excessively: 42%
 Never = 27%
 Sometimes = 31%
 Often = 20%
 Very often = 22%

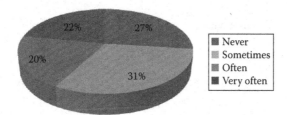

Blurts out answers to questions before they have been completed: 36%
 Never = 26%
 Sometimes = 38%
 Often − 23%
 Very often = 13%

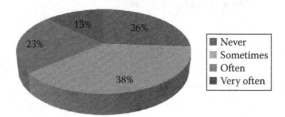

Has difficulty awaiting turn in group activities: 29%
 Never = 30%
 Sometimes = 40%
 Often = 17%
 Very often = 12%

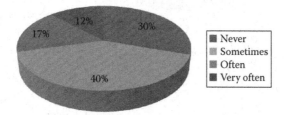

Interrupts people or butts into other children's activities: 47%
   Never = 17%
   Sometimes = 36%
   Often = 22%
   Very often = 25%

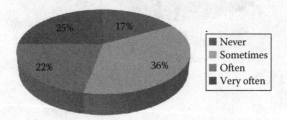

OPPOSITIONAL AND DEFIANT BEHAVIOR

Loses temper: 49%
   Never = 11%
   Sometimes = 40%
   Often = 29%
   Very often = 20%

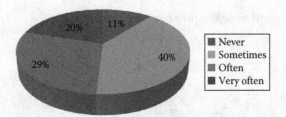

Argues with adults: 53%
   Never = 14%
   Sometimes = 33%
   Often = 29%
   Very often = 24%

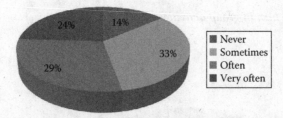

Defies or refuses what you tell him/her to do: 45%
   Never = 16%
   Sometimes = 38%
   Often = 26%
   Very often = 19%

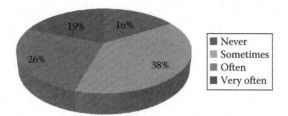

Does things to deliberately annoy others: 37%
    Never = 24%
    Sometimes = 39%
    Often = 25%
    Very often = 12%

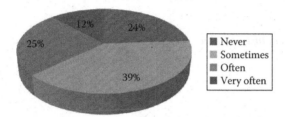

Blames others for own misbehavior or mistakes: 41%
    Never = 16%
    Sometimes = 43%
    Often − 18%
    Very often = 23%

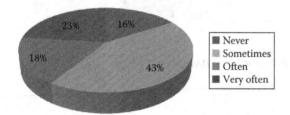

Is touchy or easily annoyed by others: 47%
    Never = 19%
    Sometimes = 34%
    Often = 29%
    Very often = 18%

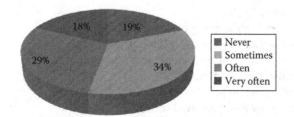

Is angry and resentful: 33%
  Never = 37%
  Sometimes = 30%
  Often = 20%
  Very often = 13%

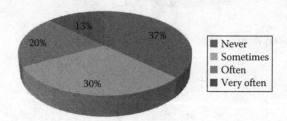

Takes anger out on others or tries to get even: 30%
  Never = 39%
  Sometimes = 31%
  Often = 19%
  Very often = 11%

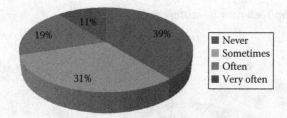

CONDUCT DISORDER, ANTISOCIAL BEHAVIOR

Symptoms seen often to very often

- Plays hookey from school: 0% often to very often
- Stays out at night when not supposed to: 0%
- Lies to get things or to avoid responsibility (cons others): 22%
- Bullies, threatens, or intimidates others: 13%
- Starts physical fights: 10%
- Has run away from home overnight: 0%
- Has stolen things when others were not looking: 8%
- Has deliberately destroyed others' property: 7%
- Has deliberately started fights: 0%
- Has stolen things from others using physical force: 1%
- Has broken into someone else's house, building, or car: 0%
- Has used a weapon when fighting (bat, brick, bottle, etc.): 0%
- Has been physically cruel to animals: 1%
- Has been physically cruel to people: 3%
- Has been preoccupied with or involved in sexual activity: 1%

Symptoms of Anxiety

Is overconcerned about abilities in academic, athletic, or social activities: 16% often and very often
Never = 51%
Sometimes = 33%
Often = 7%
Very often = 9%

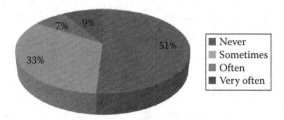

Has difficulty controlling worries: 32%
Never = 32%
Sometimes = 36%
Often = 18%
Very often = 14%

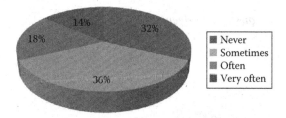

Acts restless or edgy: 31%
Never = 33%
Sometimes = 36%
Often = 22%
Very often = 9%

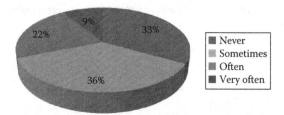

Is irritable for most of the day: 15%
Never = 50%
Sometimes = 35%
Often = 10%
Very often = 5%

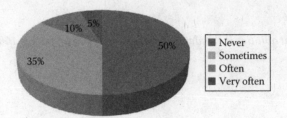

Is extremely tense or unable to relax: 23%
    Never = 48%
    Sometimes = 29%
    Often = 19%
    Very often = 4%

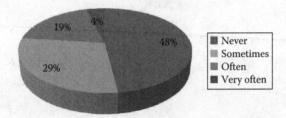

Has difficulty falling asleep or staying asleep: 25%
    Never = 34%
    Sometimes = 40%
    Often = 13%
    Very often = 12%

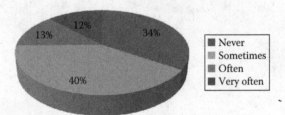

Complains about physical problems (headaches, upset stomach, etc.) for which there is no apparent cause: 21%
    Never = 48%
    Sometimes = 32%
    Often = 11%
    Very often = 10%

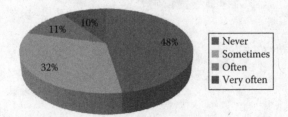

OBSESSIVE–COMPULSIVE SYMPTOMS

Shows excessive fear of specific objects or situations: 17% often and very often
Never = 50%
Sometimes = 33%
Often = 11%
Very often = 6%

Cannot get distressing thoughts out of his/her mind: 18%
Never = 55%
Sometimes = 27%
Often = 16%
Very often = 2%

Feels compelled to perform unusual habits: 7%
Never = 82%
Sometimes = 11%
Often = 5%
Very often = 2%

Has experienced an extremely upsetting event and continues to be bothered by it: 11%
Never = 65%
Sometimes = 25%
Often = 10%
Very often = 1%

Does unusual movements for no apparent reason: 9%
Never = 77%
Sometimes = 14%
Often = 5%
Very often = 4%

Makes vocal sounds for no apparent reason: 10%
Never = 74%
Sometimes = 16%
Often = 7%
Very often = 3%

FRAGILE EMOTIONALITY

- Has strange ideas or beliefs that are not real: 2% often and very often
- Has auditory hallucinations—hears voices talking to or telling him/her to do things: 0%
- Has extremely strange and illogical thoughts and ideas: 3%
- Laughs or cries at inappropriate times or shows no emotion in situations where most others of the same age would react: 6%
- Does extremely odd things: 1%

SYMPTOMS OF DEPRESSION

Is depressed most of the day: 6%
  Never = 73%
  Sometimes = 21%
  Often = 5%
  Very often = 1%

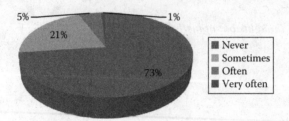

Shows little interest in pleasurable activities: 8%
  Never = 65%
  Sometimes = 27%
  Often = 7%
  Very often = 1%

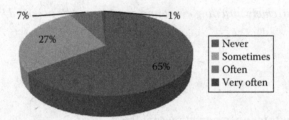

Has recurrent thoughts of death or suicide: 4%
  Never = 87%
  Sometimes = 9%
  Often = 3%
  Very often = 1%

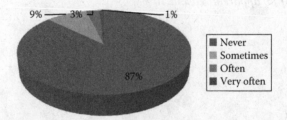

Feels worthless or guilty: 11%
  Never = 68%
  Sometimes = 22%
  Often = 7%
  Very often = 4%

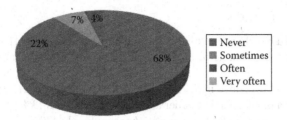

Has low energy level or is tired for no apparent reason: 9%
    Never = 72%
    Sometimes = 19%
    Often = 8%
    Very often = 1%

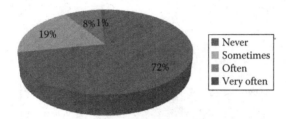

Has little confidence or is very self conscious: 37%
    Never = 29%
    Sometimes = 33%
    Often = 28%
    Very often = 9%

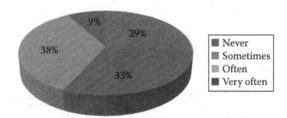

Feels that things never work out right: 22%
    Never = 48%
    Sometimes = 30%
    Often = 13%
    Very often = 9%

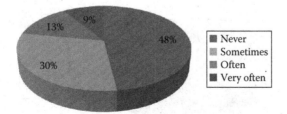

SYMPTOMS OF PHYSICAL CHANGES

- Has experienced a big change in his/her normal appetite or weight: 11%
- Has experienced a big change in his/her normal sleeping habits—cannot sleep or sleeps too much: 9%
- Has experienced a big change in his/her normal activity level—overactive or inactive: 5%
- Has experienced a big change in his/her ability to concentrate: 13%
- Has experienced a big drop in school grades or schoolwork: 17%

SYMPTOMS OF ASPERGER'S DISORDER AND AUTISM SPECTRUM

Has a peculiar way of relating to others: 16% often and very often
    Never = 54%
    Sometimes = 30%
    Often = 10%
    Very often = 6%

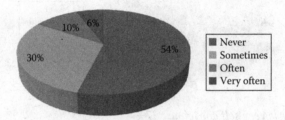

Does not play or relate well with other children: 13%
    Never = 39%
    Sometimes = 49%
    Often = 8%
    Very often = 5%

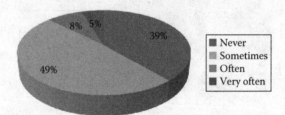

Not interested in making friends: 6%
    Never = 64%
    Sometimes = 30%
    Often = 3%
    Very often = 3%

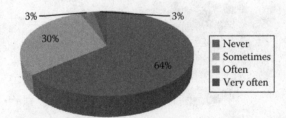

Is unaware or takes no interest in other people's feelings: 12%
   Never = 58%
   Sometimes = 30%
   Often = 10%
   Very often = 2%

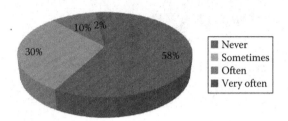

Has difficulty making socially appropriate conversation: 12%
   Never = 58%
   Sometimes = 30%
   Often = 5%
   Very often = 7%

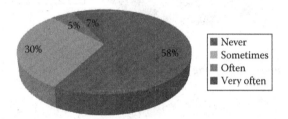

Has a significant problem with language: 7% often and very often
   Never = 81%
   Sometimes = 12%
   Often = 3%
   Very often = 4%

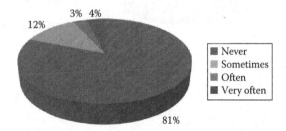

Talks in a strange way: 8%
   Never = 70%
   Sometimes = 23%
   Often = 2%
   Very often = 6%

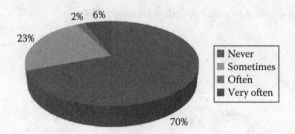

Is unable to pretend or make believe when playing: 0%
    Never = 90%
    Sometimes = 10%
    Often = 0%
    Very often = 0%

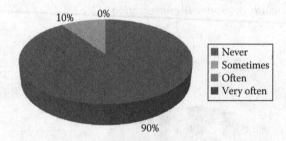

Shows excessive preoccupation with one topic: 14%
    Never = 62%
    Sometimes = 24%
    Often = 11%
    Very often = 3%

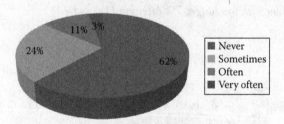

Gets very upset over small changes in routine or surroundings: 19%
    Never = 53%
    Sometimes = 28%
    Often = 15%
    Very often = 4%

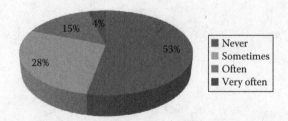

Makes strange repetitive movements: 7%
    Never = 84%
    Sometimes = 9%
    Often = 4%
    Very often = 3%

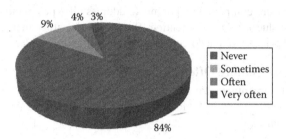

Has strange fascination for parts of objects: 3%
    Never = 88%
    Sometimes = 9%
    Often = 2%
    Very often = 1%

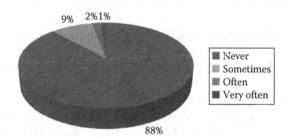

SYMPTOMS OF SOCIAL PHOBIA

- Tries to avoid contact with strangers, abnormally shy: 11%.
- Is excessively shy with peers: 7%.
- Is generally warm and outgoing with family members and familiar adults: 81%.
- When put in uncomfortable social situations, child cries, freezes, or withdraws from interacting: 14%.

SEPARATION ANXIETY SYMPTOMS

- Gets very upset when child expects to be separated from home or parents: 8% often and very often
- Worries that parents will be hurt or leave home and not come back: 10%
- Worries that some disaster will separate child from parents: 4%
- Tries to avoid going to school in order to stay home with parents: 7%
- Worries about being left at home alone or with a sitter: 4%
- Afraid to go to sleep unless near parent: 20%
- Has nightmares about being separated from parent: 2%

- Complains about feeling sick when child expects to be separated from home or parents: 1%
- Wets bed at night: 9%
- Wets or soils underwear during daytime hours: 5%

SUMMATION OF FINDINGS

This is a self-report measure completed by parents to address all types of emotional, cognitive, and behavioral symptoms including that of attention. Similar to the other measures, parents reported symptoms revealing the primary impact of attention symptoms and secondarily symptoms of anxiety.

Symptoms That Were Seen More Often

There were very small percentages for the following symptoms where the parent reported that the symptom never occurred. Over 90 or more percent of the time, parents reported the following symptoms as being present:

- Less than 1% of the parents did not report the symptom of problem of failing to give close attention to details or making careless mistakes, and 99% reported this problem of attention to details as present.
- Only 1% did not report the symptom of difficulty paying attention to tasks or activities, and 99% reported the problem of paying attention as present.
- 5% did not report the symptom of difficulty following through on instructions and failing to finish things, and 95% reported the problem as present.
- 6% did not report difficulty organizing tasks and activities, and 94% reported the problem as present.
- 5% did not report task avoidance, and 95% reported avoidance of tasks that require a lot of mental effort such as schoolwork as present.
- 1% did not report being easily distracted, and 99% reported distractibility as present.

Symptoms Seen Less Often

Consistent with the finding of attention symptoms being seen more often and ADD/ADHD being primarily a thinking disorder as opposed to behavioral issues, symptoms of oppositional or overactive were more often reported as never occurring or if they did occur, not very often:

- 30% reported difficulty awaiting turn in group activities as never occurring, and 12% reported this symptom as occurring very often.
- 32% reported the symptom of difficulty playing quietly as never occurring, and 12% reported this symptom as occurring very often.
- 33% reported the symptoms of running about or climbing on things as never occurring, and only 13% reported this symptom as occurring often.
- 37% reported the symptom of being angry and resentful as never occurring, and 13% reported this symptom as occurring very often.
- 39% reported the symptom of taking anger out on others or trying to get even as never occurring, and 11% reported this symptom as occurring very often.
- 49% reported the symptom of lying to get things or avoid responsibility, and 6% reported this symptom as occurring very often.
- 50% reported being irritable for most of the day as never occurring, and 5% as occurring very often.
- 69% reported the symptom of bullying, threatening, or intimidating others as never occurring, and 2% reported this symptom as occurring very often.
- 74% reported the symptom of starting physical fights as never occurring, and 2% reported this symptom as occurring very often.

This measure allows for the examination of other disorders or symptoms parents think are present in their child in addition to attention problems. Symptoms that were either endorsed as never occurring or not seen were the following: playing hookie from school, running away from home, deliberately starting fights, stealing things, being physically cruel to animals (more often people) or preoccupied with sexual activity, feeling compelled to perform unusual habits, having strange ideas, laughing or crying at inappropriate times, doing extremely odd things, having recurrent thoughts of death, excessive preoccupation with one topic, repetitive movements, and strange fascination for objects. This suggests that these children diagnosed with ADHD inattentive disorder and/or ADHD plus did not present with clear-cut symptoms of other disorders such as oppositional defiant disorder, obsessive–compulsive disorder, conduct disorder, Asperger's disorder, and/or significant depression.

Symptoms of psychosis were not endorsed such as auditory hallucinations or strange beliefs or doing odd things. Symptoms of trauma did not emerge as highly significant, such as being bothered by an extremely upsetting event, although there was some indication of fearfulness of specific situations or objects or being unable to get distressing thoughts out of their mind.

There was a small percentage that did reveal symptoms of depression (but not for most of the day or indicating thoughts of death), showing little interest in pleasurable activities, or feeling guilty. Having little confidence was endorsed more often. Feeling that things will not work out right was endorsed by parents as descriptive of their child but not to an extensive degree.

Symptoms of anxiety did emerge more often; overconcern about abilities, difficulty controlling worries, acting restless or edgy, unable to relax, and difficulty falling asleep were symptoms seen some of the time. Symptoms indicated some of the time included fearfulness if separated from parents and worrying about the parent not returning home.

There was not the indication of a big physical change in area of appetite or weight and sleep habits as well as activity level, ability to concentrate, and significant problem with language or school grades, suggesting the problem is more long standing as opposed to an extreme or crisis situation that parents were responding to by seeking evaluation.

There were some indications of difficulty making friends, relating well to other children, and making social conversation, which was noted some of the time. Some difficulties of being shy and uncomfortable in social situations were noted some of the time as well.

Wetting the bed at night was indicated as never occurring 86% of the time and soiling or encopresis as never occurring 88% of the time.

CHILDREN'S PROBLEM CHECKLIST

There were a large number of parents (550) who responded to this questionnaire asking them to report areas of concern regarding their child for emotions, self-issues, people interaction, school, language/thinking, concentration/organization, actions/motor skills, behavior, values, habits, and health. On this measure, parents do not rate how bad the problem is; they respond to whether they think that the item is a concern or not.

EMOTIONS

- Frequently seems anxious or tense: 27%
- Cries easily or often: 31%
- Worries a lot: 30%
- Needs to be reassured frequently: 32%
- Feelings are easily hurt: 55%
- Feels inferior: 26%
- Is easily embarrassed: 26%
- Seems uncomfortable in new situations: 27%
- Is easily upset: 47%
- Has trouble relaxing: 25%

SELF-ISSUES

- Is self-critical: 33%
- Overreacts to small mistakes: 40%
- Gives up easily: 52%
- Worries about making mistakes: 37%
- Has little self-confidence: 38%
- Is not interested in learning: 22%
- Does not give best effort: 44%
- Appears to be uninterested: 22%

PEOPLE INVOLVEMENT

- Hurts or teases other children: 16%
- Is teased a lot by other children: 23%
- Is not liked by other children: 14%
- Has trouble making friends: 23%
- Has few friends: 33%
- Does not compromise with other children: 15%
- Is a poor loser in games: 40%
- Competes too hard in games: 15%
- Is shy: 17%
- Is socially immature: 18%

SCHOOL

- Does not finish homework: 42%
- Does not like school: 23%
- Needs too much attention from teachers: 37%
- Is a discipline problem at school: 26%
- Gets poor grades: 26%
- Is an underachiever: 23%
- Is in remedial or special education classes: 17%

LANGUAGE AND THINKING

- Has trouble understanding instructions: 43%
- Forgets things: 57%
- Has a poor memory: 27%
- Has trouble with time and date: 19%
- Has trouble right from left: 18%
- Frequently daydreams: 32%
- Does not have good common sense: 22%
- Becomes confused easily: 25%
- Has trouble reading: 40%
- Has trouble with spelling or writing: 47%

CONCENTRATION AND ORGANIZATION

- Does not pay attention: 65%
- Is easily distracted: 81%

- Has trouble finishing projects: 58%
- Acts impulsively: 53%
- Has trouble getting organized: 60%
- Has trouble planning activities: 24%
- Loses interest quickly: 51%
- Changes mind often: 30%
- Has difficulty following rules: 47%

ACTIONS AND MOTOR

- Is uncoordinated: 13%
- Bumps into things: 13%
- Is clumsy: 14%
- Has trouble throwing or catching a ball: 13%
- Is overactive: 28%
- Is frequently hurt or injured: 12%
- Is restless: 30%
- Has trouble sitting still at dinner: 49%
- Is always climbing or running: 24%

BEHAVIOR AND EMOTIONS

- Often interrupts adults or children: 60%
- Is uncooperative: 28%
- Frequently argues or disagrees: 57%
- Is disobedient: 33%
- Refuses to listen: 36%
- Is stubborn: 58%
- Has a bad temper: 36%
- Always has to have own way: 40%
- Frequently sulks or pouts: 26%
- Is demanding: 34%
- Does not complete chores: 45%
- Does not respond to punishment: 29%

VALUES

- Does not complete chores: 45%
- Frequently lies: 23%
- Blames others for mistakes: 44%
- Does not feel guilty after misbehaving: 21%
- Is unappreciative: 24%
- Ignores rules: 25%
- Does not respond to punishment: 29%

HABITS

- Has problem with bed-wetting: 12%
- Has trouble getting to sleep: 32%
- Has allergies: 26%

SUMMATION OF FINDINGS

Symptoms occurring most often were not paying attention (65%) and being easily distracted (81%).

Symptoms occurring 50%–60% of the time were the following: feelings easily hurt, giving up easily, forgetting things, trouble finishing projects, acting impulsively, losing interest quickly, difficulty getting organized, frequently argues or disagrees, stubborn, and often interrupting.

Symptoms occurring 40%–50% of the time were the following: becoming easily upset, overreacting to small mistakes, not giving best effort, poor loser in games (similar to being driven to win noted on another measure), not finishing homework, difficulty understanding instructions, reading difficulties, problems with spelling or writing, difficulty following rules, trouble sitting still at dinner, has to have his own way, not completing chores, and blaming others for mistakes.

Symptoms that do not occur very often: Less than 10% suggest the absence of obsessive–compulsive behavior, psychotic behavior, extensive fearfulness, social avoidance, major depression, aggressive or oppositional defiant behavior, conduct disorder, and fatigue.

This establishes the disorder of inattention as primary. The symptoms of overactivity or impulsivity that were indicated are seen as historically reflective of anxiety. Being anxious leads to less thinking and more acting, hence impulsivity as well as the tendency to interrupt (for fear of forgetting what one has to say due to being distracted).

Anxiety creates restlessness as well as the tendency to avoid things and the desire to look good and to blame others. There is a desire to win and to want to appear intact due to worrying about what others think. While difficulty following rules and wanting their own way would typically be seen as oppositional or defiant, we see these symptoms associated with ADD.

Hypothetically, the need to be right and tendency to think one is right can negate the following of rules. ADD individuals tend to think they are right, often based upon the common issue of information processing and the tendency to build logical reasoning processes to figure things out for themselves. Reliance upon one's own logic as opposed to the opinions of others may be at the base of these symptoms. Unaware that they might be missing information, those diagnosed with ADD tend to assume they are correct in their assumptions (based upon their own logical reasoning) lacking the awareness that they might be missing information leading to a faulty basis upon which to base their logical assumptions. This is a rather common phenomenon in the ADD household and may mask itself as symptoms of some defiant behavior.

Social issues are a common theme seen initially in childhood, continuing through adolescence and into adulthood. There are parent concerns of their child being shy and having few friends. The social problems tend to result from anxiety and being overly concerned about their appearance resulting in feeling socially uncomfortable leading to the development of fewer friendships. Social discomfort does not foster involvement in social activities. The tendency to be competitive with themselves (or self-critical) tends to result in being competitive with everyone else as well, which is not always conducive to making friendships.

CHILDREN'S NEUROPSYCHOLOGICAL HISTORY

The Children's Neuropsychological History provided demographic information about the parents as well as their child and the child's symptomatology. This measure was in use from 2006 to 2008 and replaced the Developmental History form. Ninety-eight parents completed this form about their child providing historical and family information as well as their current and past symptoms. Symptoms were reported as historical, as new, or as both new and historical. Parents reported more historical than new problems consistent with the lifelong diagnosis of ADD. The following are the responses to specific questions about the child's functioning in the areas of problem solving, language (speech and math skills), spatial skills, concentration and awareness, memory, motor and coordination, sensory, physical issues, emotions, and behavior. Percentages are provided for the new and old presence of symptoms. Parents were also able to mark if a symptom did not exist or if the problem was both new and old. Very small percentages of items were indicated as both new and old; therefore, results from this category are not provided.

PROBLEM SOLVING

Easily frustrated, 81%
  New = 9%
  Old = 72%

Difficulty completing an activity in a reasonable period of time, 69%
  New = 6%
  Old = 63%

Disorganized in his/her approach to problems, 56%
  New = 2%
  Old = 54%

Difficulty understanding explanations, 56%
  New = 6%
  Old = 50%

Difficulty planning ahead, 52%
  New = 2%
  Old = 50%

Difficulty doing things in the right order, 43%
  New = 3%
  Old = 40%

Difficulty verbally describing the steps involved in doing something, 39%
  New = 4%
  Old = 35%

Difficulty making decisions, 48%
  New = 4%
  Old = 44%

Difficulty changing a plan or activity when necessary, 47%
  New = 4%
  Old = 43%

Difficulty switching from one activity to another activity, 28%
  New = 2%
  Old = 26%

Difficulty figuring how to do new things, 42%
  New = 4%
  Old = 38%

Is slow to learn new things, 26%
New = 4%
Old = 22%

Difficulty solving problems that a younger child can do, 25%
New = 7%
Old = 18%

SPEECH, LANGUAGE, AND MATH SKILLS

Difficulty understanding what he/she is reading, 30%
New = 3%
Old = 27%

Difficulty reading letters or words, 36%
New = 7%
Old = 29%

Difficulty with spelling, 45%
New = 6%
Old = 39%

Difficulty writing letters or words, 37%
New = 7%
Old = 30%

Difficulty with math, 37%
New = 5%
Old = 32%

Difficulty speaking clearly, 30%
New = 1%
Old = 29%

Difficulty finding the right word to say, 36%
New = 5%
Old = 31%

Not talking, 8%
New = 2%
Old = 6%

Rambles on and on without saying much, 30%
New = 1%
Old = 29%

Jumps from one topic to another, 37%
New = 2%
Old = 35%

Odd or unusual language or vocal sounds, 18%
    New = 3%
    Old = 15%

Difficulty understanding what others are saying, 20%
    New = 2%
    Old = 18%

SPATIAL SKILLS

Confusion telling right from left, 6%
    New = 5%
    Old = 1%

Has difficulty with puzzles, LEGO®s, blocks, or similar games, 6%
    New = 5%
    Old = 1%

Problems drawing or copying, 12%
    New = 2%
    Old = 10%

Doesn't know his/her colors, 3%
    New = 3%
    Old = 0%

Difficulty dressing (not due to physical difficulty), 6%
    New = 0%
    Old = 6%

Problems finding his/her way around places he/she has been to before, 2%
    New = 1%
    Old = 1%

Difficulty recognizing objects, 1%
    New = 0%
    Old = 1%

Seems unable to recognize facial or body expressions of disapproval or emotions, 6%
    New = 1%
    Old = 5%

Gets lost easily, 3%
    New = 1%
    Old = 2%

CONCENTRATION AND AWARENESS

Easily distracted by sounds, 74%
    New = 4%
    Old = 70%

Attention starts out OK but can't keep it up, 66%
New = 3%
Old = 63%

Difficulty concentrating on what others say but sits in front of a TV for long periods, 64%
New = 6%
Old = 58%

Mind appears to go blank at times, 51%
New = 7%
Old = 44%

Loses train of thought easily, 49%
New = 5%
Old = 44%

MEMORY

Forgetting where he/she leave things, 53%
New = 4%
Old = 49%

Forgets what he/she is supposed to be doing, 61%
New = 5%
Old = 56%

Forgets school assignments, 46%
New = 8%
Old = 38%

Forgets instructions, 57%
New = 8%
Old = 49%

Forgets events that happened quite recently, 23%
New = 5%
Old = 18%

Forgets things that happened days/weeks ago, 2%
New = 1%
Old = 1%

Forgets names more than most people do, 9%
New = 1%
Old = 8%

MOTOR AND COORDINATION

Clumsy, 26%
New = 1%
Old = 25%

Poor fine motor control skills, 20%
    New = 1%
    Old = 19%

Weakness, 5%
    New = 1%
    Old = 4%

Tremor, 1%
    New = 0%
    Old = 1%

Muscle tics or spastic, 1%
    New = 0%
    Old = 1%

Odd movements, 6%
    New = 0%
    Old = 6%

Drops things more than most children, 5%
    New = 1%
    Old = 4%

Has an unusual walk, 5%
    New = 4%
    Old = 1%

Balance problems, 6%
    New = 1%
    Old = 5%

SENSORY

Needs to squint or move closer to page to read, 7%
    New = 3%
    Old = 4%

Problems seeing objects, 2%
    New = 0%
    Old = 2%

Loss of feeling, 1%
    New = 0%
    Old = 1%

Problems hearing sounds, 5%
    New = 2%
    Old = 3%

Difficulty telling hot from cold, 1%
    New = 0%
    Old = 1%

Difficulty smelling odors, 0%
    New = 0%
    Old = 0%

Difficulty tasting food, 1%
    New = 0%
    Old = 1%

Overly sensitive to touch, 14%
    New = 2%
    Old = 12%

PHYSICAL

Frequently complains of headaches or nausea, 27%
    New = 10%
    Old = 17%

Has dizzy spells, 4%
    New = 4%
    Old = 0%

Has pains in joints, 13%
    New = 7%
    Old = 6%

Excessive tiredness, 15%
    New = 6%
    Old = 9%

Frequent urination or drinking, 17%
    New = 4%
    Old = 13%

BEHAVIOR

Emotional, 46%
    New = 6%
    Old = 40%

Immature, 45%
    New = 4%
    Old = 41%

Dependent, 22%
    New = 3%
    Old = 19%

Depressed, 18%
  New = 5%
  Old = 13%

Fearful, 33%
  New = 6%
  Old = 27%

Nervous, 15%
  New = 1%
  Old = 14%

Quiet, 11%
  New = 5%
  Old = 6%

Unmotivated, 27%
  New = 11%
  Old = 16%

Shy and withdrawn,.7%
  New = 3%
  Old = 4%

Aggressive, 41%
  New = 10%
  Old = 31%

Attached to things, not people, 14%
  New = 3%
  Old = 11%

Bizarre behavior, 10%
  New = 6%
  Old = 4%

Resists change, 22%
  New = 3%
  Old = 19%

Risk-taking, 28%
  New = 6%
  Old = 22%

Self-mutilates, 12%
  New = 5%
  Old = 7%

Self-stimulates, 15%
  New = 4%
  Old = 11%

Swears a lot, 19%
  New = 4%
  Old = 15%

Bed-wetting, 14%
  New = 2%
  Old = 12%

Bowel movements in underwear, 6%
  New = 2%
  Old = 4%

Eating habits are poor, 27%
  New = 3%
  Old = 24%

Nightmares, night terrors, sleepwalks, 22%
  New = 6%
  Old = 16%

Sleeping habits are poor, 27%
  New = 5%
  Old = 22%

SUMMATION OF FINDINGS

This is a self-report measure completed by the parents with the goal of providing an historical overview of all aspects of the child's functioning. This measure is consistent with the general information reported on the Developmental History form, which this form replaced in 2006.

Symptoms are divided up into areas of problem solving, speech, language, math skills, nonverbal skills, concentration and awareness, memory, motor and coordination, sensory, physical, and behavior. All of the frequencies for newly acquired symptoms were nonsignificant and within the 10% marker or below. This means that mostly historical symptoms were reported, which is consistent with the impact of a long-term genetic attention disorder.

Historical symptoms most prevalent in the area of *problem solving* were difficulty completing an activity within a reasonable period of time (63%) and being easily frustrated (72%). Symptoms noted by parents as present approximately 50% of the time as historical issues were the following: difficulty making decisions and planning ahead, disorganization in the approach to problems, and difficulty understanding explanations.

In the area of *speech, language, and math skills*, the majority of the responses were indicated as not applicable. Once again, new symptoms fell at or below 10%. Difficulty writing letters or words was seen 30% of the time, and difficulty reading letters or words were seen 29% of the time as historical symptoms. Difficulty with spelling was seen 39% of the time and difficulty with math 32% of the time.

Nonverbal skills did not reveal any symptoms seen as new or historical, and much of the time (between 80% and 90% or above), symptoms were not seen.

The highest percentages were in the area of *concentration and awareness*. Symptoms of being easily distracted (historically present 70% of the time) and poor sustained attention (present historically 63% of the time) were more often seen as problematic. Other symptoms such as mind appearing to go blank at times or losing train of thought easily were historically present 44% of the time.

Consistent with the idea that *memory* is a positive strength that ADD children rely upon for learning, there were only a few symptoms indicated as occurring most of the time, which is could be consistent with the effects of being distracted. Symptoms such as forgetting where things were left (49%), forgetting what they are supposed to be doing (56%), forgetting school assignments (38%), and forgetting instructions (49%) were seen more often and could be related to distractibility. In comparison, the presence of more pure memory symptoms was seen far less, such as forgetting names (seen 8% of the time) or things that happened days or weeks ago (seen 2% of the time). Once again, symptoms are not new and instead historical and reflect issues that are more suggestive of attention symptoms than actual problems of retrieval or recall of newly learned information.

The area of *motor and coordination* did not reveal any symptoms above 5% other than poor fine motor skills (19%) and clumsy (25%). Sensory symptoms were not present more than 5% of the time other than being overly sensitive to touch (12%). In the physical area, there were historical complaints of headaches or nausea (17%); otherwise, symptoms were less than 10%.

Behavior revealed higher percentages in areas of aggression (31%) being more emotional (40%) and immature (41%). Being fearful was 27%, being nervous was 14%, and having nightmares and night terrors or sleepwalking was 16%. Risk-taking and poor sleep habits were 22%.

Behavioral descriptions for the last 6 months more often included symptoms of being very fidgety (50%), being highly distracted (65%), and having hard time concentrating for long periods (74%), which is more consistent with the inattentive type.

Current symptoms of not remaining seated, not following directions or instructions, frequently making noise, being rude or interrupting, and frequently losing things needed for school ranged from 40% to 50%, while items of not finishing tasks, continual talking, not waiting their turn, not listening, easily lying, and answering before hearing the whole question ranged from 30% to 40%. Symptoms around 20% or less were not typically symptomatic of the inattentive type: doing dangerous things and stealing. Symptoms of running away from home, destroying property, and oppositional behaviors were seen less than 10% of the time. Starting fights was indicated 11% of the time. There were symptoms of behavior that could be reflective of anxiety such as continually talking, difficulty listening, answering before hearing the whole question, and lying easily to avoid someone becoming angry or upset with them.

9 Results of the Adolescent Self-Report Measure/ Checklists

The total sample size for this group was 402 adolescents from the age of 12 to 17 years. Of these 68% were males compared to 32% females. Seventy-four percent were diagnosed with attention deficit hyperactivity disorder (ADHD) inattentive type and 26% with ADHD plus suggesting an additional disorder).

The following pages reveal the statistics derived from the numerous checklists that were administered. There were checklists given to the subject's parents to complete, to their teacher(s) (scores were averaged when there were multiple teachers), and checklists completed by the adolescent.

Checklists that the teacher or teachers completed are as follows:

- Academic Performance Rating Scale
- Child Attention Profile
- Social Situations Questionnaire
- ACTeRS

Checklists that the parents completed are as follows:

- Home Situations Questionnaire
- ADHD Rating Scale
- ADDES Home Version
- Children's Problems Checklist
- Child Behavior Checklist
- Child Symptom Inventory
- Children's Neuropsychological History
- Developmental History Checklist

Checklists that the adolescent completed are as follows:

- Patient Behavior Checklist
- Beck Anxiety Inventory
- Physical Complaints Checklist
- Beck Depression Inventory
- Personal Problems Checklist for Adolescents
- Personal History Checklist for Adolescents

ACADEMIC PERFORMANCE RATING SCALE

This is a measure completed by the classroom teacher. There was an average of 133 classroom teachers who completed this measure. Teachers rated the academic work completed as well as the child's attention (following directions and instruction)and learning skills, academic development, work characteristics (quality versus quantity), and overall behavior in class.

Percentages of written math work completed relative to classmates: 45% are average and above:
   27% responded with 0%–49%.
   28% responded with 50%–69%.
   9% responded with 70%–79%.
   14% responded with 80%–89%.
   22% responded with 90%–100%.

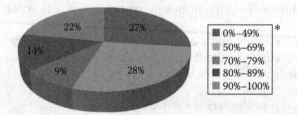

Accuracy of completed written math work: 46% are average and above:
   29% responded with 0%–49%.
   25% responded with 50%–69%.
   18% responded with 70%–79%.
   24% responded with 80%–89%.
   4% responded with 90%–100%.

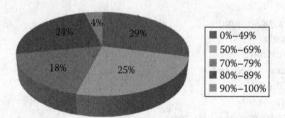

Percentage of written language arts work completed relative to classmates: 58% are average and above:
   28% responded with 0%–49%.
   15% responded with 50%–69%.
   12% responded with 70%–79%.
   18% responded with 80%–89%.
   28% responded with 90%–100%.

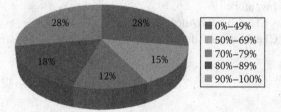

* The pie graphs range from 99 to 100 to 101 due to rounding.

Accuracy of completed written language arts work: 61% are average and above:

25% responded with 0%–49%.

15% responded with 50%–69%.

32% responded with 70%–79%.

22% responded with 80%–89%.

7% responded with 90%–100%.

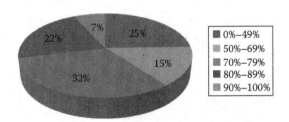

How consistent has the quality of this child's academic work been over the past week? 60% said variable to consistently poor:

14% responded with consistently poor.

23% responded with more poor than successful.

23% responded with variable.

30% responded with more successful than poor.

10% responded with consistently successful.

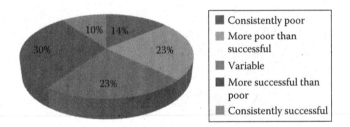

How frequently does the student accurately follow teacher instructions and/or class discussion during large group instruction? 71% said never to sometimes:

2% responded with never.

25% responded with rarely.

44% responded with sometimes.

20% responded with often.

9% responded with very often.

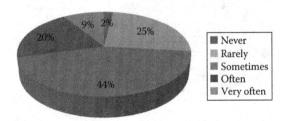

How frequently does the student accurately follow teacher instructions and/or class discussion during small group instruction? 66% said never to sometimes:
   3% responded with never.
   18% responded with rarely.
   45% responded with sometimes.
   28% responded with often.
   6% responded with very often.

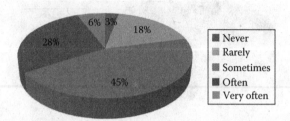

How quickly does this child learn new material? 81% said never to sometimes:
   10% responded with never.
   28% responded with rarely.
   43% responded with sometimes.
   18% responded with often.
   1% responded with very often.

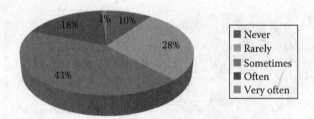

What is the quality or neatness of this child's handwriting? 42% said poor to fair:
   23% responded with poor.
   19% responded with fair.
   38% responded with average.
   18% responded with above average.
   2% responded with excellent.

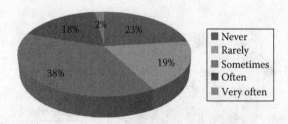

What is the quality of this child's reading skills? 33% said poor to fair:
    12% responded with poor.
    21% responded with fair.
    47% responded with average.
    16% responded with above average.
    4% responded with excellent.

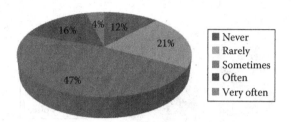

What is the quality of this child's speaking skills? 21% said poor to fair:
    7% responded with poor.
    14% responded with fair.
    42% responded with average.
    31% responded with above average.
    6% responded with excellent.

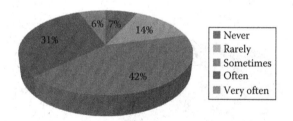

How often does the child complete written work in a careless, hasty fashion? 83% said sometimes to very often:
    1% responded with never.
    17% responded with rarely.
    35% responded with sometimes.
    27% responded with often.
    21% responded with very often.

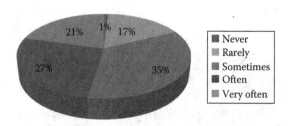

How frequently does the child take more time to complete work than his or her classmates? 71%
said sometimes to very often:

    7% responded with never.

    22% responded with rarely.

    36% responded with sometimes.

    23% responded with often.

    12% responded with very often.

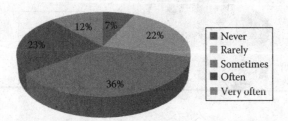

How often is the child able to pay attention without you promoting him or her? 26% said often to
very often:

    4% responded with never.

    30% responded with rarely.

    40% responded with sometimes.

    21% responded with often.

    5% responded with very often.

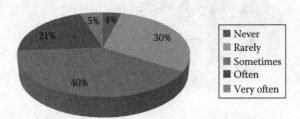

How frequently does the child require your assistance to accurately complete his or her academic
work? 78% said sometimes to very often:

    2% responded with never.

    20% responded with rarely.

    39% responded with sometimes.

    24% responded with often.

    15% responded with very often.

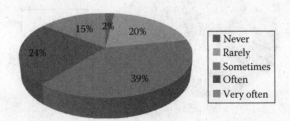

How often does the child begin written work prior to understanding the directions? 52% said sometimes to very often:

 13% responded with never.
 35% responded with rarely.
 31% responded with sometimes.
 19% responded with often.
 2% responded with very often.

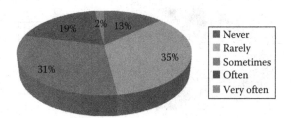

How frequently does this child have difficulty recalling material from a previous day's lesson? 74% said sometimes to very often:

 5% responded with never.
 21% responded with rarely.
 31% responded with sometimes.
 32% responded with often.
 11% responded with very often.

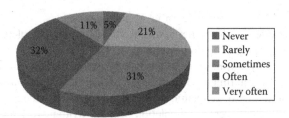

How often does the child appear to be staring excessively or "spaced out"? 68% said sometimes to very often:

 9% responded with never.
 23% responded with rarely.
 37% responded with sometimes.
 17% responded with often.
 14% responded with very often.

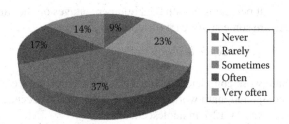

How often does the child appear withdrawn or tend to lack an emotional response in a social situation? 42% said sometimes to very often:

22% responded with never.

36% responded with rarely.

22% responded with sometimes.

15% responded with often.

5% responded with very often.

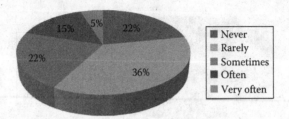

SUMMATION OF FINDINGS

This self-report measure is completed by teachers addressing the child's academic work as well as their behavior in the classroom setting. Primary issues indicated by the teacher or teachers related to the completion of work being turned in, work being accurate, as well as difficulties learning. This would be consistent with the diagnosis being made in adolescence as a result of the need for intervention, new treatment, or diagnostic answers due to continued unresolved academic problems.

Severity of problems in school includes the following:

- 81% never learned or had variable learning of new material.
- 78% required some degree of teacher assistance to accurately complete work.
- 74% required teacher prompting to pay attention.
- 71% were never or only at times able to follow teacher instruction in a large group setting.
- 66% were never or only at times able to follow teacher instruction in a small group setting.
- 60% reported that quality of academic work ranged from consistently poor to variable.
- 55% reported well below average completion of math written work and 54% of the math work was well below average.

Overall problems were noted with the ability to learn, to pay attention, to follow instruction, and to complete work independently. Math emerged as more problematic. Work continued to be completed in a careless manner likely due to increased frustration and/or hopelessness, and the quality of completed work was poor or variable. There may be increased learning difficulties due to sleep problems. The material learned is certainly more complex at this age and may reflect earlier learning difficulties due to the absence of basic concepts.

Comparison to the Children

In comparing the adolescent percentages with the child percentages on the same measure (the child sample was larger), there are some significant differences.

Change from childhood to adolescence is as follows:

- The amount of math work completed declined by 31% in adolescence.
- The accuracy of completed math work declined by 34% in adolescence.
- Reading skills improved by 12% in adolescence.

There was a decline of less than 10%, meaning the problems remained the same for the following:

- Written language work
- Quality of academic work
- Following teacher instruction in large group setting
- Speaking skills
- Completing work in a careless and hasty manner
- Taking more time to complete work
- Paying attention without prompting
- Requiring teacher assistance to complete work

There was an increase of 10% or more problems with the following:

- Beginning work prior to instruction
- Staring or spaced out
- Withdrawn

There was improvement of 10% or less problems in the following:

- Following teacher instruction in small group setting
- Quickly learning new material

Comparisons suggest that attention symptoms are following the child through time into adolescence and that some areas are becoming more problematic such as math. There was improved ability to learn new material and to follow instruction in a small group setting. Reading skills improved. There were increased problems of being withdrawn, staring episodes, or spaciness as well as the tendency to begin work prior to receiving teacher direction.

CHILD ATTENTION PROFILE

This is a measure completed by the classroom teacher to describe attention and behavioral symptoms in the classroom setting. One hundred and thirty-six classroom teachers completed this measure addressing attention symptoms seen in the adolescent. There are 12 symptoms ranked as not being true, sometimes being true, or very often or often true.

Fails to finish things he or she starts: 85% said somewhat or often true:
Not true = 14%
Somewhat true = 45%
Very true or often true = 40%

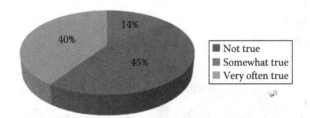

Can't concentrate, can't pay attention for long: 90% said somewhat or often true:
Not true = 10%
Somewhat true = 37%
Very true or often true = 53%

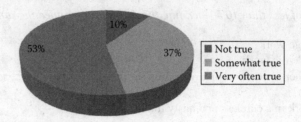

Can't sit still, restless, or hyperactive: 58% said somewhat or often true:
  Not true = 42%
  Somewhat true = 28%
  Very true or often true = 30%

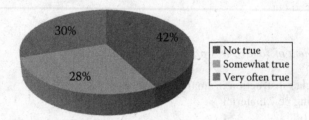

Fidgets: 57% said somewhat or often true:
  Not true = 43%
  Somewhat true = 26%
  Very true or often true = 31%

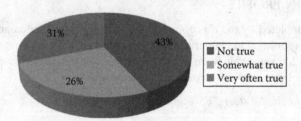

Daydreams or gets lost in his or her thoughts: 67% said somewhat or often true:
  Not true = 33%
  Somewhat true = 66%
  Very true or often true = 1%

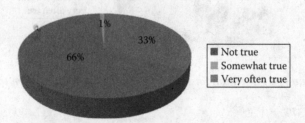

Impulsive or acts without thinking: 69% said somewhat or often true:
    Not true = 31%
    Somewhat true = 38%
    Very true or often true = 31%

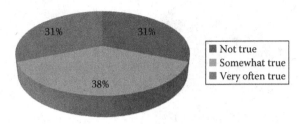

Difficulty following directions: 84% said somewhat or often true:
    Not true = 16%
    Somewhat true = 49%
    Very true or often true = 35%

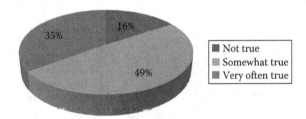

Talks out of turn: 62% said somewhat or often true:
    Not true = 38%
    Somewhat true = 33%
    Very true or often true = 29%

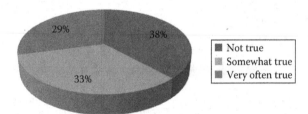

Messy work: 73% said somewhat or often true:
    Not true = 27%
    Somewhat true = 45%
    Very true or often true = 28%

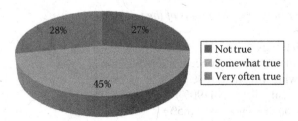

Inattentive, easily distracted: 90% said somewhat or often true:
Not true = 10%
Somewhat true = 40%
Very true or often true = 50%

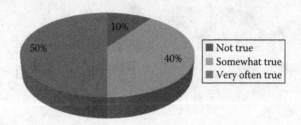

Talks too much: 64% said somewhat or often true:
Not true = 36%
Somewhat true = 35%
Very true or often true = 29%

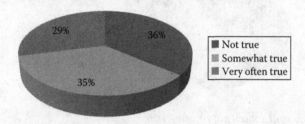

Fails to carry out assigned tasks: 85% said somewhat or often true:
Not true = 15%
Somewhat true = 37%
Very true or often true = 48%

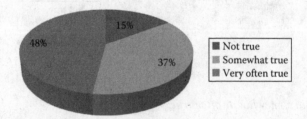

SUMMATION OF FINDINGS

More often the teacher indicated symptoms of the following:

- Failing to finish things (85%)
- Unable to sustain attention or concentration (90%)
- Difficulty following directions (84%)
- Inattentive and easily distracted (90%)
- Failing to carry out assigned tasks (85%)

Seen less often, teachers reported the following:

- Messy work (73%)
- Impulsivity (69%)
- Daydreaming (67%)
- Talking out of turn (62%)
- Talking too much (64%)
- Fidgeting (57%)

Adolescents continued to reveal more symptoms of poor sustained attention, not finishing their work, and being distracted. Attention symptoms may be increased or staying the same for the adolescent due to additional factors of emotionality and poor sleep habits.

Comparison to the Children

When symptoms are compared to the larger child sample on this self-report measure, the shift into adolescence is bringing improvement with less restlessness, fidgeting, and daydreaming, while other attention symptoms remained essentially the same.

Symptoms reported frequently that remained the same for the children and adolescents are as follows:

- Failing to finish things and carry out assigned tasks
- Concentration
- Following directions
- Messy work
- Inattentiveness

Symptoms that decreased for the adolescents include the following:

- Fidgeting by 18%
- Inability to sit still by 10%
- Daydreaming by 15%

There was no difference in symptoms seen less often:

- Talking out of turn
- Talking too much
- Impulsivity

SCHOOL SITUATIONS QUESTIONNAIRE

104 teachers provided responses to this measure asking about the adolescent's behavior in specific situations occurring in the school setting as well as to and from the school setting (if riding the bus). This is a measure designed to identify the problem settings and reflects more behavioral issues. The following percentages indicate whether there is problematic behavior present in a specific school setting:

- While arriving at school: 19%
- During individual desk work: 59%
- During small group activities: 56%
- During free play time in class: 37%

- During lectures to the class: 55%
- At recess: 10%
- At lunch: 22%
- In the hallways: 24%
- In the bathroom: 4%
- On field trips: 8%
- During special assemblies: 17%
- On the bus: 7%

SUMMATION OF FINDINGS

Adolescents did not present with the same degree of behavioral issues seen in the children.

Comparison to the Children

When compared to the child sample on this measure, there were decreases for the adolescent population of 10%–20% for the following situations:

- Arriving at school
- Free play time
- Field trips
- Special assemblies
- In the hallways

A decrease of over 20% for the adolescent versus the children was seen for the following situations:

- Recess (decrease of 27%)
- Bathroom

Behavior for the adolescents was not the primary problem. The primary problem was work productivity. Problems were indicated during times of individual desk work (59%), small group activities (56%), and during class lectures (55%).

ACTeRS

This is a measure providing descriptions of the child's behavior in the classroom falling into categories of attention, hyperactivity, social skills, and oppositional. It is completed by the adolescent's teachers who have observed the behavior of the child or adolescent in the classroom. There are a total of 24 items relevant to classroom behavior that fall into the aforementioned areas. The measure is completed by teachers who have observed the behavior of the child or adolescent in the classroom. Items are ranked from 1 to 5 (almost never to almost always seen). A total score is provided for each of the areas: attention, hyperactivity, social skills, and oppositional. There were a total of 114 teachers that completed this form.

ATTENTION

Works well independently
21% responded 1 (almost never).
27% responded 2.
31% responded 3.
16% responded 4.
5% responded 5 (almost always).

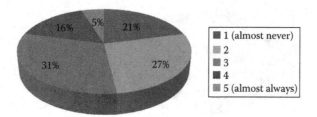

Persists with task for reasonable amount of time
   18% responded 1 (almost never).
   37% responded 2.
   32% responded 3.
   11% responded 4.
   3% responded 5 (almost always).

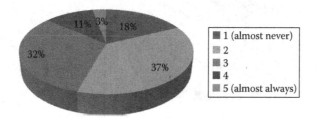

Completes assigned task satisfactorily with little additional assistance
   29% responded 1 (almost never).
   30% responded 2.
   32% responded 3.
   7% responded 4.
   2% responded 5 (almost always).

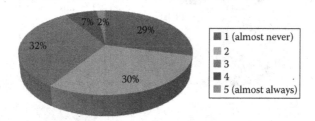

Follows simple directions accurately
   11% responded 1 (almost never).
   25% responded 2.
   35% responded 3.
   25% responded 4.
   4% responded 5 (almost always).

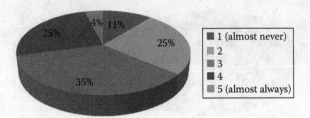

Follows a sequence of instructions
   13% responded 1 (almost never).
   35% responded 2.
   37% responded 3.
   13% responded 4.
   3% responded 5 (almost always).

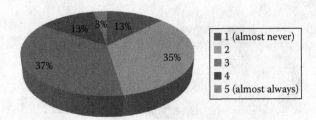

Functions well in the classroom
   13% responded 1 (almost never).
   38% responded 2.
   32% responded 3.
   14% responded 4.
   4% responded 5 (almost always).

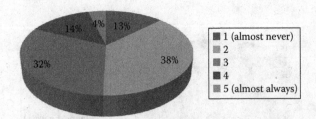

OVERACTIVITY

Extremely overactive (out of seat, on the go)
   28% responded 1 (almost never).
   25% responded 2.
   15% responded 3.
   16% responded 4.
   16% responded 5 (almost always).

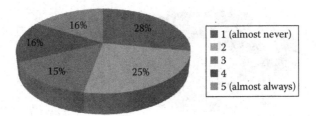

Overreacts

   30% responded 1 (almost never).
   20% responded 2.
   20% responded 3.
   15% responded 4.
   15% responded 5 (almost always).

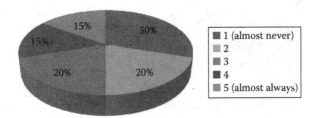

Fidgety (hands always busy)

   25% responded 1 (almost never).
   22% responded 2.
   18% responded 3.
   17% responded 4.
   18% responded 5 (almost always).

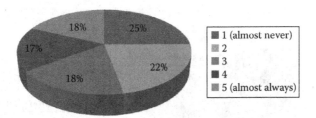

Impulsive (acts or talks without thinking)

   25% responded 1 (almost never).
   16% responded 2.
   17% responded 3.
   21% responded 4.
   21% responded 5 (almost always).

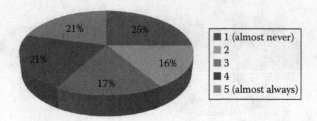

Restless (squirms in seat)
   26% responded 1 (almost never).
   26% responded 2.
   13% responded 3.
   17% responded 4.
   19% responded 5 (almost always).

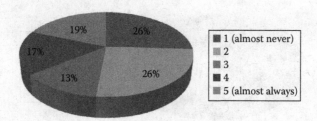

SOCIAL SKILLS

Behaves positively with peers/classmates
   6% responded 1 (almost never).
   18% responded 2.
   32% responded 3.
   30% responded 4.
   14% responded 5 (almost always).

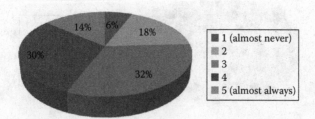

Verbal communication clear and connected
   2% responded 1 (almost never).
   21% responded 2.
   29% responded 3.
   33% responded 4.
   15% responded 5 (almost always).

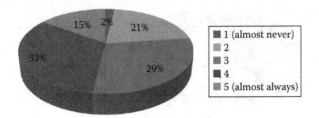

Nonverbal communication clear and connected
5% responded 1 (almost never).
13% responded 2.
40% responded 3.
29% responded 4.
12% responded 5 (almost always).

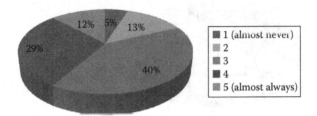

Follows group norms and social rules
15% responded 1 (almost never).
16% responded 2.
23% responded 3.
33% responded 4.
13% responded 5 (almost always).

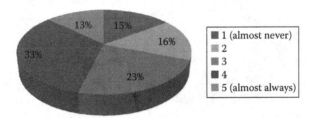

Cites general rule when criticizing
28% responded 1 (almost never).
17% responded 2.
29% responded 3.
22% responded 4.
5% responded 5 (almost always).

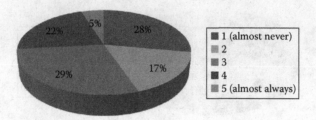

Skillful at making new friends
13% responded 1 (almost never).
23% responded 2.
36% responded 3.
20% responded 4.
9% responded 5 (almost always).

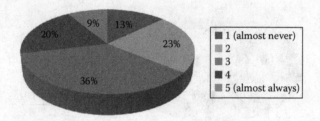

Approaches situations carefully
16% responded 1 (almost never).
32% responded 2.
33% responded 3.
14% responded 4.
5% responded 5 (almost always).

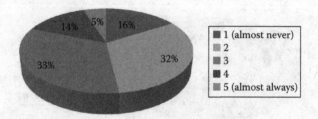

OPPOSITIONAL

Tries to get others into trouble
51% responded 1 (almost never).
13% responded 2.
19% responded 3.
10% responded 4.
8% responded 5 (almost always).

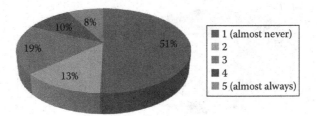

Starts fights over nothing
    61% responded 1 (almost never).
    14% responded 2.
    11% responded 3.
    4% responded 4.
    10% responded 5 (almost always).

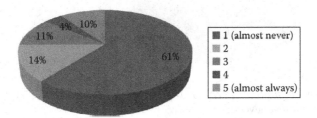

Makes malicious fun of people
    54% responded 1 (almost never).
    18% responded 2.
    13% responded 3.
    7% responded 4.
    8% responded 5 (almost always).

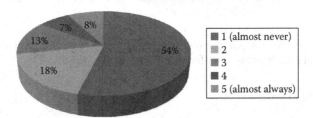

Defies authority
    59% responded 1 (almost never).
    10% responded 2.
    13% responded 3.
    8% responded 4.
    11% responded 5 (almost always).

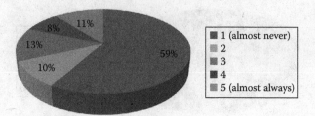

Picks on others
   51% responded 1 (almost never).
   19% responded 2.
   13% responded 3.
   9% responded 4.
   9% responded 5 (almost always).

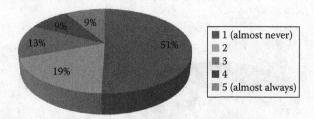

Mean and cruel to other children
   63% responded 1 (almost never).
   13% responded 2.
   13% responded 3.
   7% responded 4.
   4% responded 5 (almost always).

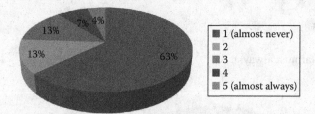

Profile scores for each of the four categories are scored for how severe the problem is and if it is seen as representing a problem. Scoring is different for boys versus girls.

MALES COMPARED TO FEMALES

Attention

Population: 26% girls and 74% boys
   Girls: 70% had significant attention problems:

- 26% of the girls had the most severe possible score for attention.
- 44% had the next most severe score.
- 15% were borderline significant for attention problems.
- 15% were not significant for attention.

Boys: 71% had significant attention problems:

- 36% of the boys had the most severe possible score for attention.
- 35% had the next most severe score.
- 27% were borderline significant for attention problems.
- 3% were not significant for attention.

Hyperactivity

Population: 27% girls and 73% boys
Girls: 44% had significant hyperactivity problems:

- 7% of the girls had the most severe possible score for hyperactivity.
- 37% had the next most severe score.
- 37% were borderline significant for hyperactivity problems.
- 20% were not significant for hyperactivity.

Boys: 55% had significant hyperactivity problems:

- 33% of the boys had the most severe possible score for hyperactivity.
- 22% had the next most severe score.
- 14% were borderline significant for hyperactivity problems.
- 31% were not significant for hyperactivity.

Social Skills

Population: 28% girls and 72% boys
Girls: 41% had significant problems with social skills:

- 8% of the girls had the most severe possible score for social skills.
- 33% had the next most severe score.
- 46% were borderline significant for social skills problems.
- 13% were not significant for social skills.

Boys: 45% had significant problems with social skills:

- 20% of the boys had the most severe possible score for social skills.
- 25% had the next most severe score.
- 34% were borderline significant for social skills problems.
- 21% were not significant for social skills.

Oppositional

Population: 30% girls and 70% boys
Girls: 34% had significant oppositional problems:

- 24% of the girls had the most severe possible score for oppositional behavior.
- 10% had the next most severe score.
- 21% were borderline significant for oppositional behavior.
- 45% were not significant for oppositional behavior.

Boys: 25% had significant oppositional problems:

- 6% of the boys had the most severe possible score for oppositional behavior.
- 19% had the next most severe score.
- 26% were borderline for oppositional behavior.
- 49% were not significant for oppositional behavior.

Summation of Findings
- Girls and boys were equal for attention symptoms.
- Boys were seen as more hyperactive than girls.
- Girls and boys had the same degree of social problems; girls were slightly less.
- Oppositional behavior was seen the least; girls were slightly higher than boys.

When compared to the child data, attention problems were slightly increased by adolescence. Boys had more hyperactivity, and girls declined slightly for social problems, while oppositional behavior remained the same. By the time of adolescence, the problem seems to be increased attention issues observed in the classroom prompting parents to seek evaluation. Increased hyperactivity for boys may be the result of increased anxiety as school continues to be difficult for them.

Another method of examining the results of this measure is to look at individual items and symptoms for all of the children.

More problems were seen for attention than any other category. Attention was problematic over one-half of the time for task persistence, ability to complete work without teacher assistance, and overall classroom function. These symptoms were seen almost never to only some of the time. The teacher(s) reported the following symptoms for the adolescents:

- 48% almost never or only some of the time worked independently (children were 55% of the time).
- 55% almost never or only some of the time persisted with a task for a reasonable amount of time (children were 51% of the time).
- 59% almost never or only some of the time completed an assigned task without assistance from the teacher (children were 58%).
- 36% almost never or only some of the time followed simple directions accurately (children were 40%).
- 48% almost never or only some of the time followed a sequence of instructions (children were 54%).
- 51% almost never or only some of the time functioned well within the classroom (children were 48%).

Hyperactive behavior was primarily seen in the form of impulsivity occurring less than 50% of the time. Other symptoms occurred about one-third of the time. Symptoms seen almost always to most of the time are as follows:

- 32% were out of their seat and on the go (children were 37%).
- 30% were overreactive (children were 34%).
- 35% were fidgety (children were 48%).
- 42% were impulsive (children were 47%).
- 36% were restless (children were 43%).

Social skills were primarily a problem for approaching a situation carefully and citing a general rule when criticizing, which still occurred slightly less than 50% of the time. (Don't understand the statement.) Other symptoms were one-third or less. Symptoms seen almost never to only some of the time are as follows:

- 24% almost never or only some of the time had positive peer interactions (children were 21%).
- 23% almost never or only some of the time had verbal communication that was clear and connected (children were 22%).
- 18% almost never or only some of the time had nonverbal communication that was clear and connected (children were 21%).
- 31% almost never or only some of the time followed group norms and social rules (children were 31%).
- 45% almost never or only some of the time cited a general rule when criticizing (children were 25%).
- 36% almost never or only some of the time were skillful at making new friends (children were 33%).
- 48% almost never or only some of the time approached social situations carefully (children were 40%).

Oppositional behavior was seen less than one-quarter of the time. Symptoms seen almost always to most of the time are as follows:

- 18% tried to get others into trouble (children were seen 18% of the time).
- 14% started fights over nothing (children were seen 7% of the time).
- 15% made malicious fun of people (children were seen 9% of the time).
- 19% defied authority (children were seen 19% of the time).
- 18% picked on others (children were seen 11% of the time).
- 11% were mean or cruel (children were seen 10% of the time).

It is apparent that oppositional behavior is not observed very often and that the problem is more one of inattention (task completion, independent work, following instructions). The same pattern was noted for the children on this measure. Teachers saw far less oppositional behavior and far more attention problems. Half of the time it was reported that more often the adolescent was not working independently, remaining focused on the task to completion, or following instruction.

With regard to oppositional behavior, there was the report of symptoms seen more often in adolescence that could be related to bullying, starting fights over nothing, making malicious fun of people, and picking on others.

Social skills remained problematic for the adolescents in terms of their ability to make friends. There was more of a problem with not approaching situations carefully and not citing a general rule when criticizing. Anxiety can often result in behavior that occurs without careful consideration of the consequences. Having the skill and ability to easily make friends had not resolved by the time of adolescence according to teacher reports.

The presence of impulsivity, fidgeting, and restlessness was seen with more regularity, (although fidgeting and restlessness had more of a decline in symptoms when compared to the children) and can be related to anxiety. The adults reported these symptoms more often as well. When considering if the symptom is present at all, adults reported impulsivity 87% of the time, physical restlessness 86% of the time, and mental restlessness 91% of the time.

HOME SITUATIONS QUESTIONNAIRE

There are a total of 16 specific situations occurring in and out of the home setting that the parent is asked to indicate whether the child's behavior is problematic. One hundred and seventy parents of adolescents completed this measure. The percentage of parents reporting problem behaviors in adolescents in these settings is indicated in the following:

- Playing alone: 13%
- Playing with other children: 37%
- Mealtimes: 32%
- Getting dressed/undressed: 17%
- Washing and bathing: 20%
- When you are on the telephone: 42%
- Watching television: 27%
- When visitors are in your home: 31%
- When you are visiting someone's home: 24%
- In public places: 33%
- When father is home: 29%
- When asked to do chores: 85%
- When asked to do homework: 83%
- At bedtime: 47%
- While in the car: 27%
- When with a babysitter: 14%

SUMMATION OF FINDINGS

Most problematic for the adolescent was when asked to do chores (85%) and homework (83%).

Comparisons to the Children

Adolescents did not present with the same behavioral issues seen in the children.

When compared to the child sample on this measure, there were decreases for the adolescents of 10%–20% for the following situations:

- Playing alone
- Playing with other children
- Watching television
- When visiting outside the home
- When father is home
- Bedtime
- In the car
- Washing and bathing

A decrease of over 20% was seen for the following situations:

- When visitors are in the home
- Mealtimes
- With babysitters
- Public places
- When parent is on the phone (decrease of 28%)
- Dressed and undressed (decrease of 35%)

Behavior for the adolescents was not the primary problem. The primary problem was work productivity similar to that seen in the school setting. The two highest problematic situations are the following: when asked to perform chores and to do homework, which did not change much from the children to the adolescents. This suggests that these two areas remain problematic from childhood to adolescence for those diagnosed with an attention disorder.

ADHD RATING SCALE

This is a measure completed by the parent regarding attention problems seen in their child. There are a total of 14 items that the parent can respond to as not present, or seen just a little, pretty much, or very much of the time that address symptoms of inattention, hyperactivity, and impulsivity. A total of 175 parents responded and reported on attention symptoms about their adolescent child. The following percentages report how often the problem exists as well as the severity of the problem.

Often fidgets or squirms in seat: 68% exist:
    Not at all = 32%
    Just a little = 35%
    Pretty much = 18%
    Very much = 15%

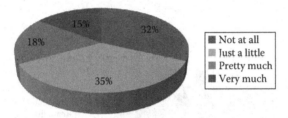

Has difficulty remaining seated: 58%
    Not at all = 41%
    Just a little = 30%
    Pretty much = 19%
    Very much = 9%

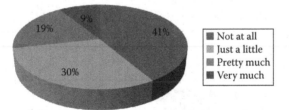

Is easily distracted: 95%
    Not at all = 5%
    Just a little = 18%
    Pretty much = 39%
    Very much = 38%

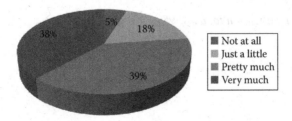

Has difficulty awaiting turn in groups: 59%
    Not at all = 41%
    Just a little = 31%
    Pretty much = 18%
    Very much = 10%

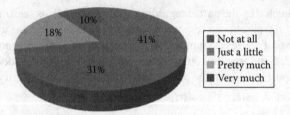

Often blurts out answers to questions: 61%
    Not at all = 39%
    Just a little = 30%
    Pretty much = 17%
    Very much = 14%

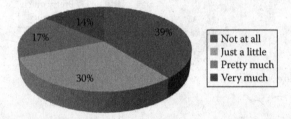

Has difficulty following instructions: 91%
    Not at all = 8%
    Just a little = 28%
    Pretty much = 29%
    Very much = 34%

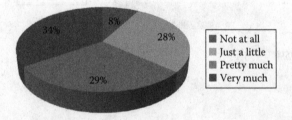

Has difficulty sustaining attention to tasks: 95%
    Not at all = 6%
    Just a little = 16%
    Pretty much = 37%
    Very much = 42%

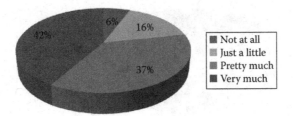

Often shifts from one uncompleted activity to another: 81%
    Not at all = 18%
    Just a little = 23%
    Pretty much = 33%
    Very much = 25%

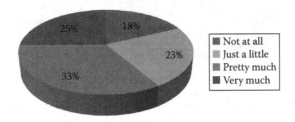

Has difficulty playing quietly: 48%
    Not at all = 52%
    Just a little = 30%
    Pretty much = 11%
    Very much = 7%

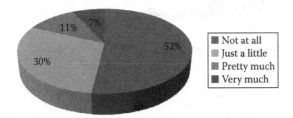

Often talks excessively: 55%
    Not at all = 44%
    Just a little = 22%
    Pretty much = 20%
    Very much = 13%

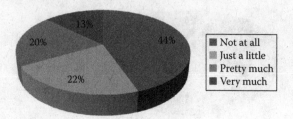

Often interrupts or intrudes on others: 73%
    Not at all = 27%
    Just a little = 30%
    Pretty much = 22%
    Very much = 21%

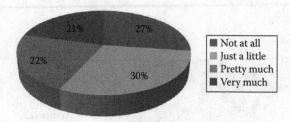

Often does not seem to listen: 94%
    Not at all = 6%
    Just a little = 30%
    Pretty much = 34%
    Very much = 30%

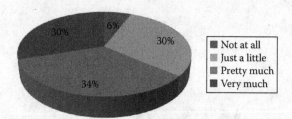

Often loses things necessary for tasks: 88%
    Not at all = 12%
    Just a little = 30%
    Pretty much = 31%
    Very much = 27%

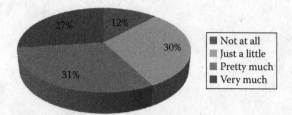

Often engages in physically dangerous activities without considering consequences: 47%
Not at all = 54%
Just a little = 29%
Pretty much = 13%
Very much = 5%

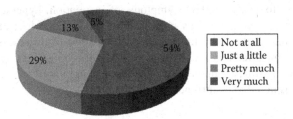

Symptoms occurring pretty much or very much of the time were the following:

- Being easily distracted (77%)
- Difficulty sustaining attention (79%)
- Difficulty following instructions (63%)
- Often not seeming to listen (64%)
- Often losing things necessary to complete tasks (58%)
- Shifting from one uncompleted task to another (58%).

SUMMATION OF FINDINGS

Report by parents using this index of attention suggests primary symptoms of inattention, distractibility, and difficulty following directions.

Comparisons to the child sample using the same measure revealed symptoms that were worse (more prevalent) as well as those that were better (seen less often).

Comparisons to the Children

Symptoms revealing a 10%–20% decline for the adolescents versus the children include the following:

- Fidgets
- Talks excessively
- Interrupts

Symptoms showing a greater than 20% decline include the following:

- Difficulty remaining seated

Symptoms seen often that remained the same include the following:

- Difficulty following instructions
- Sustained attention
- Shifting from uncompleted activities
- Easily distracted
- Not listening
- Losing things necessary for task completion

The largest decline was on the task of remaining seated, which declined by 21 points for the adolescents versus the children.

ADDES: HOME VERSION

This is a measure used to assess ADHD, symptoms of inattention, hyperactivity, and combined subtype (impulsivity) that is completed by parents. Two hundred and fourteen parents completed this measure. Results include both the first and second versions of this measure. Parents rate the symptoms based upon how often it is occurring as well as if it is not occurring at all. Symptoms are assigned a score from 0 to 4 based upon how often the symptom is observed in the home setting. Severity of symptoms is noted in occurrence of hourly to daily.

DISTRACTIBILITY AND LISTENING

Is easily distracted by other things happening in the home (e.g., other kids, TV, radio): 63% occurring hourly to daily
   8% do not engage in the behavior.
   10% engage in the behavior one to several times per month.
   19% engage in the behavior one to several times per week.
   44% engage in the behavior one to several times per day.
   19% engage in the behavior one to several times per hour.

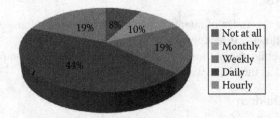

Does not listen to what others are saying: 47% occurring hourly to daily
   8% do not engage in the behavior.
   15% engage in the behavior one to several times per month.
   29% engage in the behavior one to several times per week.
   39% engage in the behavior one to several times per day.
   8% engage in the behavior one to several times per hour.

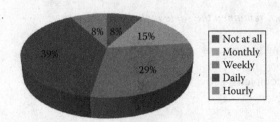

Does not direct attention or fails to maintain attention to important sounds in the immediate environment: 47% occurring hourly to daily
    18% do not engage in the behavior.
    15% engage in the behavior one to several times per month.
    20% engage in the behavior one to several times per week.
    38% engage in the behavior one to several times per day.
    9% engage in the behavior one to several times per hour.

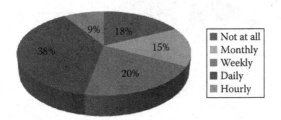

Is unsuccessful in activities requiring listening: 22% occurring hourly to daily
    19% do not engage in the behavior.
    22% engage in the behavior one to several times per month.
    37% engage in the behavior one to several times per week.
    18% engage in the behavior one to several times per day.
    4% engage in the behavior one to several times per hour.

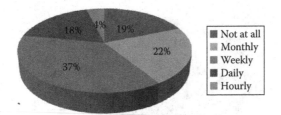

Needs oral questions and directions frequently repeated: 55% occurring hourly to daily
    7% do not engage in the behavior.
    10% engage in the behavior one to several times per month.
    28% engage in the behavior one to several times per week.
    41% engage in the behavior one to several times per day.
    14% engage in the behavior one to several times per hour.

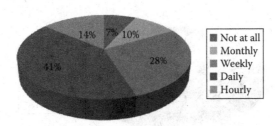

Does not listen to or follow verbal directions: 48% occurring hourly to daily
   8% do not engage in the behavior.
   12% engage in the behavior one to several times per month.
   32% engage in the behavior one to several times per week.
   39% engage in the behavior one to several times per day.
   9% engage in the behavior one to several times per hour.

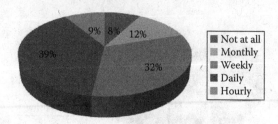

ATTENTION AND CONCENTRATION

Has difficulty concentrating: 54% occurring hourly to daily
   8% do not engage in the behavior.
   12% engage in the behavior one to several times per month.
   27% engage in the behavior one to several times per week.
   41% engage in the behavior one to several times per day.
   13% engage in the behavior one to several times per hour.

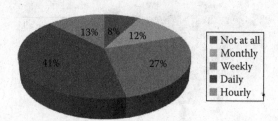

Can't concentrate, can't pay attention for long: 64% occurring hourly to daily
   6% do not engage in the behavior.
   6% engage in the behavior one to several times per month.
   25% engage in the behavior one to several times per week.
   37% engage in the behavior one to several times per day.
   27% engage in the behavior one to several times per hour.

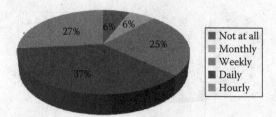

Forgets things: 52% occurring hourly to daily
  3% do not engage in the behavior.
  9% engage in the behavior one to several times per month.
  36% engage in the behavior one to several times per week.
  36% engage in the behavior one to several times per day.
  16% engage in the behavior one to several times per hour.

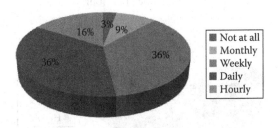

Changes from one activity to another without finishing first, without putting things away, before time to move on to next activity: 49% occurring hourly to daily
  11% do not engage in the behavior.
  10% engage in the behavior one to several times per month.
  29% engage in the behavior one to several times per week.
  11% engage in the behavior one to several times per day.
  38% engage in the behavior one to several times per hour.

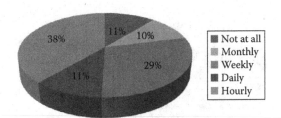

Has short attention span: 51% occurring hourly to daily
  8% do not engage in the behavior.
  8% engage in the behavior one to several times per month.
  33% engage in the behavior one to several times per week.
  32% engage in the behavior one to several times per day.
  19% engage in the behavior one to several times per hour.

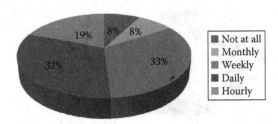

ORGANIZATION AND TASK COMPLETION

Is disorganized with possessions: 46% occurring hourly to daily
8% do not engage in the behavior.
13% engage in the behavior one to several times per month.
33% engage in the behavior one to several times per week.
29% engage in the behavior one to several times per day.
17% engage in the behavior one to several times per hour.

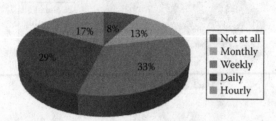

Starts but does not complete homework: 66% occurring hourly to daily
10% do not engage in the behavior.
12% engage in the behavior one to several times per month.
43% engage in the behavior one to several times per week.
23% engage in the behavior one to several times per day.
12% engage in the behavior one to several times per hour.

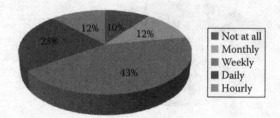

Does not independently perform chores or responsibilities: 57% occurring hourly to daily
5% do not engage in the behavior.
13% engage in the behavior one to several times per month.
26% engage in the behavior one to several times per week.
41% engage in the behavior one to several times per day.
16% engage in the behavior one to several times per hour.

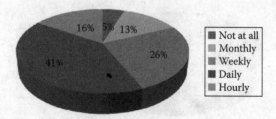

Does not remain on task to study or prepare for tests or quizzes: 46% occurring hourly to daily
8% do not engage in the behavior.
9% engage in the behavior one to several times per month.
37% engage in the behavior one to several times per week.
31% engage in the behavior one to several times per day.
15% engage in the behavior one to several times per hour.

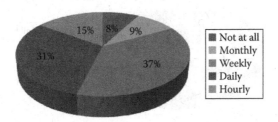

Does not organize responsibilities: 53% occurring hourly to daily
6% do not engage in the behavior.
9% engage in the behavior one to several times per month.
33% engage in the behavior one to several times per week.
35% engage in the behavior one to several times per day.
18% engage in the behavior one to several times per hour.

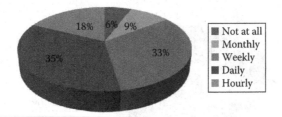

Does not prepare for school assignments: 50% occurring hourly to daily
8% do not engage in the behavior.
7% engage in the behavior one to several times per month.
34% engage in the behavior one to several times per week.
38% engage in the behavior one to several times per day.
12% engage in the behavior one to several times per hour.

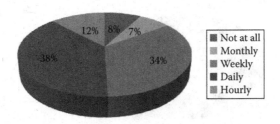

Rushes through chores or tasks with little or no regard for quality: 53% occurring hourly to daily
   8% do not engage in the behavior.
   9% engage in the behavior one to several times per month.
   29% engage in the behavior one to several times per week.
   38% engage in the behavior one to several times per day.
   15% engage in the behavior one to several times per hour.

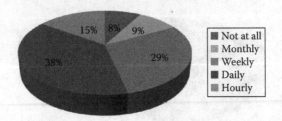

FOLLOWING DIRECTIONS

Does not read or follow written directions: 34% occurring hourly to daily
   10% do not engage in the behavior.
   18% engage in the behavior one to several times per month.
   38% engage in the behavior one to several times per week.
   25% engage in the behavior one to several times per day.
   9% engage in the behavior one to several times per hour.

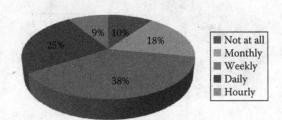

Fails to follow necessary steps in doing things: 38% occurring hourly to daily
   19% do not engage in the behavior.
   22% engage in the behavior one to several times per month.
   21% engage in the behavior one to several times per week.
   24% engage in the behavior one to several times per day.
   14% engage in the behavior one to several times per hour.

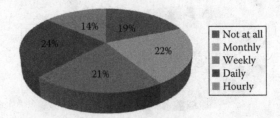

Does not follow directions from parents or other home authority figures: 11% occurring hourly to daily

48% do not engage in the behavior.
22% engage in the behavior one to several times per month.
19% engage in the behavior one to several times per week.
8% engage in the behavior one to several times per day.
3% engage in the behavior one to several times per hour.

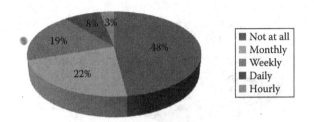

Refuses to follow requests or accept decisions made by parents: 12% occurring hourly to daily

48% do not engage in the behavior.
20% engage in the behavior one to several times per month.
20% engage in the behavior one to several times per week.
9% engage in the behavior one to several times per day.
3% engage in the behavior one to several times per hour.

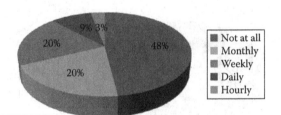

Begins things before receiving directions or instructions: 25% occurring hourly to daily

30% do not engage in the behavior.
20% engage in the behavior one to several times per month.
25% engage in the behavior one to several times per week.
19% engage in the behavior one to several times per day.
6% engage in the behavior one to several times per hour.

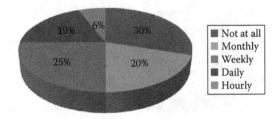

EMOTIONAL AND IMPULSIVE

Is easily frustrated: 42% occurring hourly to daily
    13% do not engage in the behavior.
    16% engage in the behavior one to several times per month.
    29% engage in the behavior one to several times per week.
    28% engage in the behavior one to several times per day.
    14% engage in the behavior one to several times per hour.

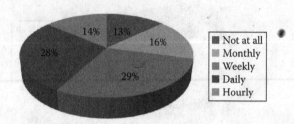

Does not wait his or her turn in activities or games: 25% occurring hourly to daily
    35% do not engage in the behavior.
    22% engage in the behavior one to several times per month.
    18% engage in the behavior one to several times per week.
    19% engage in the behavior one to several times per day.
    6% engage in the behavior one to several times per hour.

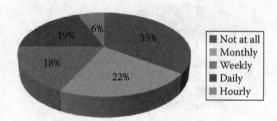

Grabs things away from others: 27% occurring hourly to daily
    33% do not engage in the behavior.
    18% engage in the behavior one to several times per month.
    23% engage in the behavior one to several times per week.
    19% engage in the behavior one to several times per day.
    8% engage in the behavior one to several times per hour.

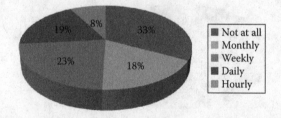

Interrupts others: 18% occurring hourly to daily
    38% do not engage in the behavior.
    23% engage in the behavior one to several times per month.
    22% engage in the behavior one to several times per week.
    13% engage in the behavior one to several times per day.
    5% engage in the behavior one to several times per hour.

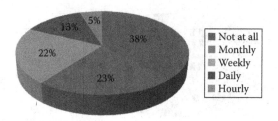

Is impulsive: 23% occurring hourly to daily
    27% do not engage in the behavior.
    27% engage in the behavior one to several times per month.
    23% engage in the behavior one to several times per week.
    15% engage in the behavior one to several times per day.
    8% engage in the behavior one to several times per hour.

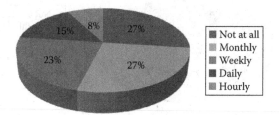

Fails to follow a routine: 44% occurring hourly to daily
    15% do not engage in the behavior.
    13% engage in the behavior one to several times per month.
    28% engage in the behavior one to several times per week.
    30% engage in the behavior one to several times per day.
    14% engage in the behavior one to several times per hour.

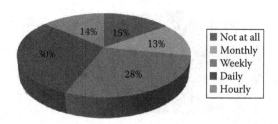

Is easily angered, annoyed, or upset: 44% occurring hourly to daily
 15% do not engage in the behavior.
 15% engage in the behavior one to several times per month.
 27% engage in the behavior one to several times per week.
 30% engage in the behavior one to several times per day.
 14% engage in the behavior one to several times per hour.

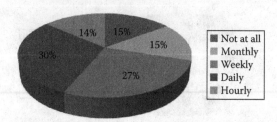

Has accidents that are the result of impulsive or careless behavior: 8% occurring hourly to daily
 47% do not engage in the behavior.
 28% engage in the behavior one to several times per month.
 17% engage in the behavior one to several times per week.
 5% engage in the behavior one to several times per day.
 3% engage in the behavior one to several times per hour.

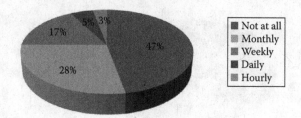

INTRUSIVE AND OPPOSITIONAL

Intrudes on others: 23% occurring hourly to daily
 27% do not engage in the behavior.
 25% engage in the behavior one to several times per month.
 26% engage in the behavior one to several times per week.
 20% engage in the behavior one to several times per day.
 3% engage in the behavior one to several times per hour.

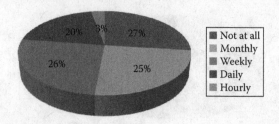

Bothers others while they are trying to work, play, etc.: 26% occurring hourly to daily
    35% do not engage in the behavior.
    18% engage in the behavior one to several times per month.
    22% engage in the behavior one to several times per week.
    22% engage in the behavior one to several times per day.
    4% engage in the behavior one to several times per hour.

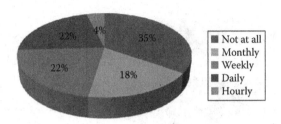

Ignores consequences of his or her behavior: 38% occurring hourly to daily
    20% do not engage in the behavior.
    20% engage in the behavior one to several times per month.
    22% engage in the behavior one to several times per week.
    23% engage in the behavior one to several times per day.
    15% engage in the behavior one to several times per hour.

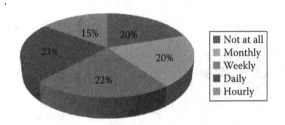

Does not follow the rules of games: 9% occurring hourly to daily
    56% do not engage in the behavior.
    21% engage in the behavior one to several times per month.
    14% engage in the behavior one to several times per week.
    8% engage in the behavior one to several times per day.
    1% engage in the behavior one to several times per hour.

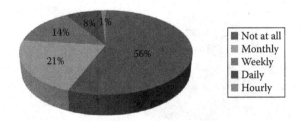

Behaves inappropriately when riding in the car: 6% occurring hourly to daily
    67% do not engage in the behavior.
    15% engage in the behavior one to several times per month.
    12% engage in the behavior one to several times per week.
    5% engage in the behavior one to several times per day.
    1% engage in the behavior one to several times per hour.

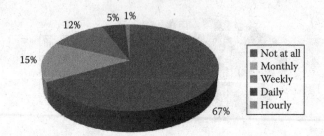

OVERACTIVE AND RESTLESS

Moves about while seated, squirms, fidgets, etc.: 27% occurring hourly to daily
    35% do not engage in the behavior.
    22% engage in the behavior one to several times per month.
    16% engage in the behavior one to several times per week.
    15% engage in the behavior one to several times per day.
    12% engage in the behavior one to several times per hour.

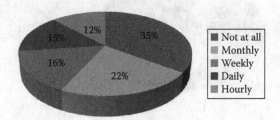

Appears restless: 29% occurring hourly to daily
    35% do not engage in the behavior.
    20% engage in the behavior one to several times per month.
    16% engage in the behavior one to several times per week.
    19% engage in the behavior one to several times per day.
    10% engage in the behavior one to several times per hour.

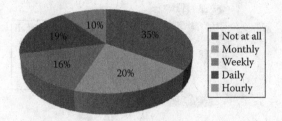

Does not remain seated: 16% occurring hourly to daily
  51% do not engage in the behavior.
  19% engage in the behavior one to several times per month.
  14% engage in the behavior one to several times per week.
  10% engage in the behavior one to several times per day.
  6% engage in the behavior one to several times per hour.

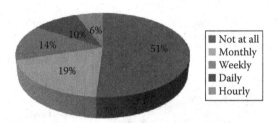

Does not adjust behavior to expectations of different situations: 16% occurring hourly to daily
  50% do not engage in the behavior.
  20% engage in the behavior one to several times per month.
  14% engage in the behavior one to several times per week.
  11% engage in the behavior one to several times per day.
  5% engage in the behavior one to several times per hour.

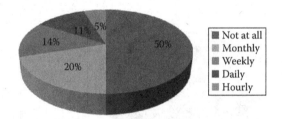

Becomes overexcited: 17% occurring hourly to daily
  49% do not engage in the behavior.
  23% engage in the behavior one to several times per month.
  11% engage in the behavior one to several times per week.
  11% engage in the behavior one to several times per day.
  6% engage in the behavior one to several times per hour.

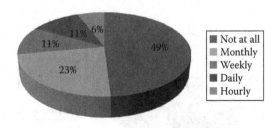

Climbs on things: 6% occurring hourly to daily
    70% do not engage in the behavior.
    14% engage in the behavior one to several times per month.
    9% engage in the behavior one to several times per week.
    5% engage in the behavior one to several times per day.
    1% engage in the behavior one to several times per hour.

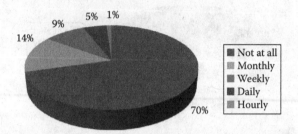

Moves about unnecessarily: 11% occurring hourly to daily
    68% do not engage in the behavior.
    14% engage in the behavior one to several times per month.
    7% engage in the behavior one to several times per week.
    9% engage in the behavior one to several times per day.
    2% engage in the behavior one to several times per hour.

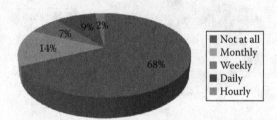

Runs in the house, does not sit appropriately on furniture: 15% occurring hourly to daily
    61% do not engage in the behavior.
    17% engage in the behavior one to several times per month.
    7% engage in the behavior one to several times per week.
    12% engage in the behavior one to several times per day.
    3% engage in the behavior one to several times per hour.

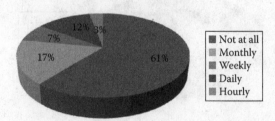

Runs in the shopping mall, pushes and makes noises in line at movies, yells in stores, etc.: 5%
occurring hourly to daily
   79% do not engage in the behavior.
   11% engage in the behavior one to several times per month.
   5% engage in the behavior one to several times per week.
   5% engage in the behavior one to several times per day.
   0% engage in the behavior one to several times per hour.

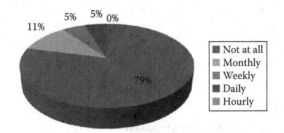

Makes excessive noise: 14% occurring hourly to daily
   65% do not engage in the behavior.
   14% engage in the behavior one to several times per month.
   7% engage in the behavior one to several times per week.
   11% engage in the behavior one to several times per day.
   3% engage in the behavior one to several times per hour.

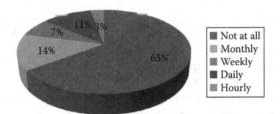

SUMMATION OF FINDINGS

Attention and not completing work are the primary issues with this group. Distractibility can easily result in forgetting things, not hearing all of the directions, and not remaining organized. Information-processing deficits and missing small pieces of information lead to confusion regarding directions. It appears to others as if the person is not listening. Distractibility and lack of eye contact can also present as not listening. Frustration can lead to not caring about how well one has performed and rushing through tasks simply to get them done.

Primary symptoms present much of the time include the following:

- Easily distracted: 92%
- Not listening to others: 92%
- Needing oral questions and directions repeated: 93%
- Not listening or following verbal directions: 92%
- Difficulty concentrating: 92%
- Cannot concentrate or pay attention for long: 94%
- Forgetting things: 97%

- Short attention span: 92%
- Disorganized: 92%
- Starting but not completing homework: 90%
- Not independently performing chores: 95%
- Not remaining on task to study: 92%
- Not organizing responsibilities: 94%
- Not preparing for school assignments: 92%
- Rushing through chores or tasks: 92%
- Does not read or follow written directions: 90%

COMPARISON TO THE CHILDREN

Increase of the following symptoms remained consistent for the children and adolescents:

- Easily distracted
- Not listening to others
- Needing oral questions and directions repeated
- Not listening or following verbal directions
- Difficulty concentrating
- Cannot concentrate or pay attention for long
- Forgetting things
- Short attention span
- Disorganized
- Not independently performing chores
- Rushing through chores or tasks

The following symptoms were increased for the adolescents when compared to the children:

- Starting but not completing homework: increase of 17%
- Not remaining on task to study: increase of 17%
- Not organizing responsibilities: increase of 13%
- Not preparing for school assignments: increase of 27%
- Does not read or follow written directions: increase of 17%

As the child ages, symptoms change. Symptoms seen in childhood are not observed to the same degree in adolescence. More cognitive and less behavioral symptoms are seen in adolescence. There were increased problems of following directions, completing homework, studying, lack of organization, and preparing for school assignments. This suggests that school is getting more difficult and adolescents are practicing more avoidance.

Children's Problem Checklist

There were 185 to 186 parents who responded to this questionnaire asking them to report areas of concern regarding their child for emotions, self-issues, people interaction, school, language/thinking, concentration/organization, actions/motor skills, behavior, values, habits, and health. Parents do not rate how bad the problem is. They respond to whether they think that the item is a concern.

Emotions
- Frequently seems anxious or tense: 35%
- Worries a lot: 35%
- Needs to be reassured frequently: 25%
- Feelings are easily hurt: 45%

- Frequently seems sad or depressed: 33%
- Feels inferior: 39%
- Is easily embarrassed: 25%
- Seems uncomfortable in new situations: 29%
- Is easily upset: 42%
- Seems withdrawn or spends a lot of time alone: 24%

When compared to the child sample, there was substantially increased depression (by 18%) increased withdrawal and feelings of inferiority as well as continued symptoms of anxiety.

Self-Issues

- Is self-critical: 36%
- Overreacts to small mistakes: 30%
- Is always a follower, never a leader: 29%
- Gives up easily: 55%
- Worries about making mistakes: 26%
- Has little self-confidence: 57%
- Is not interested in learning: 46%
- Does not give best effort: 63%
- Appears to be uninterested: 48%

When compared to the child sample, there was substantially increased problems of self-confidence (by 19%), increased lack of interest in learning (by 24%), overall lack of interest (by 26%), and lack of effort (by 19%). Consistent with the lack of interest is a decrease in over-reactivity to small mistakes and worry about making mistakes as well as an increase of being a follower and not a leader.

People Involvement

- Has trouble making friends: 21%
- Has few friends: 34%
- Is a poor loser in games: 29%
- Has friends who are a bad influence: 27%
- Is socially immature: 32%

When compared to the child sample, there was a substantial increase in friends who were a bad influence (by 17%) and social immaturity (by 14%). There was a decreased tendency to be a poor loser in games and loss of competitiveness as a result of lowered self-esteem and overall motivation.

School

- Does not finish homework: 79%
- Does not like school: 48%
- Does not get along with teachers: 27%
- Needs too much attention from teachers: 23%
- Is a discipline problem at school: 25%
- Blames teachers for problems in school: 49%
- Gets poor grades: 71%
- Is an underachiever: 61%

When compared to the child sample, there were dramatic increases in not finishing homework (by 37%), not liking school (by 25%), getting poor grades (by 45%), being an underachiever (by 38%), blaming teachers for problems in school (by 30%), and not getting along with teachers (by 17%). Needing attention from teachers decreased (by 14%) and being a discipline problem declined by 1%, suggesting that adolescents were quietly slipping away and not monitored by teachers due to their age and promotion of independent study.

Language and Thinking
- Has trouble understanding instructions: 47%
- Forgets things: 70%
- Has a poor memory: 38%
- Frequently daydreams: 37%
- Does not have good common sense: 24%
- Becomes confused easily: 27%
- Has trouble reading: 45%
- Has trouble with spelling or writing: 47%

When compared to the child sample, there was an increase in poor memory (by 11%) and forgetting things (by 13%) while symptoms of confusion, difficulty reading, and trouble with spelling and writing remained consistently problematic.

Concentration and Organization
- Does not pay attention: 62%
- Is easily distracted: 78%
- Has trouble finishing projects: 72%
- Acts impulsively: 52%
- Has trouble getting organized: 79%
- Has trouble planning activities: 35%
- Loses interest quickly: 58%
- Changes mind often: 29%
- Has difficulty following rules: 48%

When compared to the child sample, parents were no longer monitoring as well. There was an increase in difficulty finishing projects (by 14%), increase in problems of organization (by 19%), and increase in difficulty planning activities (by 11%). Other symptoms remained consistent.

Actions and Motor
- Is frequently hurt or injured: 29%
- Is restless: 29%
- Seems listless or lacks energy: 21%

When compared to the child sample, there was an increased frequency of becoming hurt or injured (by 16%) and listlessness or lack of energy (by 13%) while restlessness remained the same.

Behavior and Emotions
- Often interrupts adults or children: 38%
- Is uncooperative: 30%
- Frequently argues or disagrees: 54%
- Is disobedient: 29%
- Refuses to listen: 29%
- Is stubborn: 52%
- Is resentful: 28%

- Is secretive: 20%
- Has a bad temper: 35%
- Always has to have own way: 34%
- Frequently sulks or pouts: 20%
- Is demanding: 35%
- Manipulates others: 29%
- Swears or uses bad language: 25%
- Is defiant: 28%
- Is irresponsible: 38%

When compared to the child sample, there were more behavioral and emotional issues; being irresponsible (by 23%), swearing or bad language (by 13%), manipulating others (by 12%), and being resentful (by 12%). Often interrupting decreased (by 22%) and other symptoms remained the same.

Values
- Does not complete chores: 65%
- Does not respond to punishment: 39%
- Frequently lies: 37%
- Blames others for mistakes: 54%
- Does not feel guilty after misbehaving: 26%
- Is unappreciative: 33%
- Ignores rules: 28%
- Is disrespectful of authority: 36%
- Does not keep agreements: 26%

When compared to the child sample, there were increased behavioral problems within the parental relationship; increase in not completing chores (by 20%), increase in lying (by 14%), increase in disrespect of authority (by 16%), not keeping agreements (by 13%), and blaming others for mistakes or not responding to punishment (by 10%).

Habits
- Does not brush teeth: 17%
- Sleeps poorly: 14%
- Is frequently tired: 24%
- Has trouble getting to sleep: 27%
- Has allergies: 27%
- Has asthma: 15%
- Has frequent headaches: 26%
- Has frequent stomach aches: 16%
- Uses sickness to avoid chores or school: 20%

When compared to the child sample, there were increased symptoms of being frequently tired (by 15%) and headaches (by 10%), with other symptoms remaining similar.

Primary Symptoms Reported by the Parents Related to School Difficulties
Over one-half of parents reported their child as not giving their best effort (63%), not finishing homework (79%), getting poor grades (71%), being an underachiever (61%), forgetting things (70%), having trouble finishing projects (72%), trouble getting organized (79%), losing interest quickly (58%), and not completing chores (65%).

Almost one-half of parents reported their child as not being interested in learning (46%), appearing to be uninterested in everything (48%), not liking school (48%), having difficulty understanding instructions (47%), trouble with reading (45%), difficulty with spelling or writing (47%), and difficulty following rules (48%). Poor memory was noted by parents as present 38% of the time.

Acting in a defiant manner or being impulsive was behavior seen as related to other variables and not necessarily as a separate symptom; it was impacted by other symptoms such as anxiety, the need to be right about things, or perhaps the presence of anger related to depression (similar to that noted on other checklists) and no longer caring about anything. The adolescent population showed an increase in depressed symptoms.

Over one-half of the adolescents were described by their parent as acting impulsively (52%), frequently arguing or disagreeing (54%), and being stubborn (52%).

One-third were seen as often interrupting (38%), always having to have their own way (34%), having a bad temper (35%), being demanding (35%), irresponsible (38%), not responding to punishment (39%), frequently lying (37%), and being disrespectful of authority (36%).

Over one-fourth of the adolescents were seen as uncooperative (30%), disobedient (29%), refusing to listen (29%), resentful (28%), manipulating others (29%), defiant (28%), ignoring rules (28%), not feeling guilty after misbehaving (26%), and not keeping agreements (26%).

Parents did not tend to report that their adolescent child was in trouble with the law (6%) or mean natured or having a bad reputation (10%) or involved in vandalism (4%). This would suggest that the problem is more an issue of feeling beaten down, so they are no longer interested in school or in anything. They fail to follow through, not caring about anything, yet are angry and frustrate, lying to get by with the goal of keeping everyone away as they avoid completion of school tasks and it spills over into life tasks.

Parents indicated some additional symptoms observed in their adolescent child: They blame others for mistakes (54%) likely avoid getting into trouble. They appear to be unappreciative (33%) because they are only momentarily happy. This would make sense and is consistent with other reported symptoms of being highly sensitive, having trouble getting to sleep (27%), and worrying about things. Allergies were reported at (27%) and headaches (26%).

Parents reported their adolescent child as having issues with their teacher or teachers:

- 27% were seen as not getting along with teachers.
- 23% were seen as needing too much attention from teachers.
- 25% were seen as a discipline problem at school.
- 49% blamed teachers for problems in school.

Attention issues were reported less than the consequences of the long-term presence of a genetic attention disorder (such as not completing schoolwork), likely the reason for evaluation. This is commonly a time that evaluation is sought, when the problem had become intolerable and the primary issues were still distractibility and inattention:

- Not paying attention was reported at 62%.
- Easily distracted was reported at 78%.
- Frequent daydreaming was reported at 37%.
- Becoming confused easily was reported at 27%.

The adolescent population emerged as being very sensitive: Almost one-half of reported feelings are easily hurt (45%) and easily upset (42%).

Anxiety was clearly a factor: One-third reported frequent anxiety or tension (35%) and worrying a lot (35%), and being restless was reported at 29%.

Self-confidence was another issue:

- Over one-half of the parents reported their child as giving up easily (55%) and having little self-confidence (57%).
- One-fourth of the parents reported that their child needed frequent reassurance (25%), became easily embarrassed (25%), and was uncomfortable in new situations (29%).
- Over one-third of the parents reported that their child feels inferior (39%) and self-critical (36%).
- Over one-fourth of the parents reported their child as overreacting to small mistakes (30%) and being a follower not a leader (29%).

Depression was indicated as follows: One-third of parents saw their child as sad or depressed (33%), appearing withdrawn (24%), having difficulty planning activities (35%), and often changing their mind (29%).

Social issues were noted as follows:

- One-third of the parents reported their child as having few friends (34%).
- Over one-fourth of the parents reported their child as being a poor loser in games (29%), having friends who are a bad influence (27%), and being socially immature (32%).
- Clumsiness may be seen in parent's report of their child being frequently hurt or injured at 29%.

CHILD BEHAVIOR CHECKLIST

This is a self-report measure completed by the parent regarding their child's emotions and behavior. There were a total of 212 parents who completed this checklist. Symptoms present in childhood seem to be following the child into adolescence. Scoring is done on a three-step response scale; not present, occurs some of the time, and occurs very often. The following is the combination of percentages for somewhat or very often true, meaning the symptom is present to some degree (whether at times or often).

DEPRESSION

Cries a lot: 26%
  Not true = 74%
  Somewhat or sometimes true = 23%
  Very true or often true = 3%

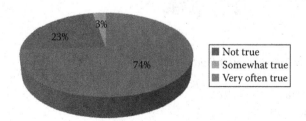

Complains of loneliness: 27%
  Not true = 73%
  Somewhat or sometimes true = 23%
  Very true or often true = 4%

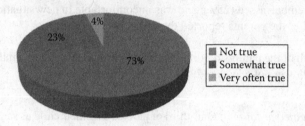

There is very little he or she enjoys: 5%
  Not true = 95%
  Somewhat or sometimes true = 5%
  Very true or often true = 0%

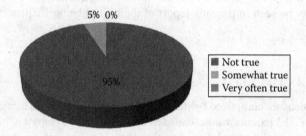

Argues a lot: 87%
  Not true = 13%
  Somewhat or sometimes true = 41%
  Very true or often true = 46%

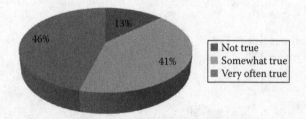

Deliberately harms self or attempts suicide: 12%
  Not true = 88%
  Somewhat or sometimes true = 10%
  Very true or often true = 2%

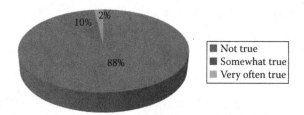

Doesn't get along with other kids: 43%
    Not true = 56%
    Somewhat or sometimes true = 38%
    Very true or often true = 5%

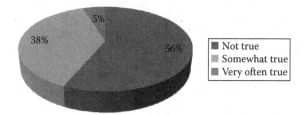

Feels or complains that no one loves him or her: 47%
    Not true = 53%
    Somewhat or sometimes true = 36%
    Very true or often true = 11%

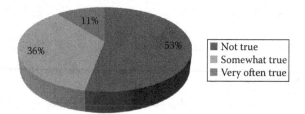

Feels worthless or inferior: 64%
    Not true = 36%
    Somewhat or sometimes true = 44%
    Very true or often true = 20%

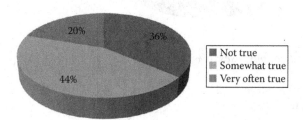

Talks about killing self: 24%
    Not true = 76%
    Somewhat or sometimes true = 19%
    Very true or often true = 5%

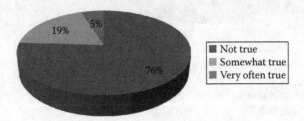

Unhappy, sad, or depressed: 53%
    Not true = 47%
    Somewhat or sometimes true = 36%
    Very true or often true = 17%

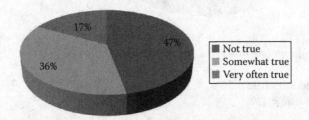

Substance Abuse

Drinks alcohol without parents' approval: 42%
    Not true = 58%
    Somewhat or sometimes true = 22%
    Very true or often true = 20%

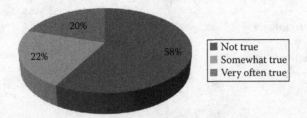

Uses drugs for nonmedical purposes: 6%
    Not true = 94%
    Somewhat or sometimes true = 4%
    Very true or often true = 2%

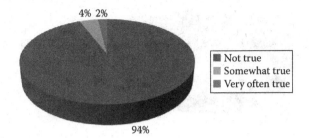

Smokes, chews, or sniffs tobacco: 7%
    Not true = 93%
    Somewhat or sometimes true = 2%
    Very true or often true = 5%

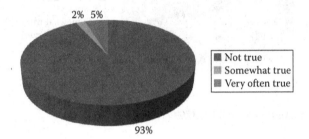

DELINQUENT AND ANTISOCIAL BEHAVIOR

Steals at home: 24%
    Not true = 76%
    Somewhat or sometimes true = 19%
    Very true or often true = 5%

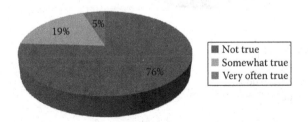

Steals outside the home: 14%
    Not true = 86%
    Somewhat or sometimes true = 12%
    Very true or often true = 2%

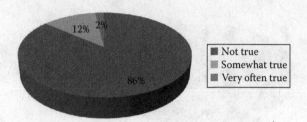

Cruel to animals: 10%
  Not true = 89%
  Somewhat or sometimes true = 8%
  Very true or often true = 2%

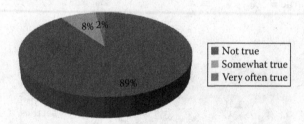

Cruelty, bullying, or meanness to others: 37%
  Not true = 63%
  Somewhat or sometimes true = 33%
  Very true or often true = 4%

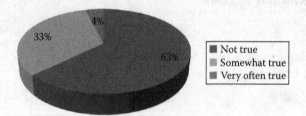

Physically attacks people: 19%
  Not true = 81%
  Somewhat or sometimes true = 15%
  Very true or often true = 4%

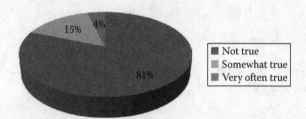

Threatens people: 26%
    Not true = 73%
    Somewhat or sometimes true = 22%
    Very true or often true = 4%

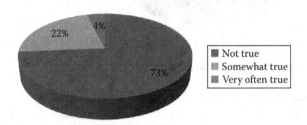

Vandalism: 7%
    Not true = 93%
    Somewhat or sometimes true = 6%
    Very true or often true = 1%

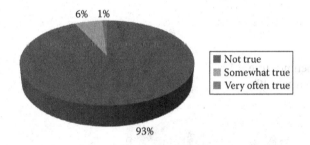

Truancy, skips school: 10%
    Not true = 90%
    Somewhat or sometimes true = 7%
    Very true or often true = 3%

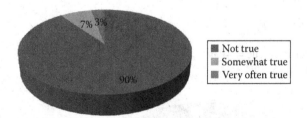

Destroys his or her things: 31%
    Not true = 69%
    Somewhat or sometimes true = 25%
    Very true or often true = 6%

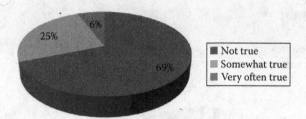

Destroys things belonging to his or her family or others: 25%
  Not true = 75%
  Somewhat or sometimes true = 19%
  Very true or often true = 6%

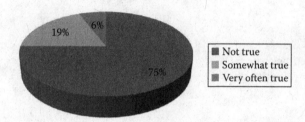

Sets fires: 13%
  Not true = 87%
  Somewhat or sometimes true = 12%
  Very true or often true = 1%

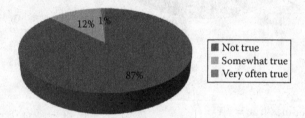

OPPOSITIONAL BEHAVIOR

Lying or cheating: 53%
  Not true = 47%
  Somewhat or sometimes true = 41%
  Very true or often true = 12%

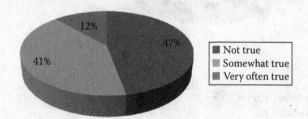

Gets in many fights: 30%
   Not true = 70%
   Somewhat or sometimes true = 25%
   Very true or often true = 5%

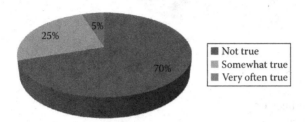

Hangs around with others who get in trouble: 40%
   Not true = 60%
   Somewhat or sometimes true = 28%
   Very true or often true = 12%

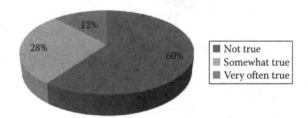

Swearing or obscene language: 40%
   Not true = 60%
   Somewhat or sometimes true = 26%
   Very true or often true = 14%

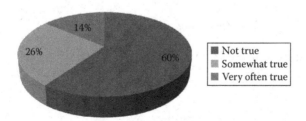

Disobedient at home: 69%
   Not true = 31%
   Somewhat or sometimes true = 43%
   Very true or often true = 26%

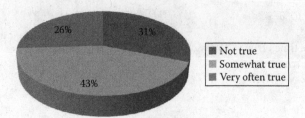

Disobedient at school: 51%
    Not true = 49%
    Somewhat or sometimes true = 32%
    Very true or often true = 19%

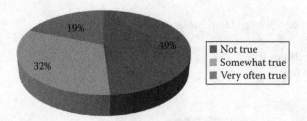

Breaks rules at home, school, or elsewhere: 3%
    Not true = 97%
    Somewhat or sometimes true = 0%
    Very true or often true = 3%

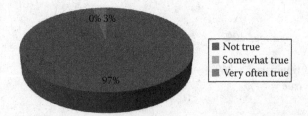

Doesn't seem to feel guilty after misbehaving: 51%
    Not true = 49%
    Somewhat or sometimes true = 31%
    Very true or often true = 20%

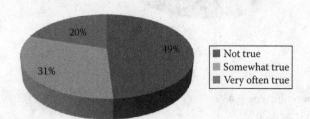

Runs away from home: 9%
    Not true = 91%
    Somewhat or sometimes true = 7%
    Very true or often true = 2%

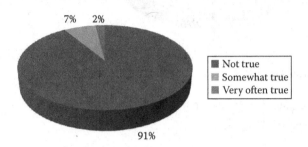

Impulsive or acts without thinking: 76%
    Not true = 24%
    Somewhat or sometimes true = 40%
    Very true or often true = 36%

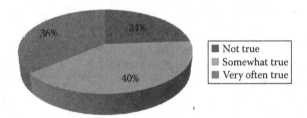

SOCIAL DIFFICULTIES

Would rather be alone than with others: 33%
    Not true = 67%
    Somewhat or sometimes true = 23%
    Very true or often true = 10%

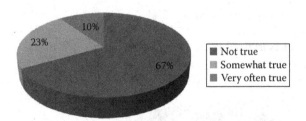

Not liked by other kids: 39%
    Not true = 61%
    Somewhat or sometimes true = 33%
    Very true or often true = 6%

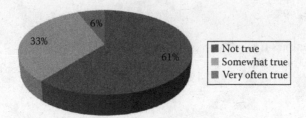

Prefers being with older kids: 36%
    Not true = 64%
    Somewhat or sometimes true = 25%
    Very true or often true = 11%

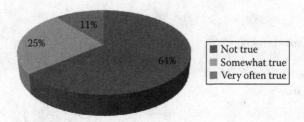

Prefers being with younger kids: 31%
    Not true = 69%
    Somewhat or sometimes true = 23%
    Very true or often true = 8%

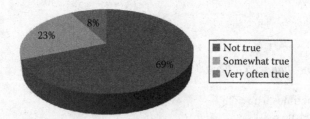

Withdrawn, doesn't get involved with others: 32%
    Not true = 68%
    Somewhat or sometimes true = 24%
    Very true or often true = 8%

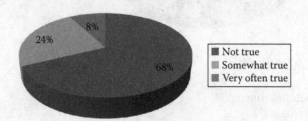

Gets teased a lot: 45%
    Not true = 55%
    Somewhat or sometimes true = 32%
    Very true or often true = 13%

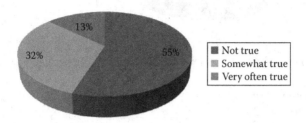

Clings to adults or too dependent: 27%
    Not true = 72%
    Somewhat or sometimes true = 21%
    Very true or often truc = 6%

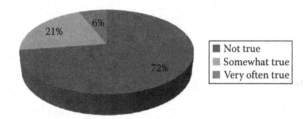

Acts too young for his or her age: 55% the problem exists:
    Not true = 44%
    Somewhat or sometimes true = 41%
    Very true or often true = 14%

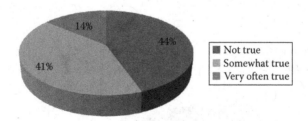

Too shy or timid: 41%
    Not true = 59%
    Somewhat or sometimes true = 32%
    Very true or often true = 9%

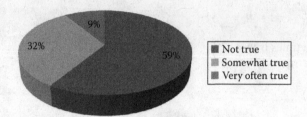

Bragging, boasting: 48%
   Not true = 52%
   Somewhat or sometimes true = 36%
   Very true or often true = 12%

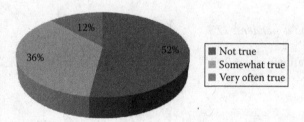

Teases a lot: 47%
   Not true = 53%
   Somewhat or sometimes true = 34%
   Very true or often true = 13%

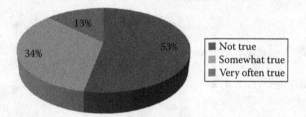

Showing off or clowning: 62%
   Not true = 38%
   Somewhat or sometimes true = 35%
   Very true or often true = 27%

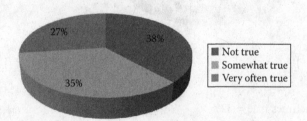

ANXIETY AND COMPULSIVE BEHAVIORS

Bites fingernails: 39%
    Not true = 61%
    Somewhat or sometimes true = 14%
    Very true or often true = 25%

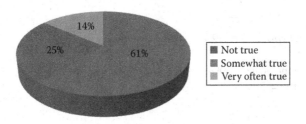

Too fearful or anxious: 29%
    Not true = 71%
    Somewhat or sometimes true = 21%
    Very true or often true = 8%

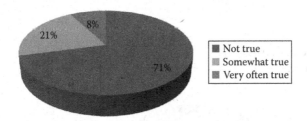

Nervous, high strung, or tense: 46%
    Not true = 54%
    Somewhat or sometimes true = 31%
    Very true or often true = 15%

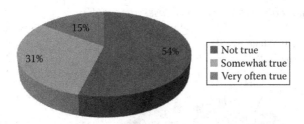

Nervous movements or twitching: 25%
    Not true = 75%
    Somewhat or sometimes true = 13%
    Very true or often true = 12%

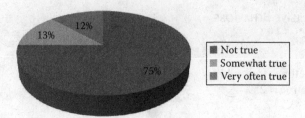

Can't sit still, restless, hyperactive: 59%
    Not true = 41%
    Somewhat or sometimes true = 39%
    Very true or often true = 20%

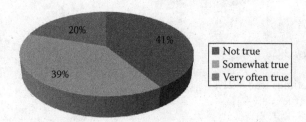

Nightmares: 18%
    Not true = 82%
    Somewhat or sometimes true = 17%
    Very true or often true = 1%

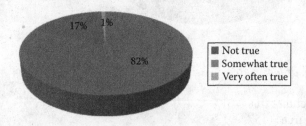

Can't get his or her mind off certain thoughts/obsessions: 46%
    Not true = 54%
    Somewhat or sometimes true = 25%
    Very true or often true = 21%

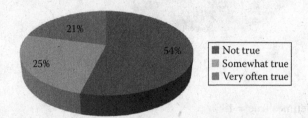

Repeats certain acts over and over: 17%
    Not true = 83%
    Somewhat or sometimes true = 7%
    Very true or often true = 10%

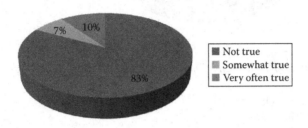

Picks nose, skin, or other parts of body: 33%
    Not true = 67%
    Somewhat or sometimes true = 19%
    Very true or often true – 14%

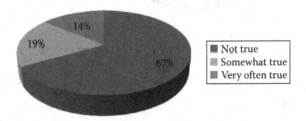

Fears certain animals, situations, or places: 19%
    Not true = 81%
    Somewhat or sometimes true = 13%
    Very true or often true = 6%

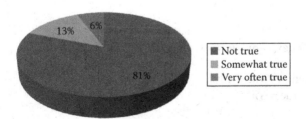

Fears going to school: 16%
    Not true = 84%
    Somewhat or sometimes true = 11%
    Very true or often true = 5%

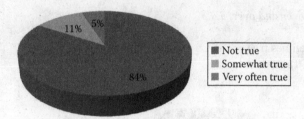

Fears he or she might think or do something bad: 24%
     Not true = 76%
     Somewhat or sometimes true = 20%
     Very true or often true = 4%

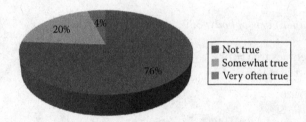

Feels he or she has to be perfect: 42%
     Not true = 58%
     Somewhat or sometimes true = 34%
     Very true or often true = 8%

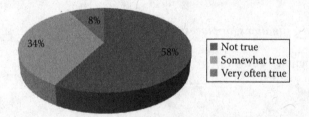

Stores up too many things he or she does not need: 18%
     Not true = 82%
     Somewhat or sometimes true = 10%
     Very true or often true = 8%

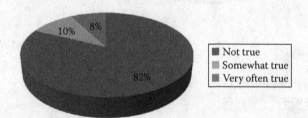

Worries: 59%
   Not true = 41%
   Somewhat or sometimes true = 40%
   Very true or often true = 19%

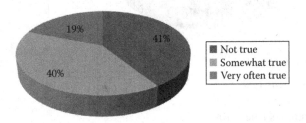

SEXUAL DIFFICULTIES

Plays with own sex parts in public: 0%
   Not true = 100%
   Somewhat or sometimes true = 0%
   Very true or often true = 0%

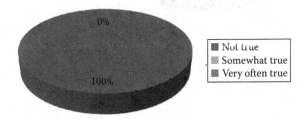

Plays with own sex parts too much: 5%
   Not true = 95%
   Somewhat or sometimes true = 5%
   Very true or often true = 0%

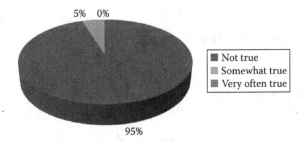

Sexual problems: 2%
   Not true = 97%
   Somewhat or sometimes true = 1%
   Very true or often true = 1%

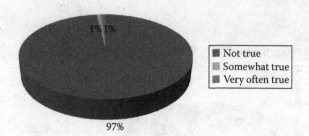

Thinks about sex too much: 12%
    Not true = 88%
    Somewhat or sometimes true = 10%
    Very true or often true = 2%

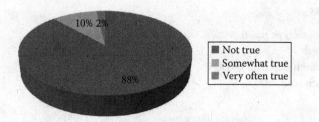

Wishes to be of opposite sex: 0%
    Not true = 100%
    Somewhat or sometimes true = 0%
    Very true or often true = 0%

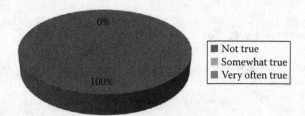

PROBLEMATIC HYGIENE, SLEEP, AND TOILET TRAINING

Gets hurt a lot, accident-prone: 25%
    Not true = 75%
    Somewhat or sometimes true = 22%
    Very true or often true = 3%

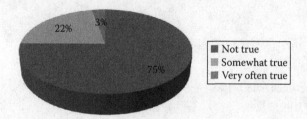

Bowel movements outside the toilet: 3%
    Not true = 97%
    Somewhat or sometimes true = 2%
    Very true or often true = 1%

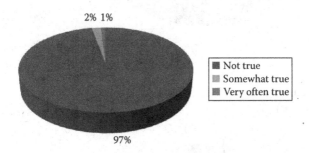

Doesn't eat well: 46%
    Not true = 54%
    Somewhat or sometimes true = 31%
    Very true or often true = 15%

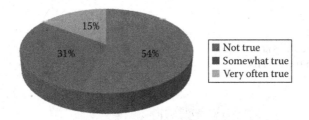

Constipated, does not move bowels: 9%
    Not true = 91%
    Somewhat or sometimes true = 7%
    Very true or often true = 2%

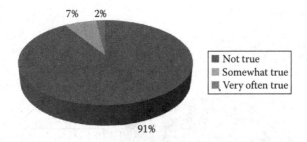

Overweight: 16%
    Not true = 84%
    Somewhat or sometimes true = 10%
    Very true or often true = 6%

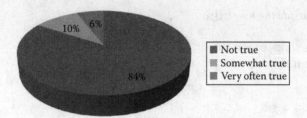

Overeating: 20%
    Not true = 80%
    Somewhat or sometimes true = 14%
    Very true or often true = 6%

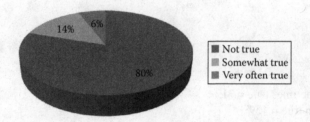

Overtired without good reason: 34%
    Not true = 66%
    Somewhat or sometimes true = 23%
    Very true or often true = 11%

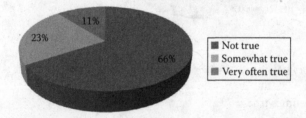

Poorly coordinated or clumsy: 27%
    Not true = 73%
    Somewhat or sometimes true = 22%
    Very true or often true = 5%

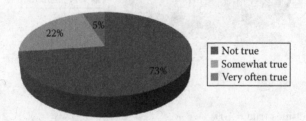

Sleeps less than most kids: 19%
   Not true = 81%
   Somewhat or sometimes true = 13%
   Very true or often true = 6%

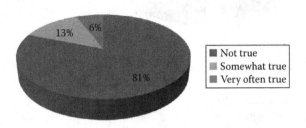

Sleeps more than most kids during day and/or night: 24%
   Not true = 75%
   Somewhat or sometimes true = 12%
   Very true or often true = 12%

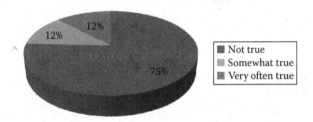

Stares blankly: 25%
   Not true = 74%
   Somewhat or sometimes true = 22%
   Very true or often true = 3%

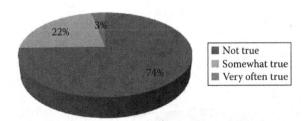

Talks or walks in sleep: 15%
   Not true = 85%
   Somewhat or sometimes true = 13%
   Very true or often true = 2%

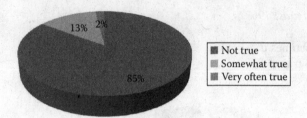

Underactive, slow moving, or lacks energy: 38%
   Not true = 62%
   Somewhat or sometimes true = 26%
   Very true or often true = 12%

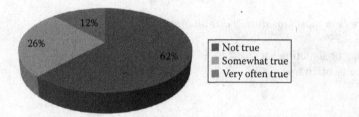

Trouble sleeping: 34%
   Not true = 65%
   Somewhat or sometimes true = 22%
   Very true or often true = 12%

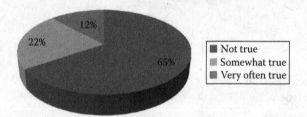

Wets the bed: 1%
   Not true = 99%
   Somewhat or sometimes true = 1%
   Very true or often true = 0%

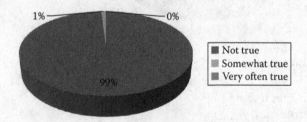

Wets self during the day: 1%
   Not true = 99%
   Somewhat or sometimes true = 1%
   Very true or often true = 0%

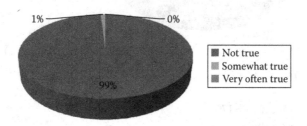

Thumb-sucking: 4%
   Not true = 96%
   Somewhat or sometimes true = 2%
   Very true or often true = 2%

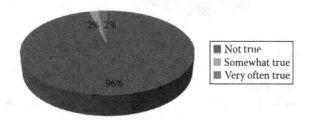

HEALTH: PHYSICAL PROBLEMS WITHOUT KNOWN MEDICAL CAUSE

Aches or pains: 29%
   Not true = 71%
   Somewhat or sometimes true = 21%
   Very true or often true = 8%

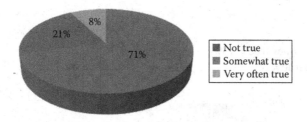

Headaches = 39%
   Not true = 61%
   Somewhat or sometimes true = 26%
   Very true or often true = 13%

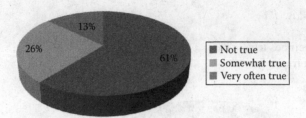

Nausea, feels sick = 21%
    Not true = 79%
    Somewhat or sometimes true = 17%
    Very true or often true = 4%

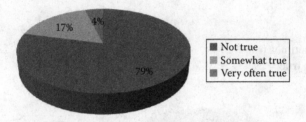

Problems with eyes = 19%
    Not true = 81%
    Somewhat or sometimes true = 14%
    Very true or often true = 5%

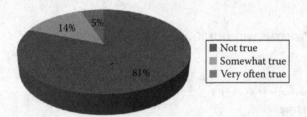

Rashes or other skin problems: 16%
    Not true = 84%
    Somewhat or sometimes true = 13%
    Very true or often true = 3%

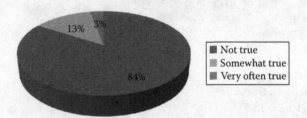

Stomach aches: 29%
    Not true = 71%
    Somewhat or sometimes true = 24%
    Very true or often true = 5%

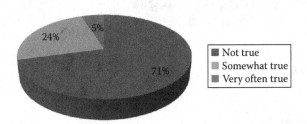

Vomiting = 3%
    Not true = 97%
    Somewhat or sometimes true = 1%
    Very true or often true = 2%

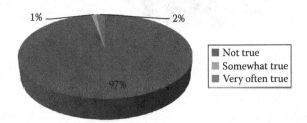

ATTENTION AND CONCENTRATION

Fails to finish things he or she starts: 19%
    Not true = 81%
    Somewhat or sometimes true = 15%
    Very true or often true = 4%

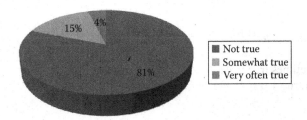

Can't concentrate, can't pay attention for long: 95%
    Not true = 5%
    Somewhat or sometimes true = 45%
    Very true or often true = 50%

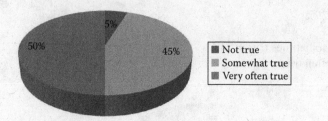

Confused or seems to be a fog: 47%
    Not true = 53%
    Somewhat or sometimes true = 35%
    Very true or often true = 12%

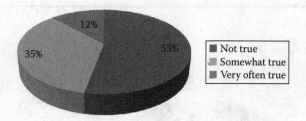

Daydreams or gets lost in his or her thoughts: 57%
    Not true = 43%
    Somewhat or sometimes true = 38%
    Very true or often true = 19%

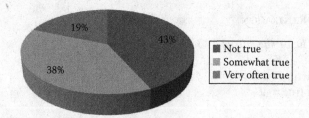

Inattentive or easily distracted: 1%
    Not true = 99%
    Somewhat or sometimes true = 1%
    Very true or often true = 0%

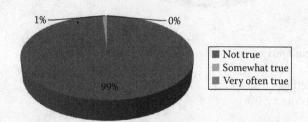

EMOTIONAL

Demands a lot of attention: 52%
   Not true = 48%
   Somewhat or sometimes true = 32%
   Very true or often true = 20%

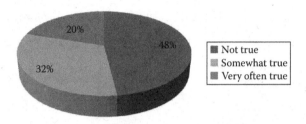

Easily jealous: 49%
   Not true = 51%
   Somewhat or sometimes true = 35%
   Very true or often true = 14%

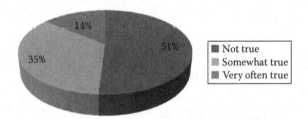

Feels too guilty: 19%
   Not true = 81%
   Somewhat or sometimes true = 15%
   Very true or often true = 4%

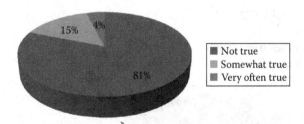

Refuses to talk: 33%
   Not true = 67%
   Somewhat or sometimes true = 27%
   Very true or often true = 6%

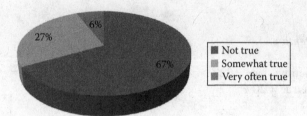

Screams a lot: 35%
  Not true = 64%
  Somewhat or sometimes true = 22%
  Very true or often true = 13%

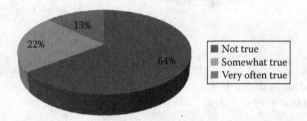

Secretive, keeps things to self: 51%
  Not true = 49%
  Somewhat or sometimes true = 34%
  Very true or often true = 17%

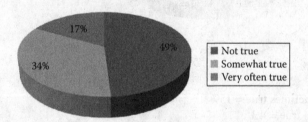

Stubborn, sullen, or irritable: 72%
  Not true = 26%
  Somewhat or sometimes true = 44%
  Very true or often true = 28%

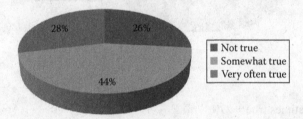

Sudden changes in mood or feelings: 67%
    Not true = 33%
    Somewhat or sometimes true = 43%
    Very true or often true = 24%

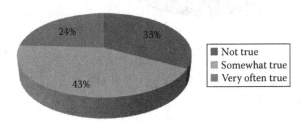

Sulks a lot: 46%
    Not true = 54%
    Somewhat or sometimes true = 32%
    Very true or often true = 14%

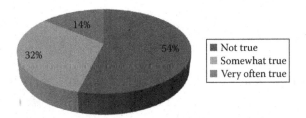

Temper tantrums or hot temper: 58%
    Not true = 42%
    Somewhat or sometimes true = 28%
    Very true or often true = 30%

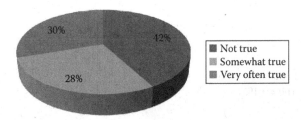

Unusually loud: 39%
    Not true = 61%
    Somewhat or sometimes true = 26%
    Very true or often true = 13%

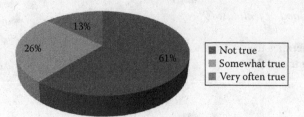

Whining: 28%
  Not true = 72%
  Somewhat or sometimes true = 21%
  Very true or often true = 7%

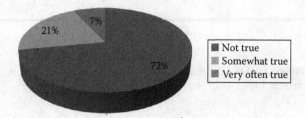

Talks too much: 45%
  Not true = 54%
  Somewhat or sometimes true = 29%
  Very true or often true = 16%

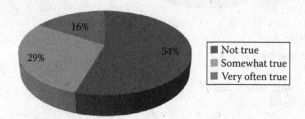

LEARNING PROBLEMS

Poor schoolwork: 86%
  Not true = 14%
  Somewhat or sometimes true = 25%
  Very true or often true = 61%

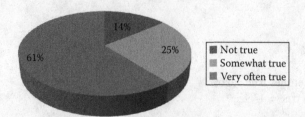

Speech problem: 8%
    Not true = 92%
    Somewhat or sometimes true = 5%
    Very true or often true = 3%

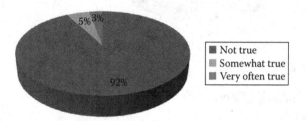

Fragile Emotionality

Hears sounds or voices that aren't there: 3%
    Not true = 97%
    Somewhat or sometimes true = 2%
    Very true or often true = 1%

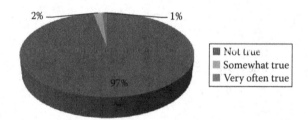

Sees things that aren't there: 3%
    Not true = 97%
    Somewhat or sometimes true = 2%
    Very true or often true = 1%

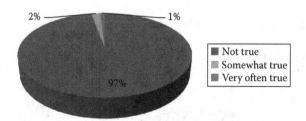

Self-conscious or easily embarrassed: 59%
    Not true = 41%
    Somewhat or sometimes true = 40%
    Very true or often true = 19%

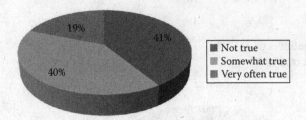

Strange behavior: 11%
    Not true = 89%
    Somewhat or sometimes true = 9%
    Very true or often true = 2%

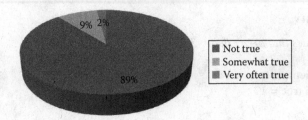

Strange ideas: 11%
    Not true = 89%
    Somewhat or sometimes true = 9%
    Very true or often true = 2%

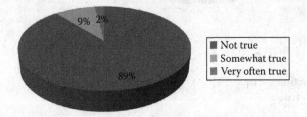

Feels others are out to get him or her: 36%
    Not true = 64%
    Somewhat or sometimes true = 28%
    Very true or often true = 8%

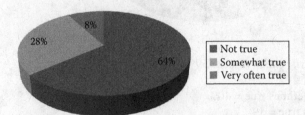

Suspicious: 24%
  Not true = 76%
  Somewhat or sometimes true = 19%
  Very true or often true = 5%

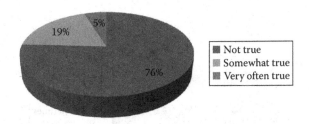

SUMMATION OF FINDINGS

Poor schoolwork: Parents reported poor schoolwork as present 86% of the time.

Attention symptoms: Parents reported becoming defensive, arguing, and generally increased emotions in connection to their adolescent child being unable to concentrate or sustain attention (95%), confused in a fog (47%), and daydreaming (57%).

Symptoms of worrying and anxiety: Parents reported that their adolescent child was unable to get his or her mind off of certain thoughts (46%) and could not sit still with symptoms of being restless (59%), nervous or tense (46%), secretive (51%), and worrying (59%).

Symptoms of depression: Parents reported that their adolescent child had feelings of being worthless or inferior (64%), stubborn or irritable (72%), sudden mood changes (67%), feeling unloved (47%), sulking a lot (46%), temper tantrums (58%), and being unhappy and sad (53%).

Response to having low self-esteem and an inability to cope with life: this may reflect their unhappiness with their life and/or this is a natural consequence of adolescence. Parents reported symptoms of arguing a lot (87%), bragging or boasting (48%), being disobedient at home (69%), not feeling guilty after misbehaving (51%), easily jealous (49%), lying or cheating (53%), self-conscious, easily embarrassed (59%), showing off or clowning (62%), and teasing a lot (47%).

Immaturity: Parents reported that their adolescent child acts too young for his or her age (55%) and demands attention (52%).

Impulsivity: Parents report that their adolescent child acts without thinking (76%).

Social issues remain: Parents report that their adolescent child is teased a lot (45%).

Some symptoms seem to be more characteristic of adolescence as opposed to being specific to a genetic attention disorder: Parents report drinking (42%) and poor eating habits (46%) as well.

CHILD SYMPTOM INVENTORY-4

The Child Symptom Inventories-4 (CSI-4) are parent-completed rating scales that allow for the screening of ADHD and other emotional and behavioral disorders. Questions are asked regarding the following types of disorders: ADHD, oppositional defiant disorder, conduct disorder, anxiety, schizophrenia, major depressive disorder, dysthymic disorder, autistic disorder, Asperger's disorder, social phobia, and separation anxiety disorder. There were 32 parents who responded to this questionnaire used between the years 2006 and 2009 and currently in use. Parents rated the symptoms as occurring never, sometimes, often, or very often. The following are the significant percentages for symptoms that parents saw as occurring often or very often.

ATTENTION–THINKING SYMPTOMS

Fails to give close attention to details or makes careless mistakes: 19% seen often and very often

Never = 19%
Sometimes = 63%
Often = 19%
Very often = 0%

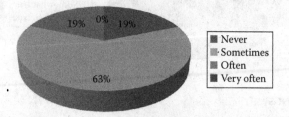

Has difficulty paying attention to tasks or activities: 56% seen often and very often
Never = 6%
Sometimes = 38%
Often = 47%
Very often = 9%

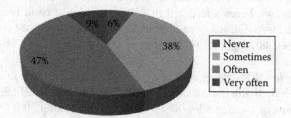

Does not seem to listen when spoken to directly: 39% seen often and very often
Never = 3%
Sometimes = 58%
Often = 26%
Very often = 13%

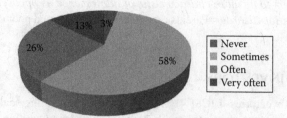

Has difficulty following through on instructions and fails to finish things: 72% seen often and very often
Never = 3%
Sometimes = 25%
Often = 50%
Very often = 22%

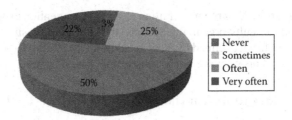

Has difficulty organizing tasks and activities: 39% seen often and very often
Never = 23%
Sometimes = 39%
Often = 39%
Very often = 0%

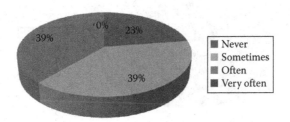

Is easily distracted by other things going on: 38% seen often and very often
Never = 19%
Sometimes = 44%
Often = 38%
Very often = 0%

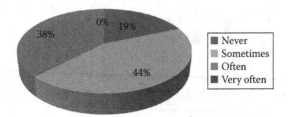

Is forgetful in daily activities: 69% seen often and very often
Never = 6%
Sometimes = 25%
Often = 38%
Very often = 31%

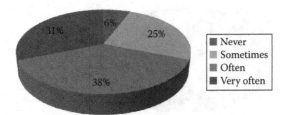

Compared to the child sample, symptoms of failing to give close attention to detail declined by 50% for the adolescents, and difficulty organizing declined by 27%. Being easily distracted declined by 44% and not appearing to listen declined by 20%. In addition, becoming forgetful in daily activities increased by 12%. Adolescents were seen as less distracted, listening more, and attending to details.

BEHAVIORAL SYMPTOMS RELATED TO ATTENTION

Avoids doing tasks that require a lot of mental effort (schoolwork, homework, etc.): 75% seen often and very often
>   Never = 3%
>   Sometimes = 22%
>   Often = 25%
>   Very often = 50%

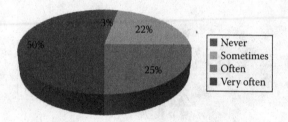

Loses things necessary for activities: 53% seen often and very often
>   Never = 9%
>   Sometimes = 38%
>   Often = 31%
>   Very often = 22%

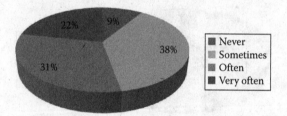

Fidgets with hands or feet or squirms in seat: 51% seen often and very often
>   Never = 23%
>   Sometimes = 26%
>   Often = 32%
>   Very often = 19%

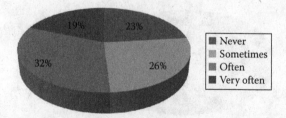

Has difficulty remaining in seat when asked to do so: 19% seen often and very often
    Never = 48%
    Sometimes = 32%
    Often = 16%
    Very often = 3%

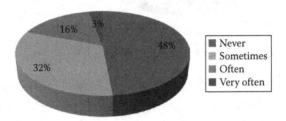

Runs about or climbs on things when asked not to do so: 0% seen often and very often
    Never = 71%
    Sometimes = 29%
    Often = 0%
    Very often = 0%

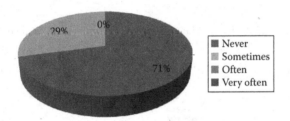

Has difficulty playing quietly: 10% seen often and very often
    Never = 57%
    Sometimes = 33%
    Often = 7%
    Very often = 3%

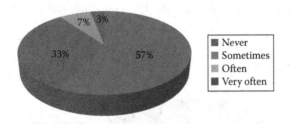

Is "on the go" or acts as if "driven by a motor": 3% seen often and very often
    Never = 58%
    Sometimes = 39%
    Often = 3%
    Very often = 0%

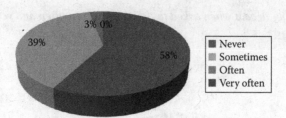

Talks excessively: 16% seen often and very often
    Never = 43%
    Sometimes = 40%
    Often = 13%
    Very often = 3%

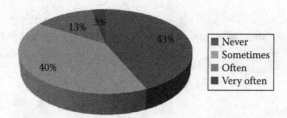

Blurts out answers to questions before they have been completed: 32% seen often and very often
    Never = 46%
    Sometimes = 21%
    Often = 25%
    Very often = 7%

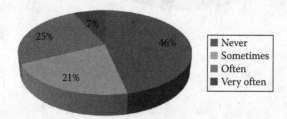

Has difficulty awaiting turn in group activities: 22% seen often and very often
    Never = 46%
    Sometimes = 32%
    Often = 18%
    Very often = 4%

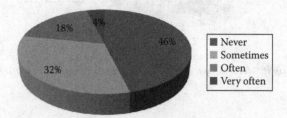

Interrupts people or butts into other children's activities: 32% seen often and very often
    Never = 42%
    Sometimes = 26%
    Often = 26%
    Very often = 6%

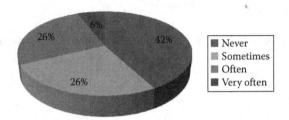

Compared to the child sample, adolescents remained in their seat, did not run or climb on things, and did not display the hyperactive symptoms seen in the child population. This may be related to the child population having almost 50%ADHD plus where there was an additional disorder diagnosed that would have contributed to symptoms of hyperactivity (sleep is a good example and failure to control anxiety can result in overly active behavior as well). Having difficulty remaining in their seat declined by 25% in adolescence. Running about or climbing on things declined by 31%. Difficulty playing quietly declined by 16%. Being "on the go" as if "driven by a motor" declined by 40%. Talking excessively declined by 26%. Interrupting people declined by 15% in adolescence.

OPPOSITIONAL AND DEFIANT BEHAVIOR

Loses temper: 39% seen often and very often
    Never = 6%
    Sometimes = 55%
    Often = 23%
    Very often = 16%

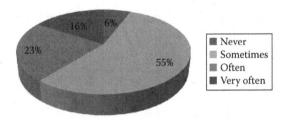

Argues with adults: 64% seen often and very often
    Never = 9%
    Sometimes = 28%
    Often = 41%
    Very often = 23%

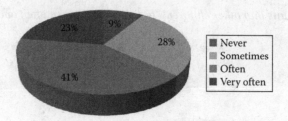

Defies or refuses what you tell him or her to do: 39% seen often and very often
    Never = 19%
    Sometimes = 42%
    Often = 26%
    Very often = 13%

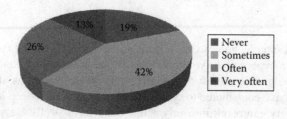

Does things to deliberately annoy others: 26% seen often and very often
    Never = 23%
    Sometimes = 50%
    Often = 13%
    Very often = 13%

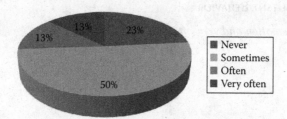

Blames others for own misbehavior or mistakes: 32% seen often and very often
    Never = 16%
    Sometimes = 52%
    Often = 19%
    Very often = 13%

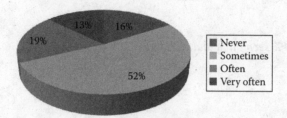

Is touchy or easily annoyed by others: 32% seen often and very often
    Never = 16%
    Sometimes = 52%
    Often = 19%
    Very often = 13%

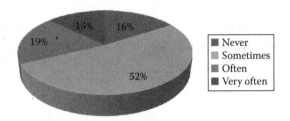

Is angry and resentful: 29% seen often and very often
    Never = 31%
    Sometimes = 41%
    Often = 13%
    Very often − 16%

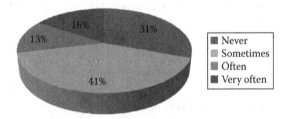

Takes anger out on others or tries to get even: 25% seen often and very often
    Never = 44%
    Sometimes = 31%
    Often = 19%
    Very often = 6%

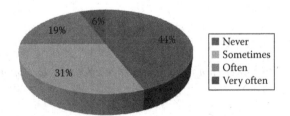

Compared to the child sample, symptoms of losing temper declined by 10% in adolescence, doing things to annoy people declined by 11%, and being touchy and easily annoyed declined by 15%; arguing with adults increased by 11%. While adolescents displayed less oppositional behavior in these areas, other areas remained the same (remaining angry and resentful) and arguing with adults increased.

CONDUCT DISORDER AND ANTISOCIAL BEHAVIOR

Plays hooky from school: 7% seen often and very often
  Never = 30%
  Sometimes = 64%
  Often = 5%
  Very often = 2%

Stays out at night when not supposed to: 3% seen often and very often
  Never = 88%
  Sometimes = 9%
  Often = 3%
  Very often = 0%

Lies to get things or to avoid responsibility (cons others): 19% seen often and very often
  Never = 53%
  Sometimes = 28%
  Often = 6%
  Very often = 13%

Bullies, threatens, or intimidates others: 6% seen often and very often
  Never = 78%
  Sometimes = 16%
  Often = 3%
  Very often = 3%

Starts physical fights: 0% seen often and very often
  Never = 75%
  Sometimes = 25%
  Often = 0%
  Very often = 0%

Has run away from home overnight: 0% seen often and very often
  Never = 97%
  Sometimes = 3%
  Often = 0%
  Very often = 0%

Has stolen things when others were not looking: 3% seen often and very often
  Never = 91%
  Sometimes = 6%
  Often = 3%
  Very often = 0%

Has deliberately destroyed others' property: 3% seen often and very often
  Never = 88%
  Sometimes = 9%
  Often = 3%
  Very often = 0%

Has deliberately started fights: 0% seen often and very often
   Never = 100%
   Sometimes = 0%
   Often = 0%
   Very often = 0%

Has stolen things from others using physical force: 0% seen often and very often
   Never = 97%
   Sometimes = 3%
   Often = 0%
   Very often = 0%

Has broken into someone else's house, building, or car: 0% seen often and very often
   Never = 97%
   Sometimes = 3%
   Often = 0%
   Very often = 0%

Has used a weapon when fighting (bat, brick, bottle, etc.): 0% seen often and very often
   Never = 97%
   Sometimes = 3%
   Often = 0%
   Very often = 0%

Has been physically cruel to animals: 0% seen often and very often
   Never = 94%
   Sometimes = 6%
   Often = 0%
   Very often = 0%

Has been physically cruel to people: 3% seen often and very often
   Never = 88%
   Sometimes = 9%
   Often = 3%
   Very often = 0%

Has been preoccupied with or involved in sexual activity: 0% seen often and very often
   Never = 91%
   Sometimes = 9%
   Often = 0%
   Very often = 0%

Compared to the child sample, symptoms for the adolescents remained similar other than starting physical fights, which decreased by 10%.

ANXIETY

Is overconcerned about abilities in academic, athletic, or social activities: 31% seen often and very often
   Never = 38%
   Sometimes = 31%
   Often = 25%
   Very often = 6%

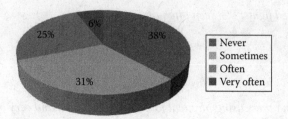

Has difficulty controlling worries: 22% seen often and very often
    Never = 31%
    Sometimes = 47%
    Often = 16%
    Very often = 6%

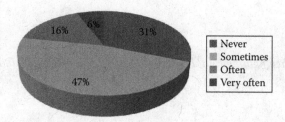

Acts restless or edgy: 32% seen often and very often
    Never = 23%
    Sometimes = 45%
    Often = 23%
    Very often = 9%

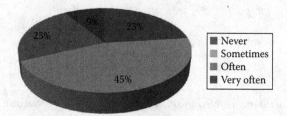

Is irritable for most of the day: 19% seen often and very often
    Never = 31%
    Sometimes = 50%
    Often = 16%
    Very often = 3%

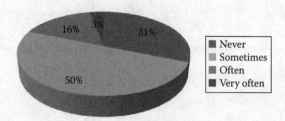

Is extremely tense or unable to relax: 13% seen often and very often
Never = 42%
Sometimes = 45%
Often = 13%
Very often = 0%

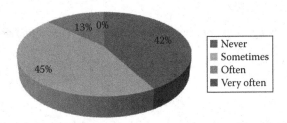

Has difficulty falling asleep or staying asleep: 44% seen often and very often
Never = 28%
Sometimes = 28%
Often = 31%
Very often = 13%

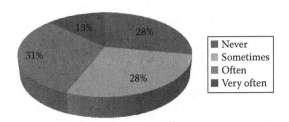

Complains about physical problems (headaches, upset stomach, etc.) for which there is no apparent cause: 15% seen often and very often
Never = 38%
Sometimes = 47%
Often = 9%
Very often = 6%

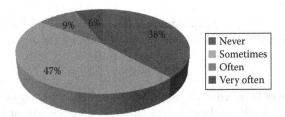

Compared to the child sample, symptoms for the adolescents remained the same for being restless, acting irritable, and physical complaints. The concern regarding their abilities increased by 15% in adolescence. Difficulty falling asleep increased by 19%. However, difficulty controlling worries and being tense declined by 10%. Adolescents, while worrying internally, may not have displayed these symptoms outwardly.

OBSESSIVE–COMPULSIVE SYMPTOMS

Shows excessive fear to specific objects or situations: 25% seen often and very often
Never = 59%
Sometimes = 16%
Often = 22%
Very often = 3%

Cannot get distressing thoughts out of his or her mind: 9% seen often and very often
Never = 69%
Sometimes = 22%
Often = 3%
Very often = 6%

Feels compelled to perform unusual habits: 6% seen often and very often
Never = 88%
Sometimes = 6%
Often = 6%
Very often = 0%

Has experienced an extremely upsetting event and continues to be bothered by it: 13% seen often and very often
Never = 75%
Sometimes = 13%
Often = 13%
Very often = 0%

Does unusual movements for no apparent reason: 13% seen often and very often
Never = 84%
Sometimes = 3%
Often = 10%
Very often = 3%

Makes vocal sounds for no apparent reason: 9% seen often and very often
Never = 75%
Sometimes = 16%
Often = 6%
Very often = 3%

Compared to the child sample, symptoms remained similar for the adolescents although distressing thoughts declined by 9%, while excessive fear to certain situations increased by 8%.

FRAGILE EMOTIONALITY

- Has strange ideas or beliefs that are not real: 0% seen often and very often
- Has auditory hallucinations—hears voices talking to or telling him or her to do things: 0% seen often and very often
- Has extremely strange and illogical thoughts and ideas: 0% seen often and very often
- Laughs or cries at inappropriate times or shows no emotion in situations where most others of the same age would react: 0% seen often and very often
- Does extremely odd things: 6% seen often and very often

Compared to the child sample, symptoms remained the same for adolescence.

SYMPTOMS OF DEPRESSION

Is depressed most of the day: 6% seen often and very often
   Never = 65%
   Sometimes = 29%
   Often = 6%
   Very often = 0%

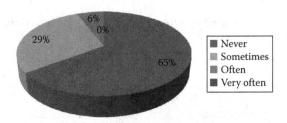

Shows little interest in pleasurable activities: 6% seen often and very often
   Never = 55%
   Sometimes = 39%
   Often = 3%
   Very often = 3%

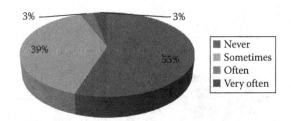

Has recurrent thoughts of death or suicide: 3% seen often and very often
   Never = 90%
   Sometimes = 6%
   Often = 3%
   Very often = 0%

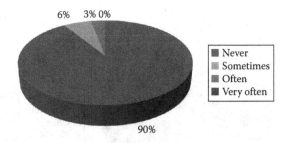

Feels worthless or guilty: 9% seen often and very often
   Never = 48%
   Sometimes = 42%
   Often = 6%
   Very often = 3%

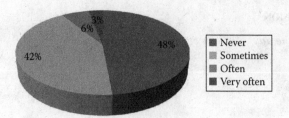

Has low energy level or is tired for no apparent reason: 25% seen often and very often
    Never = 38%
    Sometimes = 38%
    Often = 19%
    Very often = 6%

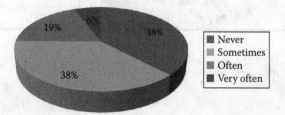

Has little confidence or is very self-conscious: 28% seen often and very often
    Never = 28%
    Sometimes = 44%
    Often = 19%
    Very often = 9%

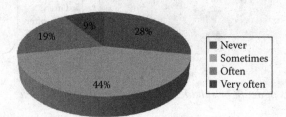

Feels that things never work out right: 12% seen often and very often
    Never = 38%
    Sometimes = 50%
    Often = 6%
    Very often = 6%

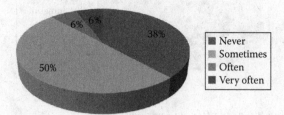

Compared to the child sample, these symptoms remained similar excluding an increase of 16% for low energy level and being tired, decrease of 9% for low self-confidence and being more self-conscious, and decrease of 10% for feeling that things won't work out.

PHYSICAL AND LIFE CHANGES

- Has experienced a big change in his or her normal appetite or weight: 21% seen often and very often
- Has experienced a big change in his or her normal sleeping habits— cannot sleep or sleeps too much: 36% seen often and very often
- Has experienced a big change in his or her normal activity level—overactive or inactive: 7% seen often and very often
- Has experienced a big change in his or her ability to concentrate: 21% seen often and very often
- Has experienced a big drop in school grades or schoolwork: 43% seen often and very often

Compared to the child sample, adolescents reported increased change in weight by 10%, increased change in sleeping habits by 27%, and increased big drop in school grades by 26%.

SYMPTOMS OF ASPERGER'S DISORDER AND AUTISM SPECTRUM

Has a peculiar way of relating to others: 16% seen often and very often
Never = 52%
Sometimes = 32%
Often = 6%
Very often = 10%

Does not play or relate well with other children: 10% seen often and very often
Never = 52%
Sometimes = 39%
Often = 10%
Very often = 0%

Not interested in making friends: 19% seen often and very often
Never = 71%
Sometimes = 10%
Often = 6%
Very often = 13%

Is unaware or takes no interest in other people's feelings: 9% seen often and very often
Never = 58%
Sometimes = 32%
Often = 3%
Very often = 6%

Has a significant problem with language: 3% seen often and very often
Never = 94%
Sometimes = 3%
Often = 3%
Very often = 0%

Has difficulty making socially appropriate conversation: 16% seen often and very often
Never = 68%
Sometimes = 16%
Often = 10%
Very often = 6%

Talks in a strange way: 0% seen often and very often
　　Never = 94%
　　Sometimes = 6%
　　Often = 0%
　　Very often = 0%

Is unable to pretend or make believe when playing: 3% seen often and very often
　　Never = 87%
　　Sometimes = 10%
　　Often = 3%
　　Very often = 0%

Shows excessive preoccupation with one topic: 3% seen often and very often
　　Never = 71%
　　Sometimes = 26%
　　Often = 3%
　　Very often = 0%

Gets very upset over small changes in routine or surroundings: 9% seen often and very often
　　Never = 71%
　　Sometimes = 19%
　　Often = 6%
　　Very often = 3%

Makes strange repetitive movements: 3% seen often and very often
　　Never = 94%
　　Sometimes = 3%
　　Often = 3%
　　Very often = 0%

Has strange fascination for parts of objects: 0% seen often and very often
　　Never = 100%
　　Sometimes = 0%
　　Often = 0%
　　Very often = 0%

Compared to the child sample, adolescents reported increased lack of interest for friends by 13% and decreased excessive preoccupation with one topic by 11%. Getting upset over changes in routine decreased by 10%; otherwise, symptoms remained similar for children and adolescents.

SYMPTOMS OF SOCIAL PHOBIA

Tries to avoid contact with strangers; abnormally shy: 16% seen often and very often
　　Never = 61%
　　Sometimes = 23%
　　Often = 13%
　　Very often = 3%

Is excessively shy with peers: 9% seen often and very often
    Never = 74%
    Sometimes = 16%
    Often = 6%
    Very often = 3%

Is generally warm and outgoing with family members and familiar adults: 71% seen often and very often
    Never = 16%
    Sometimes = 13%
    Often = 42%
    Very often = 29%

When put in uncomfortable social situations, child cries, freezes, or withdraws from interacting: 10% seen often and very often
    Never = 48%
    Sometimes = 42%
    Often = 10%
    Very often = 0%

SUMMATION OF FINDINGS

When compared to the child sample, being warm and outgoing with family decreased by 10% for the adolescents. The remainder of these symptoms was similar for children and adolescents.

Separation Anxiety

- Gets very upset when child expects to be separated from home or parents: 6% seen often and very often
- Worries that parents will be hurt or leave home and not come back: 7% seen often and very often
- Worries that some disaster will separate child from parents: 0% seen often and very often
- Tries to avoid going to school in order to stay home with parents: 0% seen often and very often
- Worries about being left at home alone or with a sitter: 3% seen often and very often
- Afraid to go to sleep unless near parent: 3% seen often and very often
- Has nightmares about being separated from parent: 0% seen often and very often
- Complains about feeling sick when child expects to be separated from home or parents: 0% seen often and very often
- Wets bed at night: 0% seen often and very often
- Wets or soils underwear during daytime hours: 0% seen often and very often

When compared to the child sample, all symptoms decreased for the adolescents to the degree that none of these symptoms are significant. Fear of going to sleep without the parent declined by 17%, wetting the bed at night declined from 9%–0%, and avoidance of school to stay home with parent declined from 7%–0%.

Comparison to the Children

In comparing symptoms for the children and the adolescents, changes primarily occurred in the areas of depression, anxiety, attention, and sleep. There was a reduction of the overactive or

hyperactive symptoms seen in childhood. Symptoms describing additional disorders such as pho-
bias, Asperger's, and fragile emotionality did not change much from the child to the adolescent
population although these issues were not highly present to begin with.

There was a smaller sample of parents that completed this checklist, yet the findings remain
similar to the other self-report measures. The differences seen when comparisons are made with the
child data are consistent despite the adolescent sample being much smaller. Another way to look at
the data is to discuss symptoms that were present versus those that were not.

Symptoms present 90% or more of the time are as follows:

- Difficulty paying attention: 94%
- Not seeming to listen when spoken to: 97%
- Difficulty following through on instructions and failing to finish things: 97%
- Forgetful in activities: 94%
- Avoidance of tasks requiring mental effort: 97%
- Losing things necessary for activities: 91%
- Loss of temper: 94%
- Arguing with adults: 91%

The aforementioned symptoms suggest the presence of inattention, avoidance of work, and the
frustration seen more in the adolescents than the children. The same issues are seen when analyzing
severity of symptoms.

Severity of Symptoms

*The highest severity of symptoms was seen in the following attention-related traits that were indi-
cated by parents as occurring often or very often*:

- Fidgeting with hands or feet or squirming in seat (which could be attributable to anxiety):
  51% of the time
- Losing things necessary for activities: 53% of the time
- Difficulty paying attention: 56% of the time
- Forgetful in daily activities: 69% of the time
- Difficulty following through on instructions and failing to finish things: 72% of the time
- Avoiding tasks that require a lot of mental effort (schoolwork or homework): 75% of the time

Inattention versus hyperactivity (seen often and very often):

- In analyzing the percentages, it can be seen that this parent population subscribed to more
  symptoms of inattention as opposed to hyperactivity or impulsivity in describing the
  behavior of their adolescent child.

Symptoms typically thought of as hyperactivity were not seen very often:

- Running about or climbing on things when asked not to do so: 0% was often or very often.
- Difficulty playing quietly: 10% were often or very often.
- On the go as if driven by a motor: 3% were often or very often.
- Blurting out answers to questions before they have been completed and interrupting: 32%
  were often and very often. Anxiety can produce these symptoms as well, which could
  explain why this symptom is seen more often.

Symptoms of anger were seen more in the adolescents than the children:

Losing one's temper, being angry, and blaming others tend to be more common traits specific to adolescence, seen often and very often:

- The highest percentage was for arguing with adults: 64% were often or very often.
- 39% indicated that their adolescent child lost their temper; 39% remained defiant, refusing to do what they were told; 29% were seen as being angry and resentful as well as blaming others; and 32% as being touchy or easily annoyed.

Antisocial behavior had percentages ranging from 0 to 10 for symptoms seen often or very often excluding lying to avoid responsibility, which was 19%.

Defiant behavior ranged from 25% to 64%.

Anxiety symptoms and somatic complaints seen often and very often had higher percentages for three items:

- Overconcern about abilities in academic, athletic, or social: 31% were often or very often.
- Acting restless or edgy: 32% were often or very often.
- Difficulty falling asleep or staying asleep: 44% were often or very often.

Obsessive symptoms and/or trauma seen often and very often revealed only one symptom that was observed more than 15% of the time. Showing excessive fear to specific objects or situations was seen 25% of the time.

Symptoms of psychiatric disorders depicting fragile emotionality, such as odd behaviors, eccentricity, and psychotic symptoms, were mostly 0% for the rating of often or very often seen. Symptoms of depression seen often or very often were under 10% for many areas (e.g., being depressed for most of the day, feeling worthless or guilty, no interest in pleasurable activities, recurrent thoughts of death). However, 25% cited low energy, 28% feeling self-conscious, and 12% feeling that things would never work out. Generally depression was seen on other checklists as more significant especially when reported by the adolescents themselves as opposed to the parents.

Social phobia, symptoms of autism spectrum, and difficulty with friendships did not present with high percentages, and symptoms were generally not reported for these disorders. It was indicated that 16% had a peculiar way of relating to others, were not interested in making friends, and had difficulty making socially appropriate conversation. Seventy-one percent of the parents indicated that often or very often their child was seen as warm and outgoing with family members and familiar adults.

Energy, confidence, sleep, and grades seen often and very often:

- 25% cited low energy level for no apparent reason (which could be sleep related) occurring often or very often.
- Little confidence or being self-conscious was seen 28% as occurring often or very often.
- Big change in normal sleeping habits: 36%.
- Big drop in grades or schoolwork: 43%.

CHILDREN'S NEUROPSYCHOLOGICAL HISTORY

The Children's Neuropsychological History provided demographic information about the parents as well as their child and the child's symptomatology. This measure was in use from 2006 to 2009 and replaced the Developmental History form. Fifty-one parents completed this form about their child providing historical and family information as well as their current and past symptoms. Symptoms were reported as historical, as new, or as both new and historical. Parents of adolescents reported more new symptoms that were different from the child sample suggesting reasons why they were seeking evaluation. Parents either saw new problems occurring that had not been seen before or an increase of problems seen prior to prompt them to get an evaluation for attention symptoms. The following are the parent responses to specific questions about their child's functioning in the following areas: problem solving, language (speech and math skills), spatial skills, concentration and awareness, memory, motor and coordination, sensory, physical issues, emotions, and behavior. Percentages are provided for new and old presence of symptoms. Very small percentages of items were indicated as both new and old; therefore, this category was not provided.

PROBLEM-SOLVING SYMPTOMS

Easily frustrated: 87% new and old symptoms
New = 16%
Old = 71%

Difficulty figuring how to do new things: 43% new and old symptoms
New = 6%
Old = 37%

Difficulty making decisions: 49% new and old symptoms
New = 12%
Old = 37%

Difficulty planning ahead: 73% new and old symptoms
New = 6%
Old = 67%

Difficulty solving problems that a younger child can do: 25% new and old symptoms
New = 4%
Old = 21%

Difficulty understanding explanations: 54% new and old symptoms
New = 6%
Old = 48%

Is slow to learn new things: 22% new and old symptoms
New = 6%
Old = 16%

Disorganized in his or her approach to problems: 73%
New = 6%
Old = 67%

Difficulty doing things in the right order: 37% new and old symptoms
New = 4%
Old = 33%

Difficulty verbally describing the steps involved in doing something: 41% new and old symptoms
New = 6%
Old = 35%

Difficulty completing an activity in a reasonable period of time: 65% new and old symptoms
New = 8%
Old = 57%

Difficulty changing a plan or activity when necessary: 42% new and old symptoms
New = 8%
Old = 34%

Difficulty switching from one activity to another activity: 26% new and old symptoms
  New = 4%
  Old = 22%

When compared to the child population using this measure, symptoms were generally similar excluding planning ahead that increased by 21% as a problem and being disorganized that increased by 17%.

SPEECH, LANGUAGE, AND MATH SKILLS

Difficulty speaking clearly: 14% new and old symptoms
  New = 2%
  Old = 12%

Difficulty finding the right word to say: 22% new and old symptoms
  New = 2%
  Old = 20%

Not talking: 8% new and old symptoms
  New = 4%
  Old = 4%

Rambles on and on without saying much: 18% new and old symptoms
  New = 2%
  Old = 16%

Jumps from one topic to another: 22% new and old symptoms
  New = 2%
  Old = 20%

Odd or unusual language or vocal sounds: 10% new and old symptoms
  New = 2%
  Old = 8%

Difficulty understanding what others are saying: 24% new and old symptoms
  New = 2%
  Old = 22%

Difficulty understanding what he or she is reading: 49% new and old symptoms
  New = 6%
  Old = 43%

Difficulty writing letters or words: 31% new and old symptoms
  New = 2%
  Old = 29%

Difficulty reading letters or words: 25% new and old symptoms
  New = 2%
  Old = 23%

Difficulty with spelling: 37% new and old symptoms
    New = 2%
    Old = 35%

Difficulty with math: 51% new and old symptoms
    New = 6%
    Old = 45%

When compared to the child population, adolescents had fewer problems with word retrieval, rambling, jumping topics, and reading. There was a decrease for finding the right word by 14%, rambling on decreased by 12%, jumping from one topic to another decreased by 15%, and difficulty reading letters or words decreased by 11%. However, adolescents had more difficulty with reading comprehension and math. Difficulty understanding what they have read increased by 19% and problems with math increased by 14%.

SPATIAL SKILLS SYMPTOMS

Confusion telling right from left: 42% new and old symptoms
    New = 0%
    Old = 42%

Has difficulty with puzzles, LEGO®s, blocks, or similar games: 10% new and old symptoms
    New = 0%
    Old = 10%

Problems drawing or copying: 12% new and old symptoms
    New = 2%
    Old = 10%

Doesn't know his or her colors: 2% new and old symptoms
    New = 0%
    Old = 2%

Difficulty dressing (not due to physical difficulty): 8% new and old symptoms
    New = 4%
    Old = 4%

Problems finding his or her way around places he or she has been to before: 4% new and old symptoms
    New = 0%
    Old = 4%

Difficulty recognizing objects: 2% new and old symptoms
    New = 2%
    Old = 0%

Seems unable to recognize facial or body expressions of disapproval or emotions: 8% new and old symptoms
    New = 2%
    Old = 6%

Gets lost easily: 6% new and old symptoms
New = 0%
Old = 6%

When compared to the child population, symptoms for adolescents were basically similar excluding right left confusion, which increased by 36%. The problem may have become more noticeable by adolescence.

CONCENTRATION AND AWARENESS

Easily distracted by sounds: 78% new and old symptoms
New = 4%
Old = 74%

Mind appears to go blank at times: 47% new and old symptoms
New = 4%
Old = 43%

Loses train of thought easily: 55% new and old symptoms
New = 2%
Old = 53%

Difficulty concentrating on what others say but sits in front of a TV for long periods: 60% new and old symptoms
New = 3%
Old = 57%

Attention starts out OK but can't keep it up: 74% new and old symptoms
New = 6%
Old = 68%

When compared to the child population, symptoms remained generally the same for adolescence; sustained attention issues increased by 8%.

MEMORY SYMPTOMS

Forgetting where he or she leaves things: 55% new and old symptoms
New = 2%
Old = 53%

Forgets events that happened quite recently: 29% new and old symptoms
New = 8%
Old = 21%

Forgets things that happened days/weeks ago: 37% new and old symptoms
New = 8%
Old = 29%

Forgets what he or she is supposed to be doing: 63% new and old symptoms
New = 8%
Old = 55%

Forgets names more than most people do: 10% new and old symptoms
    New = 2%
    Old = 8%

Forgets school assignments: 75% new and old symptoms
    New = 4%
    Old = 71%

Forgets instructions: 69% new and old symptoms
    New = 67%
    Old = 2%

When compared to the child population, there was an increase of 35% for the symptom of forgetting things that happened days or weeks ago. In this segment, forgotten school assignments increased by 29% and forgotten instructions by 12%. Forgetting things may be due to poor sleep and/or dislike of school.

MOTOR AND COORDINATION SYMPTOMS

Poor fine motor control skills: 28% new and old symptoms
    New = 26%
    Old = 2%

Clumsy: 20% new and old symptoms
    New = 0%
    Old = 20%

Weakness: 8% new and old symptoms
    New = 0%
    Old = 8%

Tremor: 8% new and old symptoms
    New = 4%
    Old = 4%

Muscle tics or spastic: 10% new and old symptoms
    New = 4%
    Old = 6%

Odd movements: 8% new and old symptoms
    New = 2%
    Old = 6%

Drops things more than most children: 6% new and old symptoms
    New = 0%
    Old = 6%

Has an unusual walk: 8% new and old symptoms
    New = 2%
    Old = 6%

Balance problems: 6% new and old symptoms
   New = 0%
   Old = 6%

When compared to the child population, symptoms remained fairly consistent. There was a 9% increase for muscle tics or spastic muscles for the adolescents. Poor fine motor skills revealed an increase of 8% when compared to the child population parental responses.

SENSORY SYMPTOMS

Needs to squint or move closer to page to read: 14% new and old symptoms
   New = 2%
   Old = 12%

Problems seeing objects: 8% new and old symptoms
   New = 2%
   Old = 6%

Loss of feeling: 2% new and old symptoms
   New = 2%
   Old = 0%

Problems hearing sounds: 4% new and old symptoms
   New = 0%
   Old = 4%

Difficulty telling hot from cold: 0% new and old symptoms
   New = 0%
   Old = 0%

Difficulty smelling odors: 2% new and old symptoms
   New = 0%
   Old = 2%

Difficulty tasting food: 0% new and old symptoms
   New = 0%
   Old = 0%

Overly sensitive to touch: 22% new and old symptoms
   New = 4%
   Old = 18%

When compared to the child population, most of the sensory issues were consistent with a few exceptions. Being overly sensitive to touch increased by 8%, needing to squint to see the page increased by 7%, and problems seeing objects increased by 6% for the adolescents.

PHYSICAL SYMPTOMS

Frequently complains of headaches or nausea: 39% new and old symptoms
   New = 6%
   Old = 33%

Has dizzy spells: 6% new and old symptoms
   New = 4%
   Old = 2%

Has pain in joints: 27% new and old symptoms
   New = 4%
   Old = 23%

Excessive tiredness: 36% new and old symptoms
   New = 19%
   Old = 17%

Frequent urination or drinking: 6% new and old symptoms
   New = 6%
   Old = 0%

When compared to the child population using this measure, three out of the four symptoms revealed an increase for the adolescents. Headache complaints increased by 12%, joint pain increased by 14%, and excessive tiredness increased by 21%. Frequent urination decreased by 11%.

BEHAVIOR SYMPTOMS

Aggressive: 40% new and old symptoms
   New = 18%
   Old = 22%

Attached to things, not people: 12% new and old symptoms
   New = 4%
   Old = 8%

Bizarre behavior: 10% new and old symptoms
   New = 6%
   Old = 4%

Resists change: 18% new and old symptoms
   New = 4%
   Old = 14%

Risk-taking: 26% new and old symptoms
   New = 6%
   Old = 20%

Self-mutilates: 18% new and old symptoms
   New = 8%
   Old = 10%

Self-stimulates: 8% new and old symptoms
   New = 6%
   Old = 2%

Swears a lot: 26% new and old symptoms
   New = 10%
   Old = 16%

When compared to the child population using this measure, behavioral symptoms remained generally consistent. Self-stimulation decreased by 7%, while swearing increased by 7% for the adolescents.

Daily Routine/Habits

Bed-wetting: 2% new and old symptoms
New = 0%
Old = 2%

Bowel movements in underwear: 4% new and old symptoms
New = 2%
Old = 2%

Eating habits are poor: 39% new and old symptoms
New = 6%
Old = 33%

Nightmares, night terrors, sleepwalks: 28% new and old symptoms
New = 6%
Old = 22%

Sleeping habits are poor: 24% new and old symptoms
New = 6%
Old = 18%

When compared to the child population, adolescents reported the general absence of enuresis down by 12%. Poor eating habits increased by 12%.

Emotions

Dependent: 20% new and old symptoms
New = 6%
Old = 14%

Depressed: 22% new and old symptoms
New = 16%
Old = 16%

Emotional: 37% new and old symptoms
New = 4%
Old = 33%

Fearful: 24% new and old symptoms
New = 2%
Old = 22%

Immature: 31% new and old symptoms
New = 2%
Old = 29%

Nervous: 22% new and old symptoms
New = 4%
Old = 18%

Quiet: 8% new and old symptoms
New = 0%
Old = 8%

Shy and withdrawn: 12% new and old symptoms
New = 2%
Old = 10%

Unmotivated: 39% new and old symptoms
New = 8%
Old = 31%

SUMMATION OF FINDINGS

When compared to the child population using this measure, there was a decrease in immaturity by 14% and increase in the problem of being unmotivated by 12% for the adolescents. Emotional and fearfulness were decreased by 9%.

Another way of looking at the parent responses on this measure is to discuss the primary symptoms in each category that they reported for their adolescent child.

Primary symptoms reported for problem solving include the following:

- 37% reported a historical problem of making decisions (12% reported as new symptom).
- 67% reported a historical problem of being disorganized in approach to problems (6% reported as new symptom).
- 48% reported a historical problem of difficulty understanding explanations (6% reported as new symptom).
- 57% reported a historical problem of difficulty completing an activity in a reasonable period of time (8% reported as new symptom).
- 71% reported a historical problem of becoming easily frustrated (16% reported as new symptom).

There was a substantial increase for new symptoms of making decisions and becoming easily frustrated.

Primary symptoms reported for speech, language, and math skills include the following:

- 43% reported a historical problem of difficulty understanding what they are reading (6% reported as new symptom).
- 45% reported a historical problem of math (6% reported as new symptom).

Primary nonverbal symptoms:

Parents did not report any significant nonverbal symptoms suggesting that ADD is not seen by parents as symptomatic of a nonverbal learning disorder.

Primary symptoms of concentration and awareness include the following:

- 74% reported a historical problem of becoming easily distracted (4% reported as new symptom).
- 53% reported a historical problem of easily losing train of thought (2% reported as new symptom).
- 57% reported a historical problem of difficulty concentrating (3% reported as new symptom).
- 68% reported a historical problem of poor sustained attention (6% reported as new symptom).

Primary symptoms of memory include the following:

- 53% reported a historical problem of forgetting things (2% reported as new symptom).
- 55% reported a historical problem of forgetting what they are supposed to be doing (8% reported as new symptom).
- 71% reported a historical problem of forgetting school assignments (4% reported as new symptom).
- 2% reported a historical problem of forgetting instructions (67% reported as new symptom).

Forgetting instructions as a new symptom showed the most significant increase.

Symptoms of motor and coordination include the following:

- 2% reported a historical problem of poor fine motor skills (26% reported as new symptom).

Poor fine motor skills showed a significant increase as a new symptom.

Symptoms of sensory problems:

There were no items reported occurring over 18% of the time suggesting that this is not an issue.

Physical symptoms include the following:

- 33% historical problem of headaches (6% reported as new symptom)
- 17% historical problem of excessive tiredness (19% reported as new symptom)

Excessive tiredness increased significantly as a new symptom.

Behavioral symptoms include the following:

- 22% historical problem of being aggressive (18% reported as new symptom)
- 16% historical problem of being depressed (16% reported as new symptom)
- 33% historical problem of poor eating habits (6% reported as new symptom)
- 33% historical problem of being emotional (4% reported as new symptom)
- 31% historical problem of being unmotivated (8% reported as new symptom)

Aggression (as an expression of depression) and depression increased substantially as new symptoms for adolescents.

Where the child population was referred due to historical symptoms or issues continuing to be problematic, the adolescent population was referred due to either new symptoms or an exacerbation of symptoms suggesting that this problem now needed to be addressed. This would explain why there are more newly reported symptoms in the adolescent population than the child population by the parents in completing this form.

PATIENT BEHAVIOR CHECKLIST

This is a checklist completed by 123 adolescents regarding their attention symptoms. Symptoms are rated for how much they disturb their everyday life.

Physical restlessness: 59% reported the symptom as present, and 29% as moderate to severe:
Not at all = 41%
Just a little = 30%
Pretty much = 19%
Very much = 10%

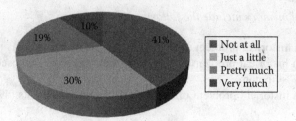

Mental restlessness: 74% reported the symptom as present, and 41% as moderate to severe:
Not at all = 26%
Just a little = 33%
Pretty much = 25%
Very much = 16%

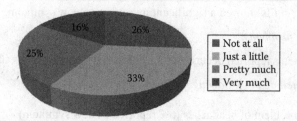

Easily distracted: 91% reported the symptom as present, and 76% as moderate to severe:
Not at all = 9%
Just a little = 15%
Pretty much = 37%
Very much = 39%

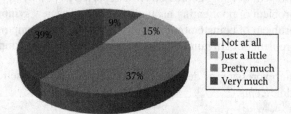

Impatient: 86% reported the symptom as present, and 63% as moderate to severe:
Not at all = 14%
Just a little = 23%
Pretty much = 31%
Very much = 32%

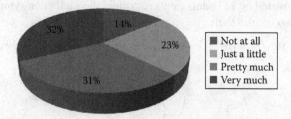

"Hot" or explosive temper: 69% reported the symptom as present, and 46% as moderate to severe:
    Not at all = 31%
    Just a little = 23%
    Pretty much = 27%
    Very much = 19%

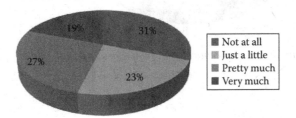

Unpredictable behavior: 62% reported the symptom as present, and 34% as moderate to severe:
    Not at all = 39%
    Just a little = 28%
    Pretty much = 17%
    Very much = 17%

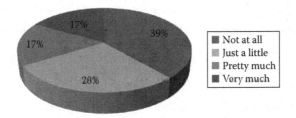

Difficulty completing tasks: 85% reported the symptom as present, and 53% as moderate to severe:
    Not at all = 15%
    Just a little = 32%
    Pretty much = 24%
    Very much = 29%

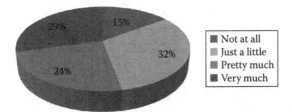

Shifting from one task to another: 80% reported the symptom as present, and 49% as moderate to severe:
    Not at all = 20%
    Just a little = 31%
    Pretty much = 28%
    Very much = 21%

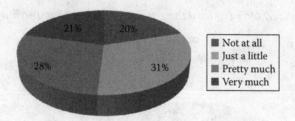

Difficulty sustaining attention: 83% reported the symptom as present, and 55% as moderate to severe:
    Not at all = 18%
    Just a little = 28%
    Pretty much = 27%
    Very much = 28%

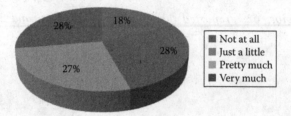

Impulsive: 69% reported the symptom as present, and 41% as moderate to severe:
    Not at all = 30%
    Just a little = 28%
    Pretty much = 23%
    Very much = 18%

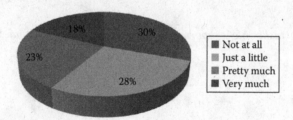

Talks too much: 71% reported the symptom as present, and 37% as moderate to severe:
    Not at all = 30%
    Just a little = 34%
    Pretty much = 26%
    Very much = 11%

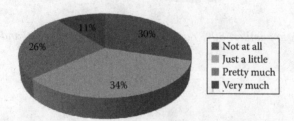

Difficulty doing tasks alone: 62% reported the symptom as present, and 28% as moderate to severe:
Not at all = 38%
Just a little = 34%
Pretty much = 14%
Very much = 14%

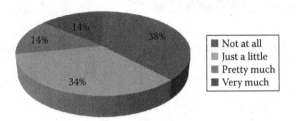

Often interrupts others: 60% reported the symptom as present, and 29% as moderate to severe:
Not at all = 40%
Just a little = 31%
Pretty much = 19%
Very much = 10%

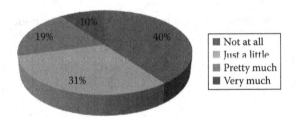

Doesn't appear to listen to others: 63% reported the symptom as present, and 31% as moderate to severe:
Not at all = 38%
Just a little = 32%
Pretty much = 20%
Very much = 11%

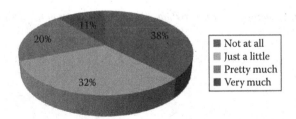

Loses a lot of things: 76% reported the symptom as present, and 39% as moderate to severe:
Not at all = 24%
Just a little = 37%
Pretty much = 19%
Very much = 20%

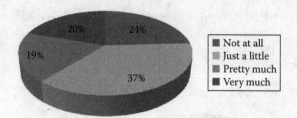

Forgets to do things: 91% reported the symptom as present, and 57% as moderate to severe:
Not at all = 10%
Just a little = 34%
Pretty much = 34%
Very much = 23%

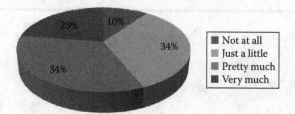

Engages in physically daring activities: 58% reported the symptom as present, and 34% as moderate to severe:
Not at all = 42%
Just a little = 24%
Pretty much = 17%
Very much = 17%

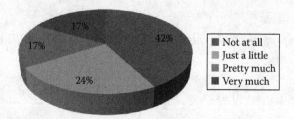

Always on the go, as if driven by a motor: 67% reported the symptom as present, and 37% as moderate to severe:
Not at all = 33%
Just a little = 30%
Pretty much = 17%
Very much = 20%

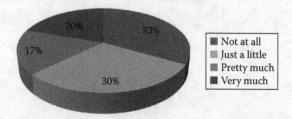

SUMMATION OF FINDINGS

The adolescents completed this checklist themselves regarding the presence of attention symptoms. *They reported the following primary attention symptoms:*

- Being easily distracted (91%).
- Impatient (86%), which likely reflects their agitation, and upset with themselves—a hot or explosive temper was seen 69%.
- Poor sustained attention (83%).
- Difficulty completing tasks (85%).
- Shifting from one task to another (80%).
- Forgetting to do things (91%).

Symptoms seen more often are those of becoming distracted and being frustrated with themselves pointing to an emotional reaction to feeling like they have failed or are disappointed in themselves as seen on the Beck inventory for depression.

BECK ANXIETY INVENTORY

This is an anxiety inventory completed by 28 adolescents. Symptoms are rated as nonexistent, mild, moderate, or severe.

Numbness or tingling: 7% indicate the symptom is present and 0% indicated moderate to severe presence:
Not at all = 93%
Mildly = 7%
Moderately = 0%
Severely = 0%

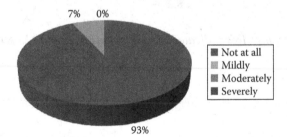

Feeling hot: 29% indicate the symptom is present and 8% indicated a moderate to severe presence:
Not at all = 68%
Mildly = 21%
Moderately = 4%
Severely = 4%

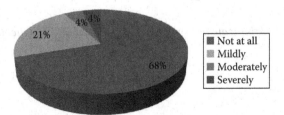

Wobbliness in legs: 26% indicate the symptom is present and 4% indicated moderate to severe presence:

    Not at all = 74%

    Mildly = 22%

    Moderately = 4%

    Severely = 0%

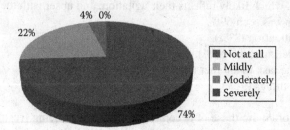

Unable to relax: 59% indicate the symptom is present and 26% indicated moderate to severe presence:

    Not at all = 41%

    Mildly = 33%

    Moderately = 15%

    Severely = 11%

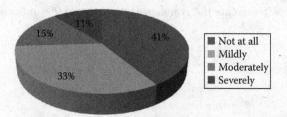

Fear of the worst happening: 48% indicate the symptom is present and 28% indicated moderate to severe presence:

    Not at all = 52%

    Mildly = 20%

    Moderately = 16%

    Severely = 12%

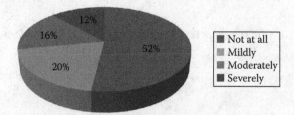

Dizzy or lightheaded: 44% indicate the symptom is present and 11% indicated moderate to severe presence:

    Not at all = 56%

    Mildly = 33%

    Moderately = 11%

    Severely = 0%

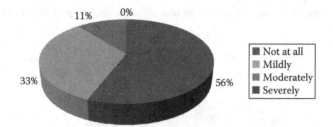

Heart pounding or racing: 41% indicate the symptom is present and 19% indicated moderate to severe presence:

    Not at all = 59%

    Mildly = 22%

    Moderately = 15%

    Severely = 4%

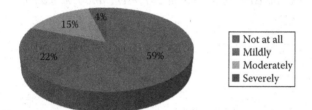

Unsteady: 26% indicate the symptom is present and 4% indicated moderate to severe presence:

    Not at all = 74%

    Mildly = 22%

    Moderately = 4%

    Severely = 0%

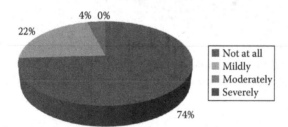

Terrified: 11% indicate the symptom is present and 7% indicated moderate to severe presence:

    Not at all = 89%

    Mildly = 4%

    Moderately = 7%

    Severely = 0%

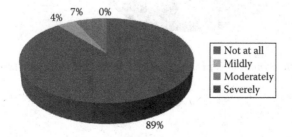

Nervous: 63% indicate the symptom is present and 30% indicated moderate to severe presence:
>   Not at all = 37%
>   Mildly = 33%
>   Moderately = 26%
>   Severely = 4%

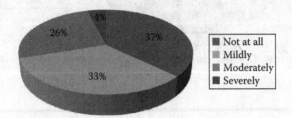

Feeling of choking: 4% indicate the symptom is present and 0% indicated moderate to severe presence:
>   Not at all = 96%
>   Mildly = 4%
>   Moderately = 0%
>   Severely = 0%

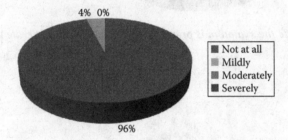

Hands trembling: 22% indicate the symptom is present and 11% indicated moderate to severe presence:
>   Not at all = 78%
>   Mildly = 11%
>   Moderately = 7%
>   Severely = 4%

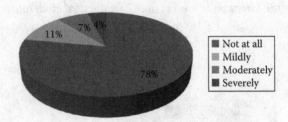

Shaky: 22% indicate the symptom is present and 11% indicated moderate to severe presence:
>   Not at all = 78%
>   Mildly = 11%
>   Moderately = 4%
>   Severely = 7%

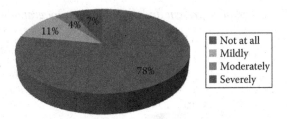

Fear of losing control: 34% indicate the symptom is present and 19% indicated moderate to severe presence:

    Not at all = 67%
    Mildly = 15%
    Moderately = 15%
    Severely = 4%

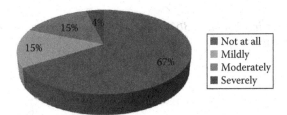

Difficulty breathing: 8% indicate the symptom is present and 4% indicated moderate to severe presence:

    Not at all = 93%
    Mildly = 4%
    Moderately = 4%
    Severely = 0%

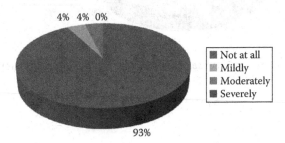

Fear of dying: 29% indicate the symptom is present and 7% indicated moderate to severe presence:

    Not at all = 70%
    Mildly = 22%
    Moderately = 7%
    Severely = 0%

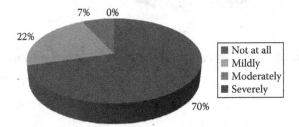

Scared: 35% indicate the symptom is present and 4% indicated moderate to severe presence:
   Not at all = 65%
   •Mildly = 31%
   Moderately = 4%
   Severely = 0%

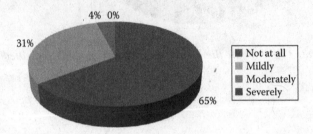

Indigestion or discomfort in abdomen: 30% indicate the symptom is present and 4% indicated moderate to severe presence:
   Not at all = 70%
   Mildly = 26%
   Moderately = 4%
   Severely = 0%

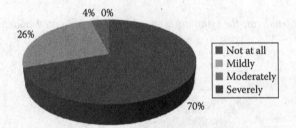

Faint: 7% indicate the symptom is present and 0% indicated moderate to severe presence:
   Not at all = 93%
   Mildly = 7%
   Moderately = 0%
   Severely = 0%

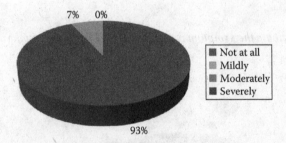

Face flushed: 4% indicate the symptom is present and 0% indicated moderate to severe presence:
   Not at all = 96%
   Mildly = 4%
   Moderately = 0%
   Severely = 0%

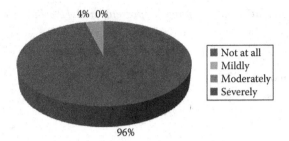

Sweating (not due to heat): 29% indicate the symptom is present and 7% indicated moderate to severe presence:
Not at all = 70%
Mildly = 22%
Moderately = 7%
Severely = 0%

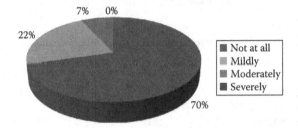

SUMMATION OF FINDINGS

While responding to other checklists on questions of anxiety, on this specific measure of anxiety, adolescents did not report as many symptoms. The following symptoms were seen more often or to a moderate to severe degree: inability to relax (26%), fear of the worst happening (28%), and nervousness (30%).

PHYSICAL COMPLAINTS CHECKLIST

Adolescents completed the Physical Complaints Checklist: 121 adolescents responded to this measure.

Headaches: 89 indicated the symptom as present, and 23% indicated as present daily to weekly:
Never = 11%
Less than 4× year = 20%
Less than once per month = 20%
Less than once per week = 26%
1–3 times per week = 14%
Nearly daily = 9%

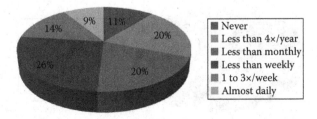

Trouble sleeping: 71 indicated the symptom as present, and 11% indicated as present daily to weekly:

Never = 29%

Less than 4× year = 19%

Less than once per month = 22%

Less than once per week = 19%

1–3 times per week = 5%

Nearly daily = 6%

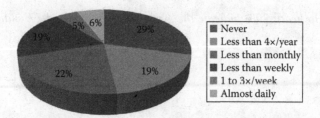

Irritable/nervous: 85 indicated the symptom as present, and 33% indicated as present daily to weekly:

Never = 16%

Less than 4× year = 15%

Less than once per month = 18%

Less than once per week = 19%

1–3 times per week = 11%

Nearly daily = 22%

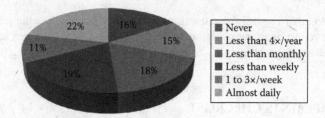

Stomach upset: 84 indicated the symptom as present, and 19% indicated as present daily to weekly:

Never = 16%

Less than 4× year = 19%

Less than once per month = 28%

Less than once per week = 18%

1–3 times per week = 12%

Nearly daily = 7%

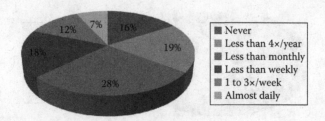

Aches and pains (not backache): 71 indicated the symptom as present, and 17% indicated as present daily to weekly:
  Never = 29%
  Less than 4× year = 19%
  Less than once per month = 21%
  Less than once per week = 14%
  1–3 times per week = 10%
  Nearly daily = 7%

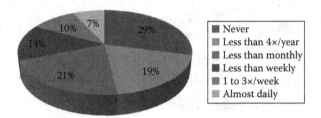

Backache: 62 indicated the symptom as present, and 16% indicated as present daily to weekly:
  Never = 39%
  Less than 4× year = 16%
  Less than once per month = 15%
  Less than once per week = 15%
  1–3 times per week = 9%
  Nearly daily = 7%

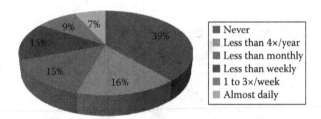

Rapid heartbeat: 48 indicated the symptom as present, and 6% indicated as present daily to weekly:
  Never = 52%
  Less than 4× year = 18%
  Less than once per month = 17%
  Less than once per week = 7%
  1–3 times per week = 4%
  Nearly daily = 2%

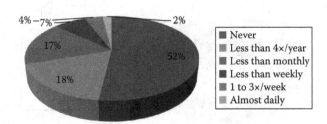

Dizziness/lightheadedness: 68 indicated the symptom as present, and 13% indicated as present daily to weekly:

    Never = 32%
    Less than 4× year = 26%
    Less than once per month = 20%
    Less than once per week = 9%
    1–3 times per week = 10%
    Nearly daily = 3%

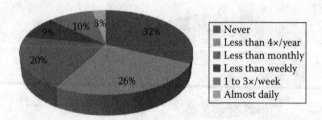

Vomiting, nausea: 53 indicated the symptom as present, and 2% indicated as present daily to weekly:

    Never = 47%
    Less than 4× year = 39%
    Less than once per month = 10%
    Less than once per week = 2%
    1–3 times per week = 2%
    Nearly daily = 0%

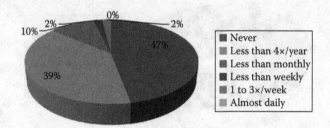

Diarrhea: 64 indicated the symptom as present, and 5% indicated as present daily to weekly:

    Never = 36%
    Less than 4× year = 34%
    Less than once per month = 21%
    Less than once per week = 4%
    1–3 times per week = 2%
    Nearly daily = 3%

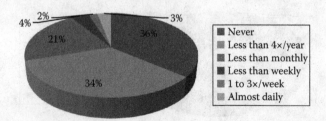

Constipation: 37 indicated the symptom as present, and 1% indicated as present daily to weekly:
  Never = 64%
  Less than 4× year = 21%
  Less than once per month = 13%
  Less than once per week = 2%
  1–3 times per week = 1%
  Nearly daily = 0%

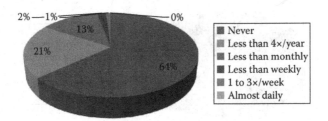

Weakness: 63 indicated the symptom as present, and 10% indicated as present daily to weekly:
  Never = 37%
  Less than 4× year = 25%
  Less than once per month = 17%
  Less than once per week = 11%
  1–3 times per week = 6%
  Nearly daily = 4%

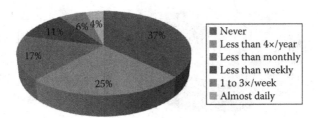

Tired during the day: 88 indicated the symptom as present, and 54% indicated as present daily to weekly:
  Never = 11%
  Less than 4× year = 3%
  Less than once per month = 15%
  Less than once per week = 16%
  1–3 times per week = 26%
  Nearly daily = 28%

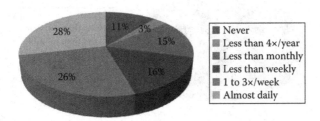

Poor appetite: 67 indicated the symptom as present, and 17% indicated as present daily to weekly:
Never = 33%
Less than 4× year = 21%
Less than once per month = 16%
Less than once per week = 13%
1–3 times per week = 8%
Nearly daily = 9%

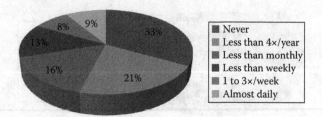

Blurred vision: 36 indicated the symptom as present, and 8% indicated as present daily to weekly:
Never = 63%
Less than 4× year = 16%
Less than once per month = 7%
Less than once per week = 5%
1–3 times per week = 4%
Nearly daily = 4%

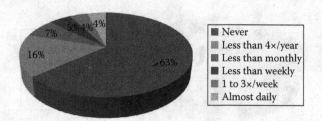

Dry mouth: 47 indicated the symptom as present, and 20% indicated as present daily to weekly:
Never = 53%
Less than 4× year = 12%
Less than once per month = 8%
Less than once per week = 7%
1–3 times per week = 11%
Nearly daily = 9%

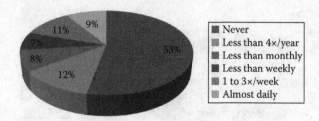

Confusion: 70 indicated the symptom as present, and 29% indicated as present daily to weekly:
Never = 30%
Less than 4× year = 15%
Less than once per month = 12%
Less than once per week = 14%
1–3 times per week = 13%
Nearly daily = 16%

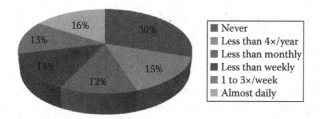

Summation of Findings

The more common complaints seen on a weekly basis are as follows:

- Headaches (23%)
- Confusion (29%)
- Being irritable or nervous (33%)

Tired during the day emerged with the highest frequency (54%). This may be the result of sleep deprivation associated with a lack of bedtime routine and poor time management.

BECK DEPRESSION INVENTORY

The individual is asked to respond to the following to describe their last 2 weeks. In this manner, this measure reports on symptoms of depression that are currently present. A total of 29 adolescents responded to this measure.

Sadness: 41% reported the symptom as present and 3% as moderate to severe:
59% indicated they do not feel sad.
38% indicated they feel sad much of the time.
3% indicated they are sad all the time.
0% indicated they are so sad or unhappy that they cannot stand it.

Pessimism: 48% reported the symptom as present, and 10% as moderate to severe:
52% indicated they are not discouraged about their future.
38% indicated they feel more discouraged about their future than they used to be.
7% indicated they do not expect things to work out for them.
3% indicated they feel that their future is hopeless and will only get worse.

Past failure: 62% reported the symptom as present, and 24% as moderate to severe:
38% indicated they do not feel like a failure.
38% indicated they have failed more than they should have.
17% indicated they look back and see a lot of failures.
7% indicated they feel a total failure.

Loss of pleasure: 31% reported the symptom as present, and 7% as moderate to severe:
    69% indicated they get as much pleasure as they ever did.
    24% indicated they don't enjoy things as much as they used to.
    7% indicated they get very little pleasure from things they enjoy.
    0% indicated they can't get any pleasure.

Guilty feelings: 34% reported the symptom as present, and 7% as moderate to severe:
    66% indicated they don't feel guilty.
    27% indicated they feel guilty over many things they have done.
    7% indicated they feel guilty most of the time.
    0% indicated they feel guilty all of the time.

Punishment feelings: 38% reported the symptom as present, and 31% as moderate to severe:
    62% indicated they don't feel they are being punished.
    7% indicated they feel they may be punished.
    17% indicated they expect to be punished.
    14% indicated they feel they are being punished.

Self-dislike: 31% reported the symptom as present, and 21% as moderate to severe:
    69% indicated they feel the same about themselves as ever.
    10% indicated they have lost confidence in themselves.
    21% indicated they are disappointed in themselves.
    0% indicated they dislike themselves.

Self-criticalness: 46% reported the symptom as present, and 14% as moderate to severe:
    54% indicated they don't criticize or blame themselves more than usual.
    32% indicated they are more critical of themselves than they used to be.
    7% indicated they criticize themselves for all of their faults.
    7% indicated they blame themselves for everything bad that happens.

Suicidal thoughts or wishes: 31% reported the symptom as present, and 7% as moderate to severe:
    69% indicated they don't have any thoughts of killing themselves.
    24% indicated they have thoughts of killing themselves but would not carry them out.
    7% indicated they would like to kill themselves.
    0% indicated they would kill themselves if they had the chance.

Crying: 37% reported the symptom as present, and 20% as moderate to severe:
    62% indicated they do not cry anymore like they used to.
    17% indicated they cry more than they used to.
    17% indicated they cry over every little thing.
    3% indicated they feel like crying but they can't.

Agitation: 57% reported the symptom as present, and 25% as moderate to severe:
    43% indicated they are no more restless or wound up than usual.
    32% indicated they feel more restless or wound up than usual.
    14% indicated they are so restless or agitated that it is hard to stay still.
    11% indicated they are so restless or agitated that they have to keep moving or doing something.

Loss of interest: 25% reported the symptom as present, and 7% as moderate to severe:
  75% indicated they have not lost interest in other people or activities.
  18% indicated they are less interested in other people or things than before.
  7% indicated they have lost most of their interest in other people or things.
  0% indicated they that it is hard to get interested in anything.

Indecisiveness: 47% reported the symptom as present, and 18% as moderate to severe:
  53% indicated they make decisions about as well as ever.
  29% indicated they find it more difficult to make decisions than usual.
  11% indicated they have much greater difficulty in making decisions than they used to.
  7% indicated they have trouble making any decisions.

Worthlessness: 25% reported the symptom as present, and 14% as moderate to severe:
  75% indicated they do not feel they are worthless.
  11% indicated they don't consider themselves as worthwhile and useful as they used to.
  14% indicated they feel more worthless as compared to other people.
  0% indicated they feel utterly worthless.

Loss of energy: 39% reported the symptom as present, and 14% as moderate to severe:
  61% indicated they have as much energy as ever.
  25% indicated they have less energy than they used to have.
  3% indicated they don't have enough energy to do very much.
  11% indicated they don't have enough energy to do anything.

Changes in sleeping pattern: 62% reported the symptom as present, and 21% as moderate to severe:
  37% indicated they have not experienced any change in their sleeping pattern.
  19% indicated they sleep somewhat more than usual.
  22% indicated they sleep somewhat less than usual.
  7% indicated they sleep a lot more than usual.
  11% indicated they sleep most of the day.
  3% indicated they wake up 1–2 h early and can't get back to sleep.

Irritability: 49% reported the symptom as present, and 30% as moderate to severe:
  52% indicated they are no more irritable than usual.
  19% indicated they are more irritable than usual.
  19% indicated they are much more irritable than usual.
  11% indicated they are irritable all the time.

Changes in appetite: 49% reported the symptom as present, and 10% as moderate to severe:
  50% indicated they have not experienced any change in appetite.
  14% indicated that their appetite is somewhat less than usual.
  25% indicated that their appetite is somewhat greater than usual.
  7% indicated that their appetite is much less than before.
  3% indicated that their appetite is much greater than usual.
  0% indicated they have no appetite at all.
  0% indicated they crave food all the time.

Concentration difficulty: 67% reported the symptom as present, and 46% as moderate to severe:
  32% indicated they cannot concentrate as well as ever.
  21% indicated they can't concentrate as well as usual.
  32% indicated that it is hard to keep their mind on anything for very long.
  14% indicated that they find they cannot concentrate on anything.

Tiredness or fatigue: 38% reported the symptom as present, and 6% as moderate to severe:
    61% indicated that they are no more tired or fatigued than usual.
    32% indicated they get more tired or fatigued more easily than usual.
    3% indicated that they are too tired or fatigued to do a lot of the things they used to do.
    3% indicated they are too tired or fatigued to do most of the things they used to do.

Loss of interest in sex: 0% reported the symptom as present, and 0% as moderate to severe:
    100% indicated they have not noticed any recent change in their interest in sex.
    0% indicated they are less interested in sex than they used to be.
    0% indicated they are much less interested in sex now.
    0% indicated they have lost interest in sex completely.

SUMMATION OF FINDINGS

Symptom severity: symptoms reported as moderate to severe are as follows:

- 31% reported feeling like they were being punished.
- 30% reported feeling irritable most of the time.
- 46% reported an inability to concentrate.

Symptoms reported more often are as follows:

- Concentration difficulty: 67%
- Past failure: 62%
- Change in sleep pattern: 62%
- Agitation: 57%

Adolescent responses to this measure support other reports of depression including parental descriptions. Depression and anger are equivalent suggesting that some of the behavioral issues of agitation and irritability that may be related to depression are seen in the adolescents and presenting as symptoms of defiance and loss of interest noted by the parents.

PERSONAL PROBLEMS CHECKLIST FOR ADOLESCENTS

This checklist had 183 adolescent responders. Adolescents were to indicate their concerns about a number of areas: social, appearance, attitude/opinions, family/home, school, money, religion, emotions, health/habits, and job.

Social:

- Being criticized by others: 31%
- Feeling uncomfortable in social settings: 17%
- Being shy: 25%
- Not having close friends: 15%
- Being taken advantage of by friends: 18%
- Not having anyone to share interests with:11%
- Feeling lonely: 25%
- Feeling unpopular: 21%
- Feeling uncomfortable when talking to people: 8%
- Feeling like people are against me: 17%
- Being let down by friends: 20%
- Feeling different from everyone else: 25%

Appearance:

- Having physical handicap: 6%
- Being too thin: 6%
- Looking too young or too old: 9%
- Looking too plain: 9%
- Not being clean and well-groomed: 5%
- Having scars: 10%
- Not being well-developed: 8%

Attitude/opinion:

- Having a poor attitude about everything: 29%
- Having no opinions about anything: 6%
- Having different opinions than others: 26%
- Having a poor attitude toward school: 42%
- Having a poor attitude toward self: 26%

Family/home:

- Brother or sister being sick: 6%
- Brother or sister having emotional problems: 7%
- Brother or sister having problem with drugs: 3%
- Brother or sister having problem with alcohol: 3%
- Being physically abused at home: 2%
- Being sexually abused at home: 1%
- Arguing with brother or sister: 32%
- Brother or sister stealing: 6%
- Being bothered by brother or sister: 28%
- Having problems with relatives: 9%
- Not having any privacy: 28%
- Not feeling close to family: 10%
- Not getting along with neighbors: 7%
- Home being dirty or run-down: 3%
- Family having a bad neighborhood: 3%
- Living in a bad neighborhood: 2%
- Not being allowed to use the car: 8%
- Not being allowed to buy a car: 6%

School:

- Getting bad grades: 68%
- Not getting along with teachers: 36%
- Not having good study habits: 59%
- Taking the wrong courses: 7%
- Not qualifying for clubs or teams: 10%
- Not having close friends at school: 12%
- School being too large: 7%
- Not understanding class material: 34%
- Not getting along with other students: 10%
- Not being interested in school: 36%

- Having a language problem in school: 3%
- Being in the wrong school: 8%
- Teachers not being interested in students: 9%
- Being bored in school: 52%
- Getting in trouble in school: 26%
- School being too far from home: 4%
- Worrying about future job or college: 30%

Money:

- Not making enough money: 27%
- Not having a steady income: 10%
- Having to spend savings: 6%
- Wasting money: 33%
- Lending money to friends or relatives: 9%
- Having to give money to parents: 7%
- Not having enough money to date: 6%
- Not having gas money: 4%

Religion:

- Feeling guilty about religion: 7%
- Not having any religious beliefs: 7%
- Arguing with parents about religious beliefs: 4%
- Failing in religious beliefs: 4%
- Boyfriend/girlfriend having a different religion: 3%
- Arguing with boyfriend/girlfriend about religion: 2%
- Not being able to get to church: 10%
- Chores interfering with church activities: 2%
- Job interfering with church activities: 2%
- Being upset by religious beliefs of others: 4%
- Being rejected by church members: 2%
- Not having friends at church: 8%

Emotions:

- Feeling anxious or uptight: 29%
- Being afraid of things: 27%
- Having the same thought over and over again: 31%
- Being tired and having no energy: 25%
- Feeling depressed or sad: 36%
- Having trouble concentrating: 58%
- Not remembering things: 53%
- Having nightmares: 9%
- Being afraid of hurting: 7%
- Feeling things are unreal: 7%
- Worrying about having a nervous breakdown: 6%
- Not being able to relax: 25%
- Not having any enjoyment in life: 9%
- Being influenced by others: 9%
- Behaving in strange ways: 10%

Health/habits:

- Not having any appetite: 7%
- Eating binges: 6%
- Frequently throwing up: 2%
- Using alcohol: 4%
- Using drugs: 4%
- Not getting enough exercise: 22%
- Not being able to sleep: 35%
- Having poor eating habits: 34%
- Having a physical problem: 5%
- Having a long-term illness: 2%
- Often being sick: 7%
- Being unhappy with doctors: 6%
- Not having any hobbies: 8%
- Not having time for interests and hobbies: 10%

Job:

- Not having a job: 32%
- Job not paying enough: 8%
- Disliking type of job: 10%
- Job being dirty: 4%
- Disliking fellow employees: 2%
- Being disliked by coworkers: 2%
- Being afraid of failing on the job: 6%
- Being afraid of being fired or laid off: 4%
- Not wanting to work: 10%
- Lacking transportation to work: 4%
- Working in unsafe conditions: 2%
- Lacking supervision on the job: 2%
- Boss being critical or unfair: 5%
- Having arguments on the job: 3%
- Working too many hours: 2%
- Job creating health problems: 2%
- Job having no future: 6%
- Being bored with job: 9%
- Lacking experience needed to get a job: 7%

SUMMATION OF FINDINGS

This is a self-report measure completed by adolescents regarding their concerns, not necessarily problems that are currently present, but concerns or worries that they have over certain issues. Problem areas are organized into individual groups of symptoms for the adolescent to read and check off what applies to them. Symptoms reported by adolescents confirm parental concerns.

Two-thirds reported bad grades.

One-half and above reported poor study habits, being bored in school, difficulty concentrating, and not remembering things.

One-third and above reported a poor attitude toward school, not getting along with teachers, not being interested in school, not understanding class material, wasting money, feeling sad or depressed, poor eating habits, and not able to sleep.

10 Results of the Adult Self-Report Measures/ Checklists

The total sample size was 1296 adults from the age of 15–80 years, respondents 36% males compared to 64% females. Of these, 75% were diagnosed with ADHD inattentive type and 25% with ADHD plus an additional disorder.

The following pages reveal the statistics on the numerous checklists that were administered. Checklists given to the adults to complete regarding their own symptoms are listed in the following:

- Physical Complaints Checklist
- Beck Depression Inventory
- Patient Behavior Checklist
- Beck Anxiety Inventory
- Quality of Life Inventory
- Personal Problems Checklist for Adults
- Sleep Disorders Questionnaire
- Adult Neuropsychological Questionnaire

ADULTS COMPLETING THE PHYSICAL COMPLAINTS CHECKLIST

1112 adults responded to this measure asking about their physical complaints.

Headaches: 93% reported as present, and 31% indicated as present daily to weekly

- 8% reported never.
- 21% report less than four times per year.
- 22% reported less than once per month.
- 19% reported less than once per week.
- 22% reported 1–3 times per week.
- 9% reported nearly daily.

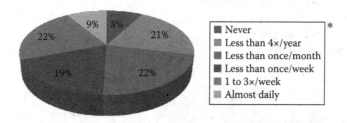

---

* The pie graphs range from 99 to 100 to 101 due to rounding.

Trouble sleeping: 88% reported as present, and 47% indicated as present daily to weekly

- 11% reported never.
- 12% report less than four times per year.
- 15% reported less than once per month.
- 14% reported less than once per week.
- 26% reported 1–3 times per week.
- 21% reported nearly daily.

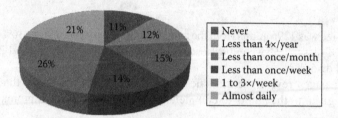

Irritable/nervous: 96% reported as present and 62% indicated as present daily to weekly

- 4% reported never.
- 8% report less than four times per year.
- 11% reported less than once per month.
- 15% reported less than once per week.
- 32% reported 1–3 times per week.
- 30% reported nearly daily.

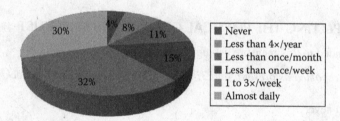

Stomach upset: 85% reported as present, and 27% indicated as present daily to weekly

- 14% reported never.
- 20% report less than four times per year.
- 21% reported less than once per month.
- 17% reported less than once per week.
- 17% reported 1–3 times per week.
- 10% reported nearly daily.

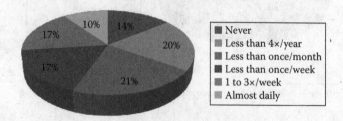

Aches and pains (not backache): 85% reported as present, and 27% indicated as present daily to weekly

- 16% reported never.
- 22% report less than four times per year.
- 20% reported less than once per month.
- 16% reported less than once per week.
- 13% reported 1–3 times per week.
- 14% reported nearly daily.

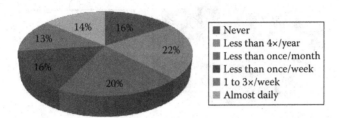

Backache: 82% reported as present, and 29% indicated as present daily to weekly

- 18% reported never.
- 20% report less than four times per year.
- 19% reported less than once per month.
- 14% reported less than once per week.
- 16% reported 1–3 times per week.
- 13% reported nearly daily.

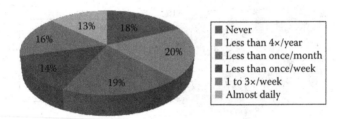

Rapid heartbeat: 62% reported as present, and 17% indicated as present daily to weekly

- 38% reported never.
- 20% report less than four times per year.
- 13% reported less than once per month.
- 12% reported less than once per week.
- 12% reported 1–3 times per week.
- 5% reported nearly daily.

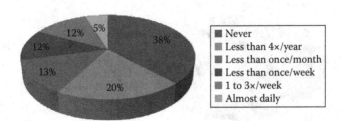

Dizziness/lightheadedness: 69% reported as present, and 15% indicated as present daily to weekly

- 31% reported never.
- 26% report less than four times per year.
- 17% reported less than once per month.
- 11% reported less than once per week.
- 10% reported 1–3 times per week.
- 5% reported nearly daily.

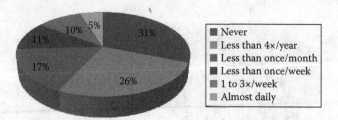

Vomiting and nausea: 50% reported as present, and 5% indicated as present daily to weekly

- 50% reported never.
- 34% report less than four times per year.
- 8% reported less than once per month.
- 3% reported less than once per week.
- 4% reported 1–3 times per week.
- 1% reported nearly daily.

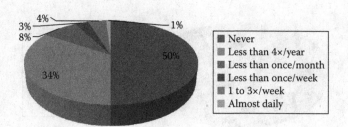

Diarrhea: 76% reported as present, and 9% indicated as present daily to weekly

- 23% reported never.
- 32% report less than four times per year.
- 23% reported less than once per month.
- 12% reported less than once per week.
- 7% reported 1–3 times per week.
- 2% reported nearly daily.

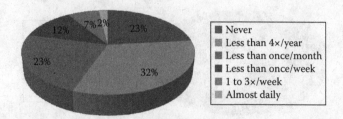

Constipation: 64% reported as present, and 9% indicated as present daily to weekly

- 37% reported never.
- 30% report less than four times per year.
- 18% reported less than once per month.
- 7% reported less than once per week.
- 5% reported 1–3 times per week.
- 4% reported nearly daily.

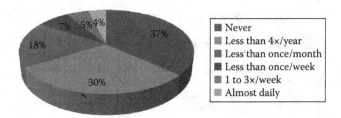

Weakness: 66% reported as present, and 15% indicated as present daily to weekly

- 34% reported never.
- 25% report less than four times per year.
- 16% reported less than once per month.
- 10% reported less than once per week.
- 10% reported 1–3 times per week.
- 5% reported nearly daily.

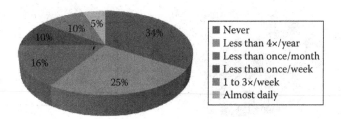

Tired during the day: 94% reported as present, and 64% indicated as present daily to weekly

- 6% reported never.
- 6% report less than four times per year.
- 9% reported less than once per month.
- 15% reported less than once per week.
- 31% reported 1–3 times per week.
- 33% reported nearly daily.

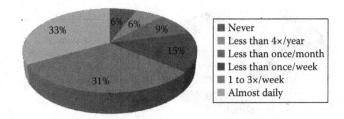

Poor appetite: 57% reported as present, and 16% indicated as present daily to weekly

- 42% reported never.
- 20% report less than four times per year.
- 12% reported less than once per month.
- 9% reported less than once per week.
- 9% reported 1–3 times per week.
- 7% reported nearly daily.

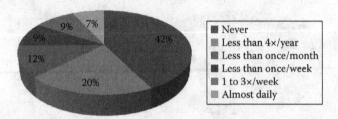

Blurred vision: 42% reported as present, and 12% indicated as present daily to weekly

- 58% reported never.
- 16% report less than four times per year.
- 7% reported less than once per month.
- 7% reported less than once per week.
- 6% reported 1–3 times per week.
- 6% reported nearly daily.

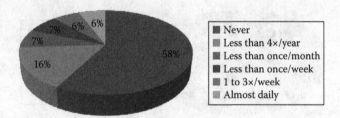

Dry mouth: 56% reported as present, and 21% indicated as present daily to weekly

- 45% reported never.
- 14% report less than four times per year.
- 11% reported less than once per month.
- 10% reported less than once per week.
- 9% reported 1–3 times per week.
- 12% reported nearly daily.

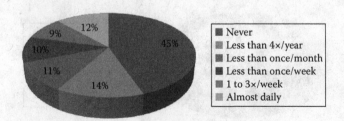

Confusion: 74% reported as present, and 37% indicated as present daily to weekly

- 25% reported never.
- 12% report less than four times per year.
- 11% reported less than once per month.
- 14% reported less than once per week.
- 16% reported 1–3 times per week.
- 21% reported nearly daily.

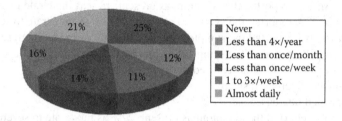

SUMMATION OF FINDINGS

A large sample of adults completed this measure asking them about common physical symptoms. The primary symptom(s) reported by almost two-thirds of the adults was anxiety and daytime fatigue. The next most often reported symptom was sleep problems. Confusion was indicated over one-third of the time. Other symptoms that were less common but still frequently reported were headaches, backaches, and/or stomach upset.

Symptoms reported one to three times per week to daily:

- 64% or almost two-thirds reported being tired during the day 1–3 times per week to daily.
- 62% or over half reported being irritable or nervous 1–3 times per week to daily.
- 47% or almost half reported trouble sleeping 1–3 times per week to daily.
- 37% or one-third reported confusion 1–3 times per week to daily.
- 31% or one-third reported headaches 1–3 times per week to daily.
- 29% reported backaches 1–3 times per week to daily.
- 27% reported stomach upset 1–3 times per week to daily.
- 27% reported aches and pains (not backaches) 1–3 times per week to daily.

In comparing the adult to the adolescent responses on this checklist, specific symptoms increase. Although the adolescent had a far smaller sample, the trend is reported as follows:

- Adults reported trouble sleeping 36% more than the adolescents.
- Being irritable and nervous was reported 29% more than the adolescents.

BECK DEPRESSION INVENTORY

Adults completed four measures to address emotional symptoms: a depression inventory, anxiety inventory, checklist of problem areas, and quality of life scale. This is a measure of depression completed by 113 adults. The individual is asked to respond to the following inventory of symptoms to describe their last 2 weeks. In this manner, this measure reports on symptoms of depression that are currently present:

- *Sadness*: 53% reported the symptom as present, 7% as moderate to severe.
- *Pessimism*: 58% reported the symptom as present, 11% as moderate to severe.
- *Past failure*: 62% reported the symptom as present, 30% as moderate to severe.

- *Loss of pleasure*: 59% reported the symptom as present, 15% as moderate to severe.
- *Guilty feelings*: 44% reported the symptom as present, 12% as moderate to severe.
- *Punishment feelings*: 23% reported the symptom as present, 11% as moderate to severe.
- *Self-dislike*: 53% reported the symptom as present, 28% as moderate to severe.
- *Self-critical*: 55% reported the symptom as present, 20% as moderate to severe.
- *Suicidal thoughts or wishes*: 21% reported the symptom as present, 1% as moderate to severe.
- *Crying*: 30% reported the symptom as present, 12% as moderate to severe.
- *Agitation*: 56% reported the symptom as present, 16% as moderate to severe.
- *Loss of interest*: 51% reported the symptom as present, 18% as moderate to severe.
- *Indecisiveness*: 53% reported the symptom as present, 23% as moderate to severe.
- *Worthlessness*: 36% reported the symptom as present, 14% as moderate to severe.
- *Loss of energy*: 71% reported the symptom as present, 20% as moderate to severe.
- *Changes in sleep pattern*: 63% reported the symptom as present.
  - 30% indicated increased sleep.
  - 34% indicated decreased sleep.
- *Irritability*: 63% reported the symptom as present, 22% as moderate to severe.
- *Changes in appetite*: 48% reported the symptom as present.
  - 27% reported decreased appetite.
  - 21% reported increased appetite.
- *Concentration difficulty*: 77% reported the symptom as present, 47% as moderate to severe.
- *Tiredness or fatigue*: 61% reported the symptom as present, 24% as moderate to severe.
- *Loss of interest in sex*: 39% reported the symptom as present, 19% as moderate to severe.

SUMMATION OF FINDINGS

Symptoms reported as moderate to severe one-fourth or more of the time:

- Past failure
- Self-dislike
- Increased sleep
- Decreased appetite

Symptoms reported almost one-third or more of the time:

- Decreased sleep

Symptoms reported almost one-half of the time:

- Poor concentration

Depression as seen in the ADD-diagnosed adult is more mild than severe but just enough to make life less enjoyable. Adults reported mild symptoms in many areas of depression. Most notable from the Beck inventory was the report of sadness, pessimism, feelings of failure, loss of pleasure, self-dislike and loss of confidence, being critical, feeling more wound up and agitated, indecisive, loss of interest, less energy, more irritable, and tired as well as a lack of concentration.

Symptoms seen more often:

- 77% reported problems with concentration.
- 71% reported diminished energy.
- 63% reported feeling more irritable.
- 63% reported change in sleep pattern.

- 62% reported awareness of past failure.
- 61% reported tiredness or fatigue.
- 58% reported feeling pessimistic about the future.
- 56% reported feeling more agitated.
- 55% reported feeling more critical of themselves.
- 53% reported feeling sad.
- 53% reported some self-dislike and loss of confidence.
- 53% reported more indecisiveness.
- 51% reported a loss of interest.

The presence of depression is seen as secondary to the lifelong attention problems. Symptoms are mild, not severe, although pervasively present, suggesting more of a reaction to life being more difficult or things not proceeding as planned. Symptoms seem to be the result of a lifetime struggle with attention issues and gradual increase in frustration over time. Symptoms of depression increased when sleep deprivation and/or insomnia or other sleep issues were present.

Mild depression symptoms:

- *Sadness*: Almost one-half or 46% of adults indicated feeling sad much of the time (as opposed to a more severe picture of feeling sad all of the time).
- *Pessimism*: Almost one-half or 47% of adults indicated feeling more discouraged about their future than they used to be (the term "used to be" as opposed to deeper emotions of not expecting things to work out or seeing the future as hopeless).
- *Loss of energy*: One-half or 51% of the time adults indicated that they had less energy than they use to feel. Either not having as much energy or the more severe picture of not having enough energy to do very much or anything at all was reported in over two-thirds of the population or 71% of the time.
- *Feelings of past failure*: Reported by 32% or almost one-third of the population. However, when the symptoms are combined with deeper feelings of failure, the percentage increases to 62% of the population and over one-half. In other words, over one-half of the adult population reported some feelings of failure.
- *Loss of pleasure*: Over one-third or 44% of the adult population indicated that they did not enjoy things as much as they used to. When combining the more serious symptoms of experiencing no pleasure or very little pleasure, the percentage increased to 59% or two-thirds of the population, meaning that two-thirds of the population reported some loss of pleasure.
- *Self-criticalness*: Seen one-third of the time or 35% of the adult population, and if all levels of severity of self-criticalness were reported, this would suggest that one-half of the population struggles with a form of this symptom or 55%.
- *Agitation*: Which could be related to anxiety or poor sleep was reported in over one-third of the adult population (40%) indicated feeling more restless or wound up than usual. However, if the additional two severity rankings are added to this item, the percentage would be 56, or slightly more than half of the population had some form of agitated feelings.
- *Loss of energy*: Which may be related directly to poor sleep was present in its mildest form, one-half or 51% of the time, in response to the question of less energy than they used to have. Adding in the more severe rankings of not having enough energy to do much or anything at all resulted in this symptom being seen in over two-thirds or 71% of the adult population.

- *Some type of sleep issue*: Seen in 63% or almost two-thirds of the adult population whether it was sleeping more or sleeping less or sleeping during the day and/or waking up too early.
- *Irritability*: Seen in 39% or a little over two-thirds of the time as reported by the adult population. When adding in reports of more severe irritability (more than usual to all of the time), the percentage increased to 63% or almost two-thirds.
- *Changes in appetite*: Whether it was wanting to eat more or less, having no appetite, or craving food, this symptom was present 48% or almost one-half of the time in the adult population.
- *Difficulty with concentration*: To a mild degree was noted to occur 30% or slightly less than one-third of the time. However, adding in the greater severity levels of having difficulty keeping their mind on anything for long or no ability to concentrate, this problem appeared 77% of the time or was reported by over two-thirds of the adult population.
- *Reporting tiredness or fatigue*: Resulted in 38% or one-third of the adult population reporting that they did not have a problem with fatigue; however, a second third or 37% felt that they were more tired or fatigued than usual. If all fatigue descriptors are used, then 61% or almost two-thirds indicated some type of fatigue.

Symptoms reported as getting worse over time:

When compared to the adolescent population (although a smaller sample), the following symptoms increased by more than 20%:

- Loss of pleasure
- Self-dislike
- Loss of interest
- Loss of energy (this was a 32% increase)
- Tiredness or fatigue
- Loss of sexual interest (this was a 39% increase)

The following symptoms increased by 10%–20% when compared to the adolescents:

- Sadness
- Pessimism
- Guilty feelings
- Worthlessness
- Irritability
- Concentration

Decrease of 10%–20% when compared to adolescents

- Punishment feelings
- Suicidal thoughts

PATIENT BEHAVIOR CHECKLIST

A large sample of adults completed this measure; 1195 responded to questions regarding their behavior and indicated the following:

Physical restlessness: 86% reported the symptom as present and 48% as moderate to severe.
   14% indicated not at all.
   38% indicated just a little.
   33% indicated pretty much.
   15% indicated very much.

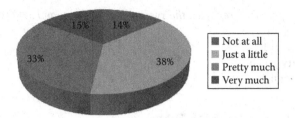

Mental restlessness: 91% reported the symptom as present and 73% as moderate to severe.

9% indicated not at all.

18% indicated just a little.

38% indicated pretty much.

35% indicated very much.

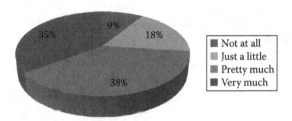

Easily distracted: 97% reported the symptom as present, and 83% as moderate to severe.

3% indicated not at all.

14% indicated just a little.

36% indicated pretty much.

47% indicated very much.

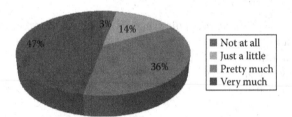

Impatient: 76% reported the symptom as present, and 37% as moderate to severe.

24% indicated not at all.

39% indicated just a little.

20% indicated pretty much.

17% indicated very much.

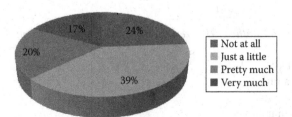

"Hot" or explosive temper: 76% reported the symptom as present, and 37% as moderate to severe.
    24% indicated not at all.
    39% indicated just a little.
    20% indicated pretty much.
    17% indicated very much.

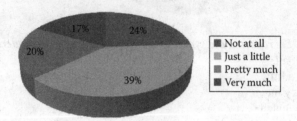

Unpredictable behavior: 68% reported the symptom as present, and 38% as moderate to severe.
    32% indicated not at all.
    40% indicated just a little.
    18% indicated pretty much.
    10% indicated very much.

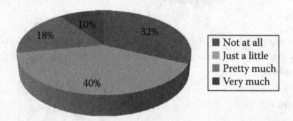

Difficulty completing tasks: 89% reported the symptom as present, and 65% as moderate to severe.
    11% indicated not at all.
    24% indicated just a little.
    30% indicated pretty much.
    35% indicated very much.

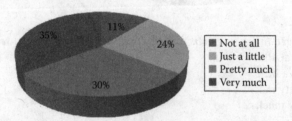

Shifting from one task to another: 91% reported the symptom as present, and 73% as moderate to severe.
    9% indicated not at all.
    18% indicated just a little.
    31% indicated pretty much.
    42% indicated very much.

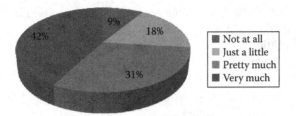

Difficulty sustaining attention: 94% reported the symptom as present, and 75% as moderate to severe.

6% indicated not at all.

19% indicated just a little.

35% indicated pretty much.

40% indicated very much.

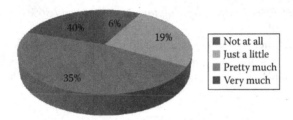

Impulsive: 87% reported the symptom as present, and 56% as moderate to severe.

14% indicated not at all.

31% indicated just a little.

30% indicated pretty much.

26% indicated very much.

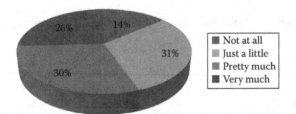

Talks too much: 65% reported the symptom as present, and 35% as moderate to severe.

35% indicated not at all.

30% indicated just a little.

20% indicated pretty much.

15% indicated very much.

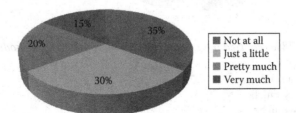

Difficulty doing tasks alone: 62% reported the symptom as present, and 32% as moderate to severe.
   39% indicated not at all.
   30% indicated just a little.
   21% indicated pretty much.
   11% indicated very much.

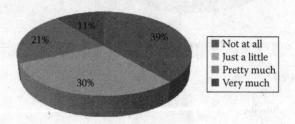

Often interrupts others: 76% reported the symptom as present, and 36% as moderate to severe.
   24% indicated not at all.
   40% indicated just a little.
   23% indicated pretty much.
   13% indicated very much.

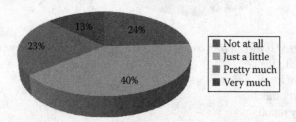

Doesn't appear to listen to others: 80% reported the symptom as present, and 44% as moderate to severe.
   20% indicated not at all.
   36% indicated just a little.
   27% indicated pretty much.
   17% indicated very much.

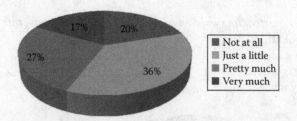

Loses a lot of things: 78% reported the symptom as present, and 47% as moderate to severe.
   23% indicated not at all.
   31% indicated just a little.
   24% indicated pretty much.
   23% indicated very much.

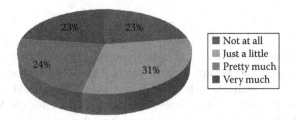

Forgets to do things: 91% reported the symptom as present, and 61% as moderate to severe.
9% indicated not at all.
30% indicated just a little.
32% indicated pretty much.
29% indicated very much.

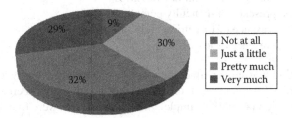

Engages in physically daring activities: 47% reported the symptom as present, and 20% as moderate to severe.
53% indicated not at all.
27% indicated just a little.
13% indicated pretty much.
7% indicated very much.

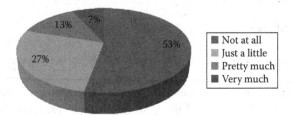

Always on the go, as if driven by a motor: 74% reported the symptom as present, and 48% as moderate to severe.
26% indicated not at all.
26% indicated just a little.
25% indicated pretty much.
23% indicated very much.

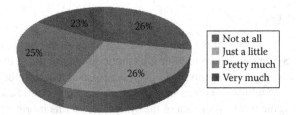

SUMMATION OF FINDINGS

Other frequently reported symptoms are as follows: mental restlessness, easily distracted, difficulty completing tasks, tending to shift from one task to another without completion, poor sustained attention, some impulsivity, and forgetting to do things. This suggests the presence of symptoms more likely attributed to an inattention disorder as opposed to what would be commonly thought of as hyperactivity. The presence of impulsivity is seen as a result of anxiety. When individuals are anxious, they think less before acting leading to impulsive behaviors.

Symptoms seen more often occurring pretty much and very much of the time were as follows:

- 83% indicated the presence of being easily distracted.
- 75% indicated the presence of poor sustained attention.
- 73% indicated the presence of difficulty shifting from one task to another.
- 73% indicated the presence of mental restlessness.
- 65% indicated the presence of difficulty completing tasks.
- 61% indicated the presence of forgetting to do things.
- 56% indicated the presence of impulsivity.

Symptoms are getting worse over time. Almost every item had some type of an increase from adolescence to adulthood. Two items remained the same and two items decreased. When compared to the adolescent population (a smaller sample), the following data were found:

Symptom that was more problematic and increased by over 20%:

- Physical restlessness

Symptoms that were more problematic and increased by 10%–20%:

- Mental restlessness
- Poor sustained attention
- Impulsivity
- Not listening to others

Symptoms that generally remained the same and were still reported frequently:

- Easily distracted (97% of the adults and 91% of the adolescents reported distractibility)
- Difficulty completing tasks (89% of the adults and 85% of the adolescents reported poor task completion)
- Forgetting to do things (91% for both the adults and adolescents reported this problem)

Symptoms that decreased through time:

- Impatience decreased by 10% for the adult population.
- Physically daring activities decreased by 11% for the adult population.

BECK ANXIETY INVENTORY

This is an inventory that inquires about the past week and as such reports only on very current symptoms of anxiety. Symptoms relate to both the emotional and physical characteristics of anxiety although individuals may have symptoms of physical issues that are not the result of anxiety symptoms. There were 125 adults that completed this measure. Subjects did endorse being unable to relax to a mild degree as the most significant of the symptoms on this inventory. Physical symptoms (such as dizzy, heart pounding, feeling unsteady) were not noted as significantly present, suggesting, similar to the depression inventory, that a full diagnosis of anxiety disorder with its autonomic, physical symptoms is not significantly present in this population. Adults identified with more of the cognitive symptoms of anxiety such as being nervous or unable to relax.

Adults did indicate a fear of the worst happening, nervousness, and some indigestion as being present to a mild to severe degree, suggesting some mild symptoms of anxiety secondarily associated with a genetic attention disorder. Adults did not tend to respond to direct questions of anxiety on this measure, although they responded to anxiety symptoms on other self-report measures:

- *Numbness or tingling*: 29% reported the symptom as present, and 15% as moderate to severe.
- *Feeling hot*: 49% reported the symptom as present, and 28% as moderate to severe.
- *Wobbliness in legs*: 28% reported the symptom as present, and 8% as moderate to severe.
- *Unable to relax*: 71% reported the symptom as present, and 38% as moderate to severe.
- *Fear of the worst happening*: 63% reported the symptom as present, and 35% as moderate to severe.
- *Dizzy or lightheaded*: 40% reported the symptom as present, and 16% as moderate to severe.
- *Heart pounding or racing*: 42% reported the symptom as present, and 15% as moderate to severe.
- *Unsteady*: 36% reported the symptom as present, and 11% as moderate to severe.
- *Feeling terrified*: 21% reported the symptom as present, and 11% as moderate to severe.
- *Being nervous*: 64% reported the symptom as present, and 34% as moderate to severe.
- *Feeling of choking*: 13% reported the symptom as present, and 2% as moderate to severe.
- *Hands trembling*: 24% reported the symptom as present, and 14% as moderate to severe.
- *Feeling shaky*: 30% reported the symptom as present, and 11% as moderate to severe.
- *Fear of losing control*: 37% reported the symptom as present, and 14% as moderate to severe.
- *Difficulty breathing*: 21% reported the symptom as present, and 7% as moderate to severe.
- *Fear of dying*: 24% reported the symptom as present, and 10% as moderate to severe.
- *Feeling scared*: 38% reported the symptom as present, and 18% as moderate to severe.
- *Indigestion or discomfort in abdomen*: 47% reported the symptom as present, and 24% as moderate to severe.
- *Feeling faint*: 13% reported the symptom as present, and 3% as moderate to severe.
- *Face flushed*: 33% reported the symptom as present, and 12% as moderate to severe.
- *Sweating (not due to heat)*: 38% reported the symptom as present, and 17% as moderate to severe.

SUMMATION OF FINDINGS

Symptoms reported as moderate to severe one-fourth or more of the time:

- Feeling hot

Symptoms reported as moderate to severe one-third or more of the time:

- Fear of the worst happening
- Being nervous
- Unable to relax

The previously mentioned symptoms reported more often are clearly compatible with a diagnosis of generalized anxiety affecting more cognitive or thinking issues as opposed to physical symptoms. This is similar to the other self-report measures and the report of feeling mentally restless 91% of the time or feeling irritable or nervous on a daily to weekly basis 77% of the time.

Symptoms of anxiety are getting worse over time. When compared to the adolescent sample (that was smaller, although trends can be seen) all of the symptoms of anxiety increased excluding fear of dying and being dizzy.

Symptoms that increased by over 20% for the adults:

- Numbness and tingling
- Face flushed

Symptoms that increased by 10%–20% for the adults:

- Feeling hot
- Feeling unsteady
- Unable to relax
- Fear of the worse happening
- Feeling terrified
- Difficulty breathing
- Indigestion

Symptoms that generally remained the same but were still seen often for the adults:

- Feeling nervous (64% adults and 63% adolescents)

Symptoms that decreased for the adults:

- Dizzy or lightheaded decreased by 4% when compared to the adolescents.
- Fear of dying decreased by 5% when compared to the adolescents.

CAARS: LONG VERSION

This was a very small sample of 22 adults. This measure was in use from 2006 to 2009 and used to measure attention symptoms.

The following are symptoms reported by the adults as occurring to a moderate to severe degree (pretty much and very much of the time):

- I like doing active things: 41%.
- I lose things necessary for tasks or activities: 45%.
- I don't plan ahead: 27%.
- I blurt out things: 18%.
- I am a risk taker or a daredevil: 33%.
- I get down on myself: 45%.
- I don't finish things I start: 55%.
- I talk too much: 46%.
- I am easily frustrated: 37%.
- I am always on the go, as if driven by a motor: 45%.
- I'm disorganized: 50%.
- I say things without thinking: 36%.
- It's hard for me to stay in one place very long: 32%.
- I have trouble doing leisure activities quietly: 23%.
- I'm not sure of myself: 37%.
- It's hard for me to keep track of several things at once: 50%.

- I'm always moving even when I should be still: 41%.
- I forget to remember things: 41%.
- I have a short fuse/hot temper: 32%.
- I am bored easily: 59%.
- I leave my seat when I am not supposed to: 10%.
- I have trouble waiting in line or taking turns with others: 19%.
- I still throw tantrums: 0%.
- I have trouble keeping my attention focused when working: 77%.
- I seek out fast-paced, exciting activities: 32%.
- I avoid new challenges because I lack faith in my abilities: 23%.
- I feel restless inside even if I am sitting still: 43%.
- Things I hear or see distract me from what I am doing: 72%.
- I am forgetful in my daily activities: 43%.
- Many things set me off easily: 33%.
- I dislike quiet introspective activities: 24%.
- I lose things I need: 38%.
- I have trouble listening to what other people are saying: 43%.
- I am an underachiever: 10%.
- I interrupt others when talking: 32%.
- I change plans/jobs midstream: 45%.
- I act okay on the outside, but inside I am unsure of myself: 27%.
- I am always on the go: 54%.
- I make comments/remarks that I wish I could take back: 32%.
- I can't get things done unless there's an absolute deadline: 59%.
- I fidget or squirm in my seat: 36%.
- I make careless mistakes or have trouble paying close attention to detail: 46%.
- I step on people's toes without meaning to: 46%.
- I have trouble getting started on a task: 54%.
- I intrude on others' activities: 45%.
- It takes a great deal of effort for me to sit still: 32%.
- My moods are unpredictable: 32%.
- I don't like homework or job activities where I have to think a lot: 18%.
- I am absent minded in daily activities: 41%.
- I am restless or overactive: 37%.
- I depend on others to keep my life in order and attend to details: 23%.
- I annoy other people without meaning to: 10%.
- Sometimes my attention narrows so much that I am oblivious to everything else, and other times it is so broad that everything distracts me: 50%.
- I tend to squirm or fidget: 28%.
- I can't keep my mind on something unless it is really interesting: 64%.
- I wish I had greater confidence in my abilities: 28%.
- I can't sit still for long: 46%.
- I give answers to questions before the questions have been completed: 41%.
- I like to be up and on the go rather than being in one place: 41%.
- I have trouble finishing job tasks or schoolwork: 63%.
- I am irritable: 28%.
- I interrupt others when they are working or playing: 14%.
- My past failures make it hard for me to believe in myself: 23%.
- I am distracted when things are going on around me: 59%.
- I have problems organizing my tasks and activities: 50%.
- I misjudge how long it takes to do something or go somewhere: 55%.

SUMMATION OF FINDINGS

Symptoms present (mild to severe) 90% or more of the time:

- Talking too much.
- Being disorganized.
- Difficulty keeping attention focused when working on a task.
- Things they see or hear distract from what they are doing.
- Interrupting others when they are talking.
- Fidgeting or squirming in their seat.
- Unable to keep their mind on something unless it is really interesting.
- Difficulty finishing job tasks or schoolwork.
- Distracted when things are going on around them.
- Misjudging how long it takes to do something or to go somewhere.

Symptoms present 80% or more of the time:

- Losing things necessary for tasks or activities.
- Blurting out things.
- Getting down on self.
- Not finishing things that are started.
- Easily frustrated.
- Not sure of self.
- Forgetting things.
- Easily bored.
- Changing jobs or plans midstream.
- Always on the go.
- Making comments or remarks they wish they could take back.
- Unable to get things done without an absolute deadline.
- Difficulty getting started on a task.
- Sometimes attention narrows so much that they are oblivious to everything else, and other times attention is so broad that everything is distracting.
- Wishing they had greater confidence in their abilities.
- Giving answers to questions before the question has been completed.
- Feeling irritable.
- Problems organizing tasks and activities.

Symptoms seen more often, from a moderate to severe degree:

- Trouble keeping attention focused when working: 77%.
- Things they see or hear distract from what they are doing: 72%.
- Cannot keep mind on something unless really interesting: 64%.
- Trouble finishing job tasks or schoolwork: 63%.
- Easily bored: 59%.
- Cannot get things done unless there is an absolute deadline: 59%.
- Distracted when things going on around them: 59%.
- Misjudging how long it takes to go somewhere or do something: 55%.
- Not finishing things: 55%.
- Always on the go: 54%.
- Trouble getting started on a task: 54%.
- Being disorganized: 50%.
- Hard to keep track of several things at once: 50%.

- Sometimes attention is too narrow or is overly broad: 50%.
- Talking too much: 46%.
- Stepping on people's toes without meaning to: 46%.
- Making careless mistakes: 46%.
- Cannot sit still for long: 46%.
- Intruding on others: 45%.
- Changing jobs/plans midstream: 45%.
- Losing things necessary for tasks or activities: 45%.
- Getting down on self: 45%.
- Always on the go as if driven by a motor: 45%.

Distractibility and focus of attention were most problematic followed by the ability to complete tasks, which is consistent with issues of avoidance and procrastination. Visual–spatial issues are seen in misjudging time or distance. Similar to other self-report measures, adults reported the tendency to be self-critical and judgmental.

QUALITY OF LIFE INVENTORY

This is a measure inquiring about sixteen life areas. Firstly, the adult is asked to rate how important each life area is to them (not important, important, or extremely important). Secondly, they are asked to rank how satisfied or dissatisfied they are for each of these areas (there is a scale for the degree of satisfaction or dissatisfaction: very satisfied, somewhat and a little satisfied, or dissatisfied). The discrepancy between importance of the life area and satisfaction provides insight into the significance of the item. Therefore, the significant items are when the person indicated that the area was very important for them and that they were dissatisfied to some degree. Seventy-five adults completed this form from the year of 2006 to 2009.

The following are percentages of adults who indicated the following life areas as being important or extremely important:

- Health: 64%
- Self-esteem: 59%
- Goals and values: 57%
- Money: 89%
- Work: 90%
- Play: 96%
- Learning: 99%
- Creativity: 92%
- Helping: 91%
- Love: 99%
- Friends: 96%
- Children: 81%
- Relatives: 95%
- Home: 98%
- Neighborhood: 87%
- Community: 92%

The percentages change when the criteria are specifically worded as extremely important:

- Health: 3%
- Self-esteem: 0%
- Goals and values: 1%

- Money: 27%
- Work: 48%
- Play: 55%
- Learning: 52%
- Creativity: 47%
- Helping: 43%
- Love: 71%
- Friends: 60%
- Children: 38%
- Relatives: 47%
- Home: 42%
- Neighborhood: 30%
- Community: 25%

SUMMATION OF FINDINGS

When using only extremely important as the criteria, it becomes readily apparent that the more important issues are love and friends, followed by play and then learning. Work, creativity, and relatives remained extremely important for almost 50 to over 50% of the adults completing this measure.

In these areas that are extremely important, adults were dissatisfied to some degree in the following life areas:

- Love: 32%
- Friends: 19%
- Play: 28%
- Learning: 38%
- Work: 43%
- Creativity: 22%
- Relatives: 31%

Very few or no individuals indicated health, self-esteem, goals, and values as extremely important. The only area indicated significantly as very important was love. While money was seen as important, it was not seen as very important. More people rated play as extremely important, rather than important. There was less of a distinction seen for work (rated almost equally as important and extremely important). Friends were more often rated as extremely important as opposed to important. Neighborhood and community were more often rated as important as opposed to not important.

A pattern begins to emerge, which helps to explain the lack of moderate to severe depression and anxiety symptoms. It seems that those with a genetic attention disorder have given up their goals and values, as well as their quest for self-esteem, and traded it in for love and friends. The question to ponder is whether values and goals became less of a priority as school became more difficult. Perhaps goals were lowered to what was felt to be possible or within one's grasp, resulting in areas of play, love, and friends being more important than self-development. This is not to say that having friends and being in love are not important, but it seems that being social took precedence over money and self-esteem or pursuit of work goals. If one is not in pursuit of difficult goals, symptoms of anxiety and depression will dissipate.

Not many indicated that they were very satisfied in anything. Areas where more people indicated that they were very satisfied were helping, love, friends, and relationships with children. No one was very satisfied with their neighborhood or community. Fewer individuals were very satisfied with money, health, work, learning, and creativity. No one indicated these areas as very important to them, raising the question of which came first, their dissatisfaction or determination of reduced importance.

The Quality of Life Scale begs the question of whether this population is truly a satisfied group or whether they have lowered their values and goals. Do they remain unsatisfied and instead turn to areas where they may have established greater success, such as their social and love life? The result is that they are not unhappy; however, they are not ecstatically happy either; the extremes have been sacrificed for comfort. This is not unlike the ADD child who avoids and procrastinates with the goal of comfort in mind as opposed to stretching their academic learning to make things work despite the difficulty or arduousness of the task.

PERSONAL PROBLEMS CHECKLIST FOR ADULTS

This checklist had 1196 responders. Adults were to indicate their concerns about a number of areas: social, appearance, vocation, family, school, finance, religion, emotions, sexuality, legal, health, attention, and crisis:

- The area reported with the highest percentage of concern was concentration (76%) followed by anxiety (63%) and not remembering things (68%).
- More than half the time, adults indicated being tired, not getting enough exercise, feeling depressed, and being uncomfortable in social settings.
- Adults reported more concerns in the area of emotions than any other area, primarily related to being unable to relax, worrying about things, and not enjoying life.
- The second area of the most reported concerns was social, which is similar to that indicated on the children and adolescent self-report measures: not feeling socially comfortable, not fitting in, shyness, feeling inferior, and lack of close relationships.
- The third area of the most reported concerns was that of health and habits: poor sleep, lack of exercise, poor eating, and overeating.
- Finances were a concern (budgeting and making enough money) and to a lesser degree, school (study habits, poor grades).
- Almost one-half of the population indicated a poor attitude toward self. A generally poor attitude and holding opinions too strongly were indicated one-quarter of the time.
- Adults did not report concerns about things such as religion, their appearance, problems with their spouse, and being unhappy with their home or their health.

Emotions:

- Having trouble concentrating: 76%.
- Feeling anxious or uptight: 63%.
- Not remembering things: 68%.
- Feeling depressed or sad: 56%.
- Getting too emotional: 44%.
- Not being able to relax: 46%.
- Feeling guilty: 39%.
- Being afraid of things: 31%.
- Having the same thought over and over again: 38%.
- Not being able to stop worrying: 33%.
- Being suspicious: 30%.
- Not having any enjoyment in life: 28%.

Social:

- Feeling uncomfortable in social settings: 50%.
- Feeling lonely: 40%.
- Being criticized by others: 43%.
- Not fitting in with peers: 30%.

- Being shy: 32%.
- Not having close friends: 32%.
- Being uncomfortable when talking to people: 33%.
- Feeling inferior: 39%.
- Feeling different from everyone else: 38%.
- Not having anyone to share interests with: 25%.
- Feeling like people are against me: 25%.

Health/habits:

- Being tired and having no energy: 55%.
- Having poor sleeping habits: 43%.
- Not getting enough exercise: 56%.
- Being overweight: 37%.
- Eating too much: 31%.
- Having poor eating habits: 37%.
- Needing a vacation: 31%.
- Not making time for leisure activities: 33%.

Attitude:

- Having a poor attitude toward self: 42%.
- Having a poor attitude about everything: 25%.
- Holding opinions too strongly: 27%.
- Having a poor attitude toward work: 25%.

Finances:

- Budgeting money: 48%.
- Not making enough money: 44%.
- Wasting money: 42%.
- Having unpaid bills: 31%.
- Having to spend savings: 26%.
- Depending on others for financial support: 25%.

Vocation:

- Being afraid of failing on the job: 37%.
- Job not paying enough: 26%.
- Job having no future: 26%.
- Being bored on the job: 27%.

School:

- Not having good study habits: 37%.
- Getting bad grades: 26%.
- Not understanding class material: 25%.

SUMMATION OF FINDINGS

This brings home the point that we tend to attribute many symptoms to ADHD when inattention remains the primary issue. Anxiety did emerge as a major symptom as well on this measure using a far larger population sample, which is consistent with what has been seen in the clinic. Anxiety is seen in children and is still observed in adults. That the symptom of not remembering things was also a primary issue points to either the presence of true memory problems or perhaps suggesting that distractibility is contributing to not remembering things and/or poor sleep. Poor sleep was noted, which can increase symptoms of depression. Depressive symptoms were seen consistent with reports from other measures completed by the adults. Executive reasoning symptoms did not emerge in the symptoms reported. Symptoms typically associated with ADHD were not endorsed by this large sample of adults such as acting overbearing or rude, acting in an immature manner, or not getting along with other people.

Adults had the most concerns in the following area:

Social issues

- One-half of the adults said they did feel socially uncomfortable.

School is problematic

- One-third of the adults endorsed not having good study habits.
- One-fourth of the adults indicated not understanding class material.

Money is an issue reported by the adults:

- Almost one-half of the adults indicated difficulty budgeting money.
- Almost one-half of the adults reported wasting money.
- Almost one-half of the adults reported not making enough money.
- Almost one-third have unpaid bills.
- One-fourth indicated depending upon others for financial support.

Anxiety is a continual factor:

- One-third of the adults indicated being afraid of things.
- One-third of the adults indicated having the same thought over and over again.
- One-third indicated that they are unable to stop worrying.
- Almost one-half indicated not being able to relax.

Poor sleep is present:

- Poor sleep habits were indicated by almost one-half.
- One-half said they were tired and had no energy.

Depression symptoms are present in this large sample but not the clinical depression:

- One-half indicated feeling depressed or sad.
- One-third indicated feeling guilty.
- One-fourth indicated not having any enjoyment in life.
- Over one-fourth indicated not making time for leisure activities.

Eating behavior:

- Over one-third indicated poor eating habits.
- Almost one-third indicate eating too much.

Attitude:

- One-quarter indicated having a poor attitude about everything.
- Almost one-quarter indicated not having any interest in things.
- Over one-quarter indicated holding opinions too strongly.
- One-fourth indicated having a poor attitude toward work.
- Almost one-half indicated having a poor attitude toward self.

Cognitive symptoms:

- Almost one-half indicated getting too emotional.
- Two-thirds indicated not remembering things.
- Two-thirds indicated having trouble concentrating.

This population is quite healthy:

- Smoking was not indicated as significant and present in less than one-fourth.
- Physical disability was not indicated as present and neither was chronic illness, recurring health problems, or having many health problems.

EPWORTH SLEEPINESS SCALE OF DAYTIME SLEEPINESS

On the Epworth Sleepiness Scale of daytime sleepiness, there are a total of 8 items, which are rated from 0 to 3 in terms of a high chance of dozing in specific situations. It is used to provide a measure of daytime sleepiness. The Epworth Sleepiness Scale asks individuals to rate the chance that they might doze off or fall asleep in eight different situations or activities that people generally engage in during daytime hours. The scale is really asking people to imagine being in a particular situation or to make a mental judgment about such a situation and to indicate whether they would doze off or not. However, individuals tend to respond with a score of 0 when they are not in the situation, which then changes the measurement. Nonetheless, it remains a valid indicator of daytime sleepiness and is used universally. The cutoff for daytime sleepiness is a score of 10. Only 20% of the general population had scores above 10. The following is based upon a far smaller sample of adults of 46 people:

- Sitting and relaxing: 60% indicated a moderate to high chance of dozing.
- Watching television: 57% indicated a moderate to high chance of dozing.
- Sitting inactive in a public place: 33% indicated a moderate to high chance of dozing.
- As a passenger in a car for an hour without a break: 54% indicated a moderate to high chance of dozing.
- Lying down to rest in the afternoon: 70% indicated a moderate to high chance of dozing.
- Sitting and talking to someone: 9% indicated a moderate to high chance of dozing.
- Sitting quietly after lunch: 42% indicated a moderate to high chance of dozing.
- In a car while stopped in traffic: 45% indicated a moderate to high chance of dozing.

SUMMATION OF FINDINGS

Notable responses on the Epworth Sleepiness Scale were when sitting and relaxing, watching television, as a passenger in a car for an hour without a break, and lying down in the afternoon to rest:

- 60% indicated a moderate to high chance of dozing when sitting and relaxing.
- 57% indicated a moderate to high chance of dozing when watching television.

- 54% indicated a moderate to high chance of dozing as a passenger in a car for an hour without a break.
- 70% indicated a moderate to high chance of dozing when lying down in the afternoon.

This suggests the presence of napping in the adult ADD population. We did not separate out ADD plus to see if the napping was the result of a sleep disorder.

SLEEP DISORDERS QUESTIONNAIRE

Approximately 48 people completed a sleep questionnaire to provide the following information:
Sleep Schedule and Sleep Hygiene

- Do you keep a fairly regular sleep/wake schedule? Only 11% responded yes.
- Do you nap during the day? 85% responded no.
- Are you refreshed by your naps? 29% responded yes.

A poor sleep schedule is a rather pronounced problem when only 11% indicated a regular sleep schedule. This does not rule out people who had jobs as shift workers. It does appear to be a primary issue for the ADD population. One way to ensure a problematic sleep schedule is to take a nap longer than a power nap of 20 min. Although the length of the naps was not a part of the response inventory, we do know that 15% reported taking naps. Of those who took naps, only 29% found them refreshing. This means that those who responded that they take naps also indicated that they do not always find these naps to be refreshing. This may suggest the tendency to nap too long, and/or the nap is being used to compensate for sleep problems and is not working as an alternative. The fact that half of the population reported insomnia symptoms suggests that the problem may be poor sleep. Anxiety and insomnia are highly related, and anxiety can be a causal factor for insomnia.

Insomnia:

- Do you often have trouble getting to sleep at night? 54% reported yes
- Do you often have awakenings during the night? 60% reported yes
- Do you have long periods when you awaken and are not able to get back to sleep? 43% reported yes
- Are you bothered by waking up too early and not being able to go back to sleep? 51% reported yes
- Do you frequently check the clock when you are unable to fall asleep? 71% reported yes

Over 54% indicated difficulty getting to sleep (which is symptomatic of sleep onset insomnia), awakening during the night, and then difficulty getting back to sleep (symptomatic of sleep maintenance insomnia). Checking of the clock was at 71%, suggesting that the presence of insomnia is a major factor in the life of an ADD adult. Likely there is a relationship to the generalized anxiety seen in all the populations (child, adolescent, adult) throughout the years and difficulty sleeping due to thinking too much and worrying about the day that's past and/or the next day.

Movement:

- Are your bed covers extremely messy when you wake up? 46% reported yes.
- Do you awaken yourself by kicking your legs during the night? 4% said yes.

There is a fair amount of research suggesting the connection of periodic leg movements (PLMD) and ADHD. In this population, almost one-half indicated sufficient movement to mess up the bed covers.

PLMD is diagnosed via a sleep study, and the diagnosis cannot be made clinically, hence the suggestion of this disorder but no proof of it. A minimal amount of people ascribed to the movement being problematic and waking them up.

Restless Legs Syndrome:

- Do you have unpleasant sensations in your legs combined with an urge to move your legs? 34% reported yes.

Not everyone responded to the following questions:

- Do these feelings in the legs occur mainly or only at rest, and do they improve with movement? 32 responded; of those, 47% said yes.
- Are these feelings in the legs worse in the afternoon, evening, or night then in the morning? 27 responded, and of those, 41% said yes.
- How often do these feelings in the legs occur? 21 responded, and of those, 33% indicated weekly (2–7 times).

Similar to PLMD, there is a plethora of research linking ADHD and RLS. Growing pains as a child can be symptomatic of RLS and result in RLS as an adult. In this sample, one-third of the subjects indicated the presence of basic symptoms of RLS. Of those that indicated basic symptoms, half indicated that the RLS symptoms are symptomatic of the disorder meeting one of the four criteria. Those individuals that indicated relief of movement went on to indicate that the problems are worse at night or lying down, again meeting criteria to establish the diagnosis of RLS. Finally, in determining whether symptoms are symptomatic of an actual disorder, only half of the original responders to this question provided further evidence of the timeliness of their symptoms. So of the half that indicated that symptoms occur in varying degrees, one-third indicated that symptoms occur weekly. The worse the symptoms become and the more they are disruptive to sleep, the greater the need for medication intervention.

Parasomnias:

- Do you currently have nightmares? 17%.
- Did you wet your bed as a child? 22%.
- Have you ever wet the bed as an adult? 15%.
- Have you ever been told that\you walk in your sleep? 15%.
- Have you recently walked in your sleep? 4%.

Having nightmares, sleep walking, sleep talking, and even bed-wetting as a child and as an adult are not highly present in this population. It is of interest that the presence of childhood enuresis is not to the degree that one would have thought, although this is reported by adults regarding their childhood and may be different for parents reporting on their children.

ADULT NEUROPSYCHOLOGICAL HISTORY

The Adult Neuropsychological History provided demographic information about the adult population as well as symptomatology and was used from 2006 to 2009. One hundred and seven adults completed this form and responded to these questions about their functioning and past history. Symptoms were reported as historical, as new, or as both new and historical. There was more indication of historical than new problems consistent with a lifelong diagnosis of ADD. The following are the responses to specific questions about the adult's functioning in the following areas: problem solving, language (speech and math skills), nonverbal skills, concentration and awareness, memory, motor and coordination, sensory, physical issues, emotions, and behavior. Percentages are provided for symptoms rated as new or old. For the adults, there were higher percentages on more items where the adult indicated the presence of *both* new and old symptoms, unlike the children or adolescents; therefore, these data have been included.

PROBLEM SOLVING

Difficulty figuring how to do new things: 34% had this symptom
  New = 9%
  Old = 25%
  Both = 0%

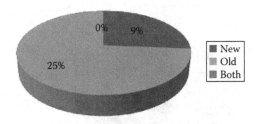

Difficulty doing more than one thing at a time: 38% had this symptom
  New = 10%
  Old = 28%
  Both = 4%

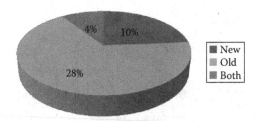

Difficulty doing things in the right order: 35% had this symptom
  New = 8%
  Old = 27%
  Both = 4%

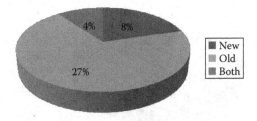

Difficulty thinking as quickly as needed: 48% had this symptom
  New = 13%
  Old = 35%
  Both = 4%

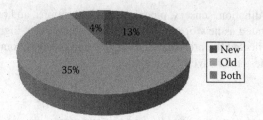

Easily frustrated: 62% had this symptom
   New = 18%
   Old = 44%
   Both = 5%

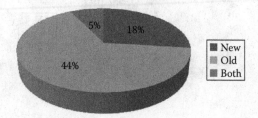

Difficulty completing an activity in a reasonable amount of time: 55% had this symptom
   New = 13%
   Old = 42%
   Both = 5%

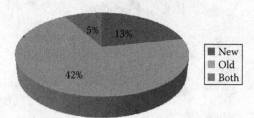

Difficulty verbally describing the steps involved in doing something: 31% had this symptom
   New = 9%
   Old = 22%
   Both = 2%

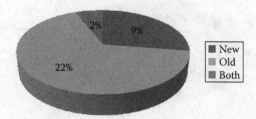

Difficulty figuring out problems that most other people can do: 27% had this symptom
   New = 6%
   Old = 21%
   Both = 2%

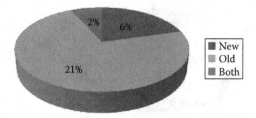

Other problem solving difficulties: 10% had this symptom
    New = 3%
    Old = 7%
    Both = 0%

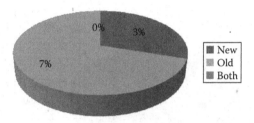

Difficulty changing a plan or activity when necessary: 21% had this symptom
    New = 5%
    Old = 16%
    Both = 1%

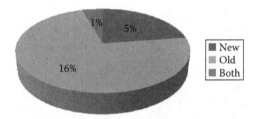

Difficulty switching from one activity to another activity: 22% had this symptom
    New = 8%
    Old = 14%
    Both = 3%

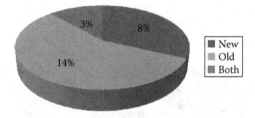

Difficulty planning ahead: 40% had this symptom
    New = 7%
    Old = 33%
    Both = 5%

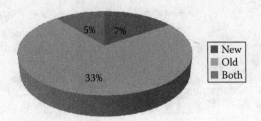

NONVERBAL SKILLS

Right–left confusion: 44% had this symptom
    New = 19%
    Old = 25%
    Both = 7%

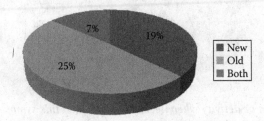

Difficulty dressing: 42% had this symptom
    New = 10%
    Old = 32%
    Both = 3%

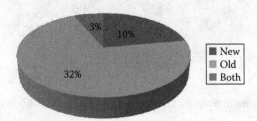

Unaware of things on one side of my body: 34% had this symptom
    New = 4%
    Old = 30%
    Both = 1%

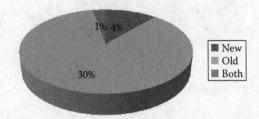

Decline in musical abilities: 45% had this symptom
    New = 7%
    Old = 38%
    Both = 6%

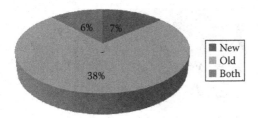

Not aware of time: 37% had this symptom
    New = 7%
    Old = 30%
    Both = 4%

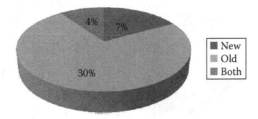

Difficulty doing things I should automatically be able to do: 18% had this symptom
    New = 10%
    Old = 8%
    Both = 3%

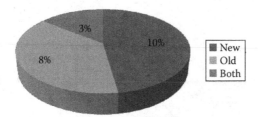

Problems drawing or copying: 11% had this symptom
    New = 7%
    Old = 4%
    Both = 2%

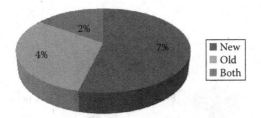

Problems finding my way around places I've been before: 15% had this symptom
    New = 5%
    Old = 10%
    Both = 2%

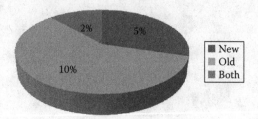

Difficulty recognizing objects or people: 13% had this symptom
    New = 7%
    Old = 6%
    Both = 1%

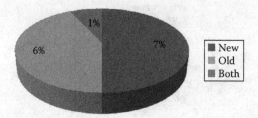

Parts of my body do not seem as if they belong to me: 6% had this symptom
    New = 4%
    Old = 2%
    Both = 0%

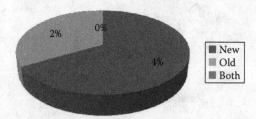

Slow reaction time: 12% had this symptom
    New = 3%
    Old = 9%
    Both = 1%

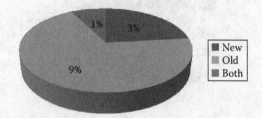

SPEECH, LANGUAGE, AND MATH SKILLS

Difficulty finding the right word to say: 11% had this symptom
    New = 2%
    Old = 9%
    Both = 4%

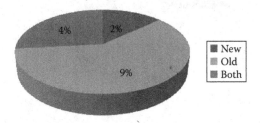

Difficulty understanding what others are saying: 8% had this symptom
    New = 3%
    Old = 5%
    Both = 0%

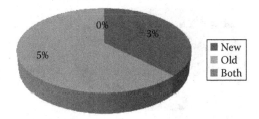

Unable to speak: 11% had this symptom
    New = 4%
    Old = 7%
    Both = 1%

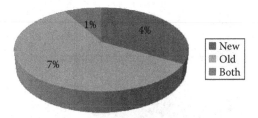

Difficulty staying with one idea: 6% had this symptom
    New = 5%
    Old = 1%
    Both = 0%

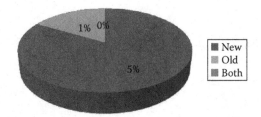

Slurred speech: 10% had this symptom
    New = 4%
    Old = 6%
    Both = 2%

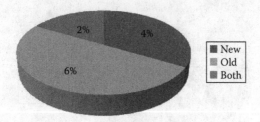

Odd or unusual speech sounds: 4% had this symptom
    New = 3%
    Old = 1%
    Both = 2%

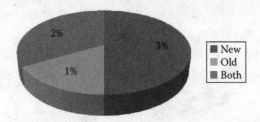

Difficulty writing letters or words: 12% had this symptom
    New = 7%
    Old = 5%
    Both = 0%

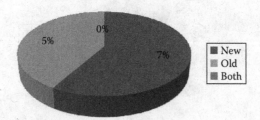

Difficulty with math: 2% had this symptom
    New = 2%
    Old = 0%
    Both = 0%

Difficulty understanding what I read: 5% had this symptom
    New = 3%
    Old = 2%
    Both = 0%

Difficulty spelling: 15% had this symptom
   New = 7%
   Old = 8%
   Both = 2%

CONCENTRATION AND AWARENESS

Highly distractible: 63% had this symptom
   New = 15%
   Old = 48%
   Both = 8%

Lose my train of thought easily: 63% had this symptom
   New = 21%
   Old = 42%
   Both = 8%

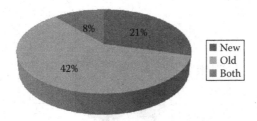

Problems concentrating: 68% had this symptom
   New = 18%
   Old = 50%
   Both = 9%

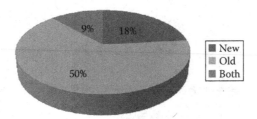

Become easily confused or disoriented: 37% had this symptom
   New = 17%
   Old = 20%
   Both = 5%

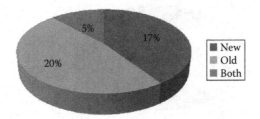

My mind goes blank: 45% had this symptom
  New = 16%
  Old = 29%
  Both = 0%

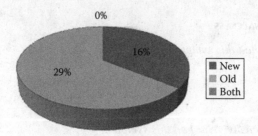

Blackout spells: 8% had this symptom
  New = 4%
  Old = 4%
  Both = 0%

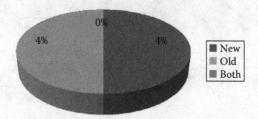

Aura: 13% had this symptom
  New = 7%
  Old = 6%
  Both = 1%

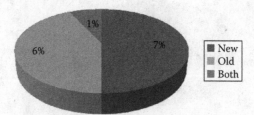

Don't feel very alert and aware of things: 27% had this symptom
  New = 16%
  Old = 11%
  Both = 4%

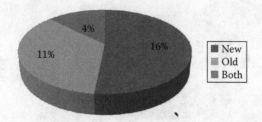

MEMORY

Forgetting where I leave things: 56% had this symptom
   New = 17%
   Old = 39%
   Both = 8%

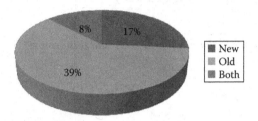

Forgetting names: 41% had this symptom
   New = 13%
   Old = 28%
   Both = 8%

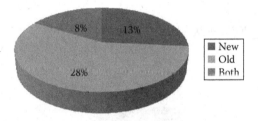

Forgetting what I should be doing: 41% had this symptom
   New = 15%
   Old = 26%
   Both = 5%

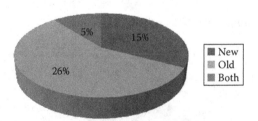

Relying more and more on notes to remember things: 43% had this symptom
   New = 28%
   Old = 15%
   Both = 3%

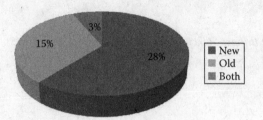

Forgetting events that happened quite recently: 32% had this symptom
    New = 21%
    Old = 11%
    Both = 2%

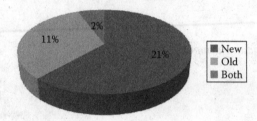

Forgetting events that happened long ago: 30% had this symptom
    New = 10%
    Old = 20%
    Both = 2%

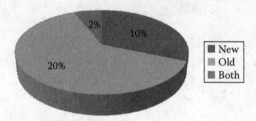

Frequently forgetting appointments: 24% had this symptom
    New = 10%
    Old = 14%
    Both = 3%

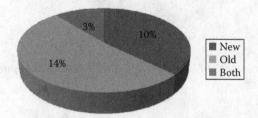

Forgetting faces of people that I know: 8% had this symptom
>New = 3%
>Old = 5%
>Both = 3%

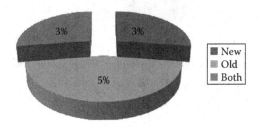

Forgetting where I am or where I am going: 13% had this symptom
>New = 8%
>Old = 5%
>Both = 4%

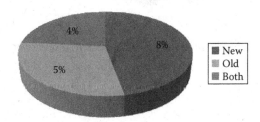

Need someone to give me a hint so I can remember things: 21% had this symptom
>New = 10%
>Old = 11%
>Both = 7%

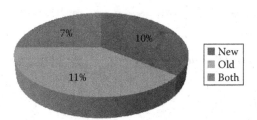

Forgetting the order of things: 15% had this symptom
>New = 9%
>Old = 6%
>Both = 1%

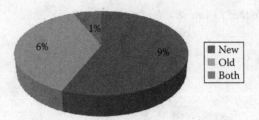

Forgetting facts, but I can remember how to do things: 26% had this symptom
New = 12%
Old = 14%
Both = 5%

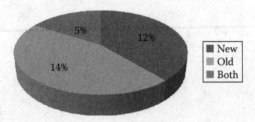

Forgetting how to do things, but I can remember facts: 8% had this symptom
New = 5%
Old = 3%
Both = 1%

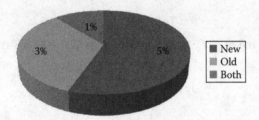

MOTOR AND COORDINATION

Fine motor control problems: 11% had this symptom
New = 7%
Old = 4%
Both = 1%

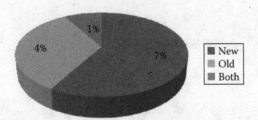

Weakness on one side of my body: 5% had this symptom
    New = 3%
    Old = 2%
    Both = 0%

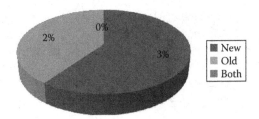

Difficulty holding onto things: 9% had this symptom
    New = 6%
    Old = 3%
    Both = 0%

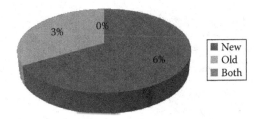

Tremor or shakiness: 13% had this symptom
    New = 7%
    Old = 6%
    Both = 0%

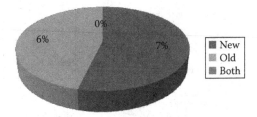

Muscle tics or strange movement: 13% had this symptom
    New = 6%
    Old = 7%
    Both = 0%

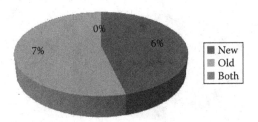

My writing is very small: 11% had this symptom
   New = 3%
   Old = 8%
   Both = 1%

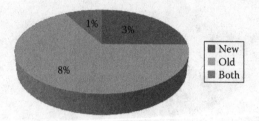

My writing is very large: 9% had this symptom
   New = 3%
   Old = 6%
   Both = 1%

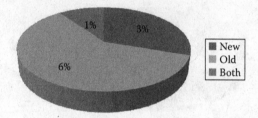

Walking more slowly than other people: 13% had this symptom
   New = 6%
   Old = 7%
   Both = 1%

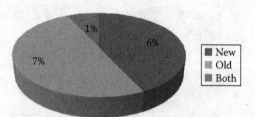

Feeling stiff: 16% had this symptom
   New = 8%
   Old = 8%
   Both = 0%

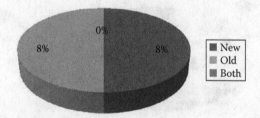

Balance problems: 12% had this symptom
    New = 8%
    Old = 4%
    Both = 1%

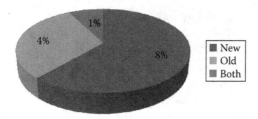

Difficulty starting to move: 7% had this symptom
    New = 4%
    Old = 3%
    Both = 0%

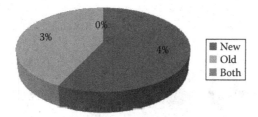

Jerky muscles: 9% had this symptom
    New = 6%
    Old = 3%
    Both = 0%

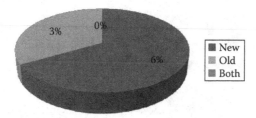

Muscles tire quickly: 17% had this symptom
    New = 10%
    Old = 7%
    Both = 0%

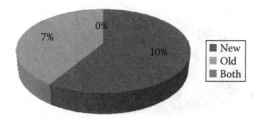

Often bumping into things: 17% had this symptom
    New = 9%
    Old = 8%
    Both = 1%

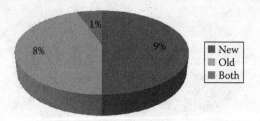

SENSORY

Loss of feeling or numbness: 17% had this symptom
    New = 11%
    Old = 6%
    Both = 1%

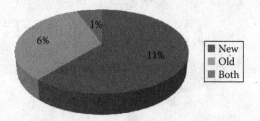

Tingling or strange skin sensations: 14% had this symptom
    New = 11%
    Old = 3%
    Both = 0%

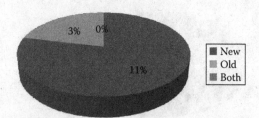

Difficulty telling hot from cold: 3% had this symptom
    New = 2%
    Old = 1%
    Both = 0%

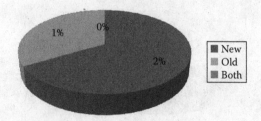

Losing hearing: 16% had this symptom
    New = 8%
    Old = 8%
    Both = 2%

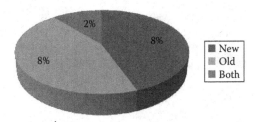

Ringing in ears or hearing strange sounds: 13% had this symptom
    New = 7%
    Old = 6%
    Both = 1%

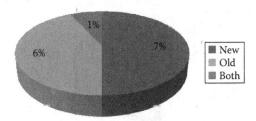

Difficulty tasting food: 4% had this symptom
    New = 3%
    Old = 1%
    Both = 0%

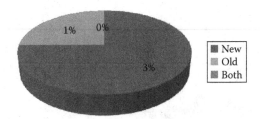

Difficulty smelling: 7% had this symptom
    New = 4%
    Old = 3%
    Both = 1%

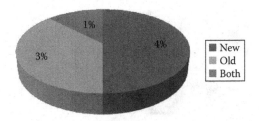

Smelling strange odors: 5% had this symptom
    New = 2%
    Old = 3%
    Both = 0%

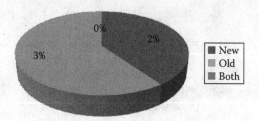

Problems seeing on one side: 2% had this symptom
    New = 1%
    Old = 1%
    Both = 0%

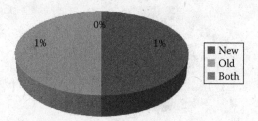

Blurred vision: 12% had this symptom
    New = 8%
    Old = 4%
    Both = 1%

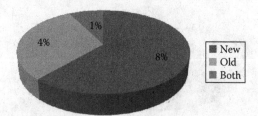

Blank spots in vision: 5% had this symptom
    New = 3%
    Old = 2%
    Both = 0%

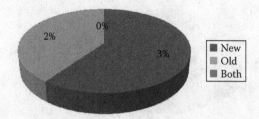

Brief periods of blindness: 2% had this symptom
 New = 1%
 Old = 1%
 Both = 0%

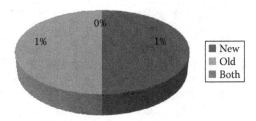

See stars or flashes of light: 13% had this symptom
 New = 6%
 Old = 7%
 Both = 0%

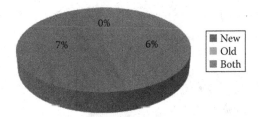

Double vision: 5% had this symptom
 New = 3%
 Old = 2%
 Both = 0%

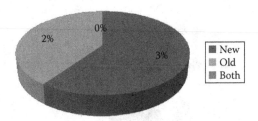

Difficulty looking quickly from one object to another object: 11% had this symptom
 New = 8%
 Old = 3%
 Both = 0%

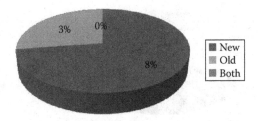

Need to squint or move closer to see clearly: 15% had this symptom
> New = 7%
> Old = 8%
> Both = 2%

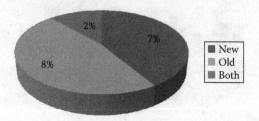

PHYSICAL

Headaches: 35% had this symptom
> New = 13%
> Old = 22%
> Both = 4%

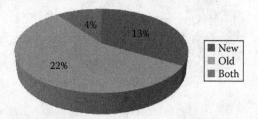

Excessive tiredness: 44% had this symptom
> New = 23%
> Old = 21%
> Both = 3%

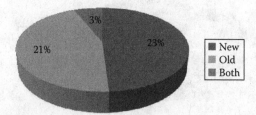

Dizziness: 14% had this symptom
> New = 9%
> Old = 5%
> Both = 1%

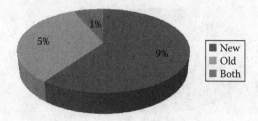

Nausea or vomiting: 15% had this symptom
    New = 6%
    Old = 9%
    Both = 0%

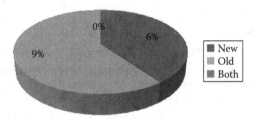

Urinary incontinence: 7% had this symptom
    New = 5%
    Old = 2%
    Both = 2%

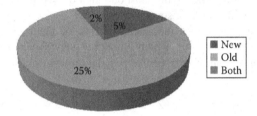

Loss of bowel control: 3% had this symptom
    New = 1%
    Old = 2%
    Both = 1%

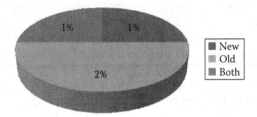

SUMMATION OF FINDINGS

Symptoms that were seen more often were in the following areas:

Problem solving:

- One-quarter of the adults indicated historical problems of difficulty figuring out how to do new things.
- One-third indicated historical problems of planning ahead.
- One-third indicated historical problems of difficulty thinking as quickly as needed.
- One-fourth indicated historical problems of difficulty doing things in the right order.
- Almost one-half indicated historical problems of difficulty completing an activity within a reasonable amount of time.
- One-fourth indicated historical problems of difficulty doing more than one thing at a time.
- Almost one-half indicated being easily frustrated.

The adults *did not* indicate difficulty changing a plan when necessary, difficulty switching from one activity to another activity, or difficulty figuring out problems or problem solving difficulties, which are typically seen symptoms when there are executive reasoning deficits or problems.

Speech, language, and math skills:

- Adults *did not* indicate a difficulty understanding what others are saying or difficulty staying with one topic in speech. These would be typical symptoms present when there is brain involvement, specifically involvement of the frontal executive reasoning processes.
- All of the symptoms in this area fell either at or below 15%, suggesting that speech, language, and math are not problematic in adulthood. It is likely that adults found jobs or work paths that did not require the skills demanded of them while in school; consequently, math or language would no longer be a problem for them in everyday situations.
- Adults *did not* indicate problems of finding the right word to express themselves (word retrieval, often thought of as an executive reasoning trait) or difficulty understanding what others are saying and problems staying with one idea or writing letters. Further, they did not specify problems with words or speech difficulties.
- There were some spelling issues indicated by 15% of the population. Seven percent indicated this as a new symptom, which could be reflective of some additional brain issue emerging given that one-fourth of this population was diagnosed with ADD plus an additional disorder.

Nonverbal skills:

- There were not enough symptoms reported to indicate that ADD is typically a nonverbal learning disorder. Problems drawing or copying were not indicated as occurring very often (4% as an old symptom and 7% as a new symptom).
- Of the nonverbal symptoms, the most prominent was right–left confusion. Almost one-half did indicate historical problems of right–left confusion. This is a problem often seen in childhood and typically regarded as related to the visual–spatial issues that accompany the long-term presence of a genetic attention disorder. One-quarter of the adult population indicated right–left confusion as a long-term, historical problem.
- Almost one-half of the adults indicated historical problems of difficulty dressing. The question asks if someone has difficulty dressing, which does not reflect a physical problem. It is meant to reference a condition typically caused by a stroke resulting in problems dressing due to a lack of awareness of the body (neglect condition). This question was probably misinterpreted (given the high response) as difficulty making a decision on what to wear each day, suggesting either the consequence of distractibility and/or just plain indecisiveness. Increased worry or concern about what other people think would make someone more indecisive regarding what to wear each day.
- Almost one-third indicated a historical lack of awareness of things on one side of their body. This item is supposed to reflect a condition called hemi-neglect occurring after a stroke when people neglect things on one side of their body (usually the result of the combined impact to parietal and visual brain processes). It is more probable that the adults interpreted this item as not being aware of situations or events occurring around them, which tends to be the result of visual–spatial issues and not always perceiving the whole picture of things.
- Over one-third indicated a historical decline in their musical abilities and almost one-half reported this as a symptom. I have no explanation for this other than to report on what people indicated.

- Almost one-third indicated a historical lack of awareness of time, which would reflect the difficulty of time management and maybe the additional impact of distractibility. Over one-third reported the problem as existing. It is typical in the ADD population that individuals lose track of time whether it is due to focusing so much on something that the result is avoidance of everything else or the typically seen problem of not adding up how much time things take. So you come up with a list of things you want to do before leaving the house but never stop to think, "Do I have enough time to get all of these things done?" This is the result of running late, poor time management, and the lack of awareness of time.
- The presence of a slow reaction time was not significantly indicated and is apparently considered separate from difficulty with timed testing. People did not see themselves as having a slowed reaction time, and typically they are not seen as having this problem. The problem of timed testing is having enough time to battle the attention symptoms of focus, distractibility, and perhaps reading the text correctly (visual–spatial issues) to perform as well as possible.
- Fifteen percent indicated difficulty finding their way around to places they had been before, which is a hallmark symptom of the beginning of Alzheimer's dementia although distractibility cannot be ruled out. Sometimes when we are distracted, we forget where we are and things look different when driving. Thirteen percent indicated difficulty recognizing objects or people, which is another strong beginning symptom of Alzheimer's disease. One-quarter of the population was diagnosed with an ADD plus an additional disorder, and about 13% of the adults were 50 years and older.

Concentration and awareness:

- Almost one-half of the adults indicated historical problems of being highly distractible, and another 15% indicated this as a new problem for a total of 63% or almost two-thirds of the population.
- Almost one-half indicated historical problems of easily losing their train of thought, and an additional 21% saw this as a new problem for a total of 63% and almost two-thirds of the population.
- One-half indicated historical issues with problems concentrating, and an additional 18% indicated this as a new problem for a total 78% or over three-quarters of the population.
- One-fourth indicated historical problems of their mind going blank, and an additional 16% saw this as a new problem for a total of 45% or almost one-half of the population.
- Using both new and old symptoms, the tendency to become confused and disoriented was one-third of the population at 37%, symptoms that were not indicated as problematic–were blackout spells, or the presence of an aura.
- Using both new and old symptoms, one-quarter of the population indicated not feeling very alert or aware of things.

Memory:

- One-third of the adults indicated historical problems of forgetting where they have left things, and an additional 17% indicated this as a new symptom resulting in over one-half of the population reporting this symptom as problematic.
- One-quarter indicated the tendency to forget names as a historical symptom, and an additional 13% indicated this as a new symptom for a combined presence of over one-third of the adults.
- One-quarter indicated the historical symptom of forgetting what they should be doing; an additional 15% reported this as a new symptom for a combined presence of over one-third reporting this symptom.

- One-quarter of the population reported the new symptom of relying more upon notes to remember things, and an additional 15% reported this as a historical symptom for a total of almost one-half of the population.
- New and historical symptoms combined and resulted in almost one-third of the population reporting forgetting recent events and events of long ago. Twenty-one percent of the adults reported new symptoms of forgetting recent events, while 10% reported new symptoms of forgetting events that happened long ago.
- Symptoms such as forgetting facts or appointments were seen about one-quarter of the time with new symptoms being reported approximately 10% of the time.
- Symptoms that clearly relate to memory problems such as forgetting how to do things but remembering facts, forgetting faces of people, forgetting where one was going, forgetting the order of things, and needing hints to remember things were seen less often (8%–21% of the time) providing confirmation that ADD is a disorder of attention processes and not memory. Historically, ADD-diagnosed individuals rely upon memory for compensation for attention symptoms.

Memory symptoms reported more often were the following: forgetting where things have been left, forgetting names or what one should be doing at the time, as well as relying upon notes to remember things, and are commonly overlapping symptoms primarily related to distractibility (anxiety and stress may be secondary factors).

While memory itself cannot be ruled out of this equation, the greater likelihood is that of attention being a primary variable given that other problems strictly related to memory were reported less often by the adults. The report of new memory symptoms may be a factor of more adults falling within the age range of 30–49 years (49%). It is well known that attention symptoms become worse with age and more noticeable. Therefore, individuals not diagnosed when younger and while in school became more aware of attention deficits as they got older as it interfered with their daily life at home or at work. Additionally, when there is the presence of a new disorder emerging (one-quarter of the adults had ADD plus an additional disorder), attention symptoms would become worse especially when sleep is an additional factor. ADD plus any additional disorder is more likely to affect memory first. Memory problems are commonly seen with sleep deprivation and/or poor restorative sleep. The adult population presented significant symptoms of being tired and having sleep difficulties.

Motor and coordination:

- None of the motor and coordination symptoms were indicated as significantly present, which has not been seen historically accompanying a genetic attention disorder.

Sensory functioning:

- None of the sensory symptoms were indicated as significantly present, which have not been historically seen accompanying a genetic attention disorder.

Physical functioning:

- Headaches were indicated as new and old symptoms in one-third of the population. Headaches may be related to tiredness and poor restorative sleep and/or a sleep-related breathing disorder.
- Excessive tiredness was indicated in almost one-half of the population for new and old symptoms. New symptoms were present in almost one-quarter of the population, which may signal the onset of sleep difficulties over time and is not part of the genetic picture of ADD.

Emotional or behavioral functioning:

Symptoms in this area reflect either accompanying reasons for the evaluation although not indicated specifically and/or the result of the long-term presence of a genetic attention disorder in one's life. The following seem to be long-standing issues that result from battling attention problems on a daily basis. There are no data to suggest whether this worsens with age, but my experience in working with this population suggests that this is the case:

- Almost two-thirds of the population reported the presence of depression, suggesting that attention symptoms can lead to depression (although depression can also create more attention problems in the form of increased distractibility and preoccupation with distressing thoughts).
- Anxiety and nervousness were similarly reported in almost two-thirds of the population. It is well documented in these results that anxiety is a comorbid or coexisting disorder with genetic ADD and becomes worse through time continually interacting with attention symptoms in a downward spiral.
- The presence of stress was reported in three-quarters of the population.
- Sleep problems were reported in one-half of the population.
- Becoming angry more easily was reported in almost one-half of the population.
- Feeling more emotional and not caring about things were reported in almost one-third of the population.
- Difficulties being spontaneous and less inhibited and/or changes in eating habits or sexual interests were not significantly reported. These symptoms are more often associated with executive reasoning deficits and are not symptoms of inattention.

Self-reported symptoms are seen as dispelling the idea that ADD is a genetic disorder involving the executive reasoning processes and instead is related to symptoms of inattention and emotional issues of anxiety.

11 Trends from the Data
What Do the Correlations Tell Us?

The following correlations are highly significant, meaning that when one symptom is present, there is a greater likelihood that the other symptom or symptoms will be present as well, or there is a significant relationship between the two symptoms. We began by determining what symptoms were related using specific items from the self-report measures or checklists. Reported correlations ranged from significant to highly significant.

ADULTS

Nine hundred and eighty-five adults completed a self-report measure: the Personal History Checklist. These adults reported themselves as a fairly healthy group. The major problem indicated was low back pain, followed by digestive system, lung, or breathing issues. These complaints could be reflective of symptoms of various other disorders such as sleep apnea, GERD, smoking, or generalized anxiety. A number of adults reported smoking, which could be a self-medicating solution for anxiety. Symptoms of anxiety can be related to a number of the problems noted in the following.

Thirty-six (35.6) percent of the adults reported receiving treatment for the following problems in adulthood. Of that, 36% of the following issues were reported:

- 8.3% indicated a diagnosis of arthritis.
- 2.5% indicated a diagnosis of cancer.
- 2.5% indicated a diagnosis of diabetes.
- 1.6% indicated a diagnosis of epilepsy.
- 5.8% indicated a diagnosis of heart problems.
- 8.9% indicated a diagnosis of hypertension.
- 33% indicated a diagnosis of low back pain.
- 13.3% indicated a diagnosis of problems with lungs and breathing.
- 21.2% indicated a diagnosis of problems with their digestive system.

ATTENTION AND SLEEP

Attention symptoms and sleep issues are related: Significant adult correlations point to the impact of the following sleep issues revealing the overlap between attention symptoms and lack of sleep or poor quality of sleep. The following are significant correlations based upon responses to questions from the Personal History Checklist as well as the Physical Complaints Checklist (completed by 1112 adults) and the Patient Behavior Checklist (completed by 1195 adults):

- Difficulty getting to sleep and mental restlessness.
- Waking up frequently at night and difficulty completing tasks.
- Waking too early in the morning and being impatient.
- Being tired and impatient.
- Being tired, trouble sleeping, and difficulty shifting tasks.
- Trouble sleeping and mental restlessness.
- Trouble sleeping and being easily distracted.

- Trouble sleeping and poor sustained attention.
- Trouble sleeping and being impulsive.

These reports by adults suggest the correlated impact of sleep upon attention. The importance of sleep is illustrated in looking at one sleep symptom reported by adult such as *being tired during the day* and its significant correlation with so many attention symptoms:

TIREDNESS

Being tired during the day was associated with

- Mental restlessness
- Easily distracted
- Difficulty completing tasks
- Impatience
- Difficulty shifting tasks
- Poor sustained attention
- Impulsivity

SCHOOL, SLEEP, AND ATTENTION

School History and Poor Sleep and Attention

When asked to report about school history, there were correlations related to being disciplined or suspended from school and poor sleep:

Adult report of *being disciplined* in school frequently was associated with

- Waking up a lot at night
- Sleeping enough but not feeling rested
- Poor sleep habits
- Trouble sleeping
- Waking up too early in the morning

Adult report of *being expelled* was associated with

- Poor sleep habits
- Trouble sleeping

Adult report of *being suspended* was associated with

- Waking up a lot at night
- Sleeping too much
- Trouble sleeping

Adult report of *being disciplined* in school frequently was correlated with

- Not having good study habits
- Not understanding class material
- Special classes for learning disability
- Repeating a grade
- Poor sustained attention
- Feeling like they are in the wrong school

Adult report of *being suspended from school* was correlated with

- Feeling out of place at school
- Not understanding class material
- Special classes for learning disability
- Repeating a grade

Adult report of *being expelled from school* was correlated with

- Repeating a grade

ANXIETY, SLEEP, AND SCHOOL

It is more likely that anxiety was related to poor school performance, which then created sleep problems. Included in this adult sample were young adults (age 15 years and up) who may have experienced sleep problems common in adults (not being tired until 11:00 or 12:00 at night and needing to get up at 5:00 or 6:00 for early school start time) or developing owl-like circadian rhythm patterns (more awake late night) or lark (early riser) or even delayed sleep phase (not being tired until 3:00 am):

Adult report of *being anxious about high school* was correlated with

- Trouble getting to sleep
- Waking up a lot at night
- Not getting enough sleep
- Sleeping too much
- Waking up too early in the morning
- Poor sleep habits
- Sleeping enough but not feeling rested
- Restlessness
- Being tired

Being anxious about high school likely increased the presence of attention symptoms and was associated with academic and behavioral difficulties at school:

Adult report of *being anxious about high school* was correlated with

- Easily distracted
- Special classes for learning disability
- Repeating a grade

Adult report of being sick often and missing a lot of school was correlated with

- Being easily distracted
- Having difficulty deciding upon the right course to study
- Concerned about taking the wrong courses

Anxiety is related to fearfulness either as a causal factor or as a product of being fearful, which then affected sleep. Social fears and concerns naturally can affect sleep through the path of anxiety, which then contributes to poor quality of sleep as well as difficulty getting to sleep. Not performing well in school promoted more anxiety and sleep issues related to anxiety:

Adult report of being *afraid of not doing well in school* was correlated with

- Waking up a lot at night
- Restlessness

- Waking up too early in the morning
- Sleeping enough but not feeling rested
- Having to repeat a grade

Adult report of the *fear of not fitting in at school* related to sleep symptoms is as follows:

- Trouble getting to sleep
- Waking up a lot at night
- Not getting enough sleep
- Sleeping too much
- Restlessness
- Waking up too early in the morning
- Sleeping enough but not feeling rested
- Being tired

Adults who reported excellent grades in high school did not report sleep problems. Enjoyment of high school was associated with good study habits, not a surprising finding.

Those who reported sleep problems also reported getting poor grades. Getting poor grades was associated with waking up too early, feelings of being in the wrong school, having special classes for a learning disability, and having to repeat a grade. As expected, special classes for a learning disability was related to having to repeat a grade, being concerned about taking the wrong courses, and feeling like they were in the wrong school. Having to repeat a grade was associated with having special classes for a learning disability and difficulty sleeping, pointing to the continual impact of sleep and anxiety. Having to repeat more than one grade was associated with being tired and difficulty getting to sleep as well as being easily distracted. Requiring special tutoring was associated with not getting along with teachers perhaps related to an overall dislike of school.

CHILDREN

Four hundred and ninety-six parents completed the Developmental History Checklist for Children. In responding to questions regarding temperament, parents described their child between the age of 2 and 5 years as generally active, happy, and content. Parents were able to choose more than one temperament to describe their child:

- 45% described temperament as being active.
- 10.7% described temperament as being passive.
- 43.9% described temperament as being happy.
- 37.9% described temperament as being content.
- Only 3.1% described temperament as being unhappy.
- Only 3.1% described temperament as being calm.

Almost one-third of the parents also described their child as being fearful, suggesting a continual overlap of anxiety seen across all ages. Children were also described as outgoing more often. Other emotional indicators are listed in the following:

- 4.7% described temperament as being nervous.
- 31.6% described temperament as being fearful.
- 13.5% described temperament as being moody.

- 39.5% described temperament as being outgoing.
- 7.7% described temperament as being shy.
- 9.1% described temperament as being quiet.
- 9.25% described temperament as being noisy.
- 6.7% described temperament as being coordinated.
- 20.3% described temperament as being clumsy.
- 4% described temperament as being intelligent.
- 6.8% described temperament as being dull.

MOOD, SLEEP, AND ATTENTION

Correlations were found for current mood, sleep, and attention using symptoms from the Developmental History for Children and the ADDES (completed by 536 parents and 84 teachers):

Parent report of *sudden change in mood or feelings* was correlated with

- Easily distracted
- Restlessness
- Refusing to get up in the morning
- Waking up frequently at night
- Not getting enough sleep

Parent report of *being impulsive* was correlated with

- Restlessness seen by parents
- Being distracted (seen by the teacher)
- Poor concentration (seen by the teacher)

Parent report of being *easily distracted* was correlated with

- Being impulsive
- Difficulty concentrating
- Restlessness
- Difficulty concentrating (seen by the teacher)

Parent report of *restlessness* was correlated with

- Being impulsive
- Distracted
- Difficulty concentrating (seen by both parent and teacher)

SLEEP, ATTENTION, AND ALLERGIES

Overall correlations suggested a relationship between these factors:

- Not getting enough sleep was correlated with being easily distracted.
- Not getting enough sleep was correlated to having an allergic reaction and difficulty concentrating.
- Refusing to go to bed was correlated to difficulty concentrating.
- Refusing to go to bed and difficulty concentrating were also correlated to having an allergic reaction.

TEMPERAMENT AND SLEEP

Temperament and Sleep Age 2–5 Years

Parent descriptions of temperament and sleep for their child during the ages 2–5 years (using the Developmental History Checklist) revealed a relationship of more negative temperament and poor sleep:

Parent description of being *calm* was correlated with

- Improvement in sleep pattern

Parent description of being *active* was correlated with

- Restlessness in bed
- Sleeping enough but still tired
- Not getting enough sleep
- Refusing to go to bed

Parent description of being *withdrawn* was correlated with

- Change in sleep pattern

Parent description of being *unhappy* was correlated with

- Waking up a lot at night

Parent description of *crying* was correlated with

- Not getting enough sleep

Parent description of being *difficult* was correlated with

- Trouble getting to sleep
- Not getting enough sleep
- Waking up too early
- Refusing to go to bed

Parent description of being *irritable* was correlated with

- Restlessness in bed
- Waking up too early
- Trouble getting to sleep

Parent description of being *angry* was correlated with

- Change in sleep pattern
- Waking up too early
- Waking up a lot at night

Parent description of being *cranky* was correlated with

- Trouble getting to sleep
- Restlessness in bed

Sleep and Temperament before Age 2 Years

Parents reported their child's temperament before the age of 2 years. Based upon parent report, sleep was found to be related to temperament:

Parent report of being *difficult* was correlated with

- Trouble getting to sleep
- Waking up too early in the morning
- Refuses to go to bed

Parent report of being *angry* was correlated with

- Not getting enough sleep

Parent report of being *withdrawn* was correlated with

- Restlessness in bed

Parent report of being *hypersensitive* was correlated with

- Waking up too early in the morning
- Restlessness in bed
- Night terrors

Parent report of *crying* was correlated with

- Waking up too early in the morning
- Sleepwalking

Parent report of being *cranky* was correlated with

- Sleepwalking

SLEEP SYMPTOMS

Based upon parent report of sleep symptoms, variables of sleep (sleep onset, sleep maintenance, not getting enough sleep, restless at night, waking up too early, and bedtime refusal) were all related with one another leading to increased tiredness, decreased energy, and difficulty getting up in the morning.

Parent report of being *underactive/slow moving/lacks energy* was correlated with

- Waking up a lot at night
- Not getting enough sleep
- Sleeping enough but still tired
- Falling asleep in school
- Refusing to get up in the morning

Parent report of *trouble getting to sleep* was correlated with

- Waking up a lot at night
- Not getting enough sleep
- Restlessness in bed

Parent report of *waking up a lot at night* was correlated with

- Change in sleep pattern
- Trouble getting to sleep
- Restlessness in bed
- Waking up too early in the morning
- Refusing to go to bed
- Refusing to get up in the morning
- Nightmares

Parent report of *not getting enough sleep* was correlated with

- Waking up too early in the morning
- Refusing to go to bed
- Refusing to get up in the morning
- Nightmares

Parent report of *restlessness in bed* was correlated with

- Change in sleep pattern
- Trouble getting to sleep
- Waking up a lot at night
- Not getting enough sleep
- Waking up too early
- Refusing to go to bed
- Refusing to get up in the morning

Parent report of *waking up too early in the morning* was correlated with

- Change in sleep pattern
- Trouble getting to sleep
- Waking up a lot at night
- Not getting enough sleep
- Restlessness in bed
- Refusing to go to bed
- Nightmares

Parent report of *refusing to go to bed* was correlated with

- Change in sleep pattern
- Trouble getting to sleep
- Waking up a lot at night
- Not getting enough sleep
- Restlessness in bed
- Waking up too early
- Refusing to get up in the morning

Parent report of *refusing to get up in the morning* was correlated with

- Change in sleep pattern
- Trouble getting to sleep
- Waking up a lot at night
- Not getting enough sleep
- Restlessness in bed

- Sleeping enough but still tired
- Change in sleep pattern
- Trouble getting to sleep
- Waking up a lot at night
- Not getting enough sleep
- Restlessness in bed
- Sleeping enough but still tired
- Refusing to go to bed
- Sleepy

Parent report of *nightmares* was correlated with

- Change in sleep pattern
- Waking up a lot at night
- Not getting enough sleep
- Restlessness in bed
- Waking up too early
- Falling asleep in school

ADOLESCENTS

Parents of 181 adolescents completed the Developmental History Checklist.

TEMPERAMENT BEFORE THE AGE OF 2 YEARS

When describing the temperament of their adolescent before the age of 2 years, parents reported their child as social, alert, happy, and affectionate as noted below.

Parents were able to choose more than one temperament to describe their child. The following is the parent's description of their adolescent child before the age of 2 years:

- 18.1% reported calm temperament.
- 24.3% reported active temperament.
- 25.1% reported sociable temperament.
- 1.3% reported withdrawn temperament.
- 37.6% reported happy temperament.
- 0.3% reported unhappy temperament.
- 25.6% reported alert temperament.
- 1.3% reported sleepy temperament.
- 30.4% reported affectionate temperament.
- 5.1% reported crying temperament.
- 4.0% reported difficult temperament.
- 3.5% reported irritable temperament.
- 1.1% reported hypersensitive temperament.
- 6% reported angry temperament.
- 1.9% reported fearful temperament.

SLEEP AND TEMPERAMENT BEFORE THE AGE OF 2 YEARS

Parents described their adolescent child's sleep and temperament prior to age 2 years. Based upon parent report, there were significant correlations for sleep and temperament factors prior to the age of 2 years. It is likely that the following descriptors were clearly present for parents to be able to recall them when their child was in adolescence which was the time period they completed this self-report measure. Correlations noted below are based upon questions from the Developmental History for Children and the Child Behavior Checklist (completed by 212 parents).

Parent report of being *withdrawn* was correlated with

- Poor sleep habits
- Change in sleep habits
- Nightmares

Parent report of being *unhappy* was correlated with

- Sleeping too much
- Change in sleep habits
- Refusing to go to bed
- Refusing to get up in the morning

Parent report of being *sleepy* was correlated with

- Poor sleep habits
- Change in sleep habits

Parent report of being *affectionate* was correlated with

- Change in sleep habits

Parent report of *crying* was correlated with

- Poor sleep habits
- Change in sleep habits
- Sleeping poorly
- Refusing to go to bed
- Trouble getting to sleep

Parent report of being *difficult* was correlated with

- Poor sleep habits
- Change in sleep habits
- Sleeping poorly
- Trouble getting to sleep
- Nightmares
- Waking up too early
- Waking up a lot at night

Parent report of being *irritable* was correlated with

- Change in sleep habits

Parent report of being *hypersensitive* was correlated with

- Poor sleep habits
- Change in sleep habits
- Trouble getting to sleep

Parent report of being *angry* was correlated with

- Poor sleep habits
- Change in sleep habits

Parent report of being *fearful* was correlated with

- Poor sleep habits
- Change in sleep habits

Parent report of being *cranky* was correlated with

- Change in sleep pattern
- Waking up too early
- Sleepwalking

TEMPERAMENT FROM AGE 2 TO 5 YEARS

Parents of adolescents reported on their child's temperament from the age of 2 to 5 years and continued to describe their child in a generally similar manner to their description of before 2 years, as active, sociable, affectionate, and alert:

- 12.5% reported calm temperament.
- 26.7% reported active temperament.
- 24.5% reported sociable temperament.
- 2.7% reported withdrawn temperament.
- 36.8% reported happy temperament.
- 1.1% reported unhappy temperament.
- 22.7% reported alert temperament.
- 5% reported sleepy temperament.
- 29.3% reported affectionate temperament.
- 2.9% reported crying temperament.
- 6.9% reported difficult temperament.
- 4.5% reported irritable temperament.
- 4% reported hypersensitive temperament.
- 4.3% reported angry temperament.
- 3.7% reported fearful temperament.

SLEEP AND TEMPERAMENT FROM AGE 2 TO 5 YEARS

Parent reported on their child's sleep and temperament from age 2 to 5 years: There were significant correlations found among the following temperament characteristics reported by parents and the development of symptoms of sleep and sleep-related physical issues over time. Tonsillitis emerged as a problem associated with sleep and temperament difficulties. Poor sleep was found to be related to mood changes and lack of energy:

Parent report of being *difficult* was correlated with

- Trouble getting to sleep
- Waking up a lot at night
- Waking up too early
- Sleeping poorly
- Trouble getting to sleep
- Poor sleeping habits

- Refusing to get to bed
- Refusing to get up in the morning
- Tonsillitis

Parent report of being *irritable* was correlated with

- Poor sleep habits

Parent report of being *hypersensitive* was correlated with

- Sleeping too much
- Trouble getting to sleep
- Poor sleep habits
- Asthma diagnosis

Parent report of *sudden changes in mood/feelings* was correlated with

- Poor sleep habits
- Nightmares
- Change in sleep habits

Parent report of being *angry* was correlated with

- Waking too early
- Sleeping poorly
- Change in sleep habits
- Poor sleep habits

Parent report of *crying* was correlated with

- Waking too early
- Poor sleep habits
- Sleeping poorly

Parent report of being *fearful* was correlated with

- Change in sleep habits
- Poor sleep habits

Parent report of being *cranky* was correlated with

- Frequently tired

Parent report of being *underactive/slow moving/lacks energy* was correlated with

- Sleeping too much
- Sleeps enough but still tired
- Refusing to go to bed
- Nightmares
- Poor sleep habits
- Sleeps poorly
- Frequently tired

Sleep, Attention, Emotions, Tonsillitis, and Ear Infections

When statistically analyzed, further tonsillitis and ear infections were seen more often and related to poor concentration/distractibility, increased emotions, and poor sleep. The following are correlations for sleep, attention, temperament, tonsillitis and ear infections:

- Refusing to go to bed, difficult temperament, and easily distracted.
- Frequently tired and ear infections.
- Frequently tired, difficult temperament, and easily distracted.
- Difficult temperament and restlessness in bed.
- Restless in bed and easily distracted.
- Restless in bed, difficult temperament, and ear infections.
- Frequently tired, irritable, tonsillitis, and difficulty concentrating.

Parent report of being *easily distracted* was correlated with

- Tonsillitis
- Difficulty concentrating
- Restlessness
- Impulsivity

Parent report of *difficulty concentrating* was correlated with

- Being impulsive
- Restlessness
- Impulsive

Parent report of being *impulsive* was correlated with

- Distracted
- Restlessness

Parent report of *restlessness* was correlated with

- Being impulsive
- Distracted
- Difficulty concentrating
- Impulsive

Overall, these statistically significant correlations suggest the continual cyclical relationship between emotions, sleep, and attention factors. The question is whether the finding of ear infections (seen more often in this sample) and tonsillitis is related to sleep-disordered breathing problems. What is clear is that poor sleep predisposes individuals for more attention issues. Anxiety seems to be another rather powerful mediating factor affecting sleep and attention. Poor school performance certainly increases anxiety, and anxiety through the path of avoidance can lead to poor school performance.

12 Published Research Resulting from This Study

Two research studies are currently in preparation for publication using the data presented in this book.

The first is the study of adults: *Sleep disturbances and executive function in adults with attention deficit/hyperactivity disorder* (Yoon et al., in preparation). Sleep disturbances and the impact of sleep on attention were assessed using neuropsychological testing for a 20 year period (1989–2009) with an adult population of 958 subjects. Findings of the study suggested the most significant difficulty with sleep was sleep initiation as well as sleep maintenance and overall quality of sleep. A considerable number of adults reported more than one ongoing sleep problem, and approximately half of the subjects indicated the presence of fatigue. The frequency of fatigue was correlated with the frequency of sleep problems.

Sustained attention was found to be affected by both gender and fatigue. Performance was worse for females suffering from severe fatigue. Differences were not seen between subjects with no or mild sleep problems and those with severe sleep problems, suggesting that compensation occurs with severe but not moderate sleep problems. Gender and the experience of fatigue were found to be important factors affecting neuropsychological performance. Sleep disorders and fatigue were found to be an important clinical consideration in ADD/ADHD.

A large percentage of adults diagnosed with an attention disorder reported sleep problems, and of those sleep problems, approximately 75% had one to three concurrent sleep problems, and 25% had four to seven concurrent sleep problems. Approximately half of the ADD adults reported having sleep problems at least once per week. Fatigue was found to be correlated with sleep problems; the greater the fatigue, the more sleep problems that were reported.

Women were found to be more vulnerable to the development of sleep problems, reporting more fatigue than males. Suggested is the possibility of gender differences relating to sleep that may be hormonally related.

Neuropsychological tests were found to be significantly impacted by gender and fatigue severity but not by sleep problems indicating that fatigue seems to be a different phenomenon on testing than a sleep problem.

Females performed better than males on the written portion of the measure of whole-brain functioning (SDMT). Both males and females performed poorly on the Paced Addition Serial Attention Test (PASAT), a measure of paced addition assessing information processing.

The second research article used all of the subjects, children, adolescents, and adults, and compared their performance on the self-report measures and neuropsychological testing. It is entitled *Gender Differences in Neuropsychological Testing Performance across the Lifespan in a Diagnosed ADD/ADHD Population from the Years 1989 to 2009* (Fisher et al., in preparation).

Test results for 1828 children (ages 5–11 years), adolescents (12–17 years), and adults evaluated between the years 1989 and 2009 were analyzed. Results revealed that age, in combination with inattentive ADD/ADHD versus ADHD plus an additional disorder, was associated with numerous sleep and anxiety issues.

The progression from childhood to adolescence and adulthood revealed increased report of anxiety and fatigue symptoms. A higher report of daytime fatigue was seen in comparing the children, adolescents, and adult; fatigue steadily increased as the subject(s) age increased. Adult males reported more fatigue than females.

The diagnosis of ADHD versus ADHD plus an additional disorder, gender, age, as well as anxiety and sleep factors (problems with sleep onset, maintenance, and restive sleep) were significant variables impacting neuropsychological test performance and functioning.

Children diagnosed with ADHD plus had more difficulty on tests of sequencing and cognitive flexibility, while those with inattentive ADHD performed worse on a task of slow-paced verbal input. Adolescents and adults diagnosed with ADHD plus an additional disorder performed worse on tests of distractibility, whole-brain functioning (timed measure), and cognitive flexibility.

On the oral portion of the speeded measure of whole-brain functioning, those with no sleep problems or fatigue performed better than those with moderate to severe fatigue. This portion can be impacted by distractibility and tendency to lose one's place when not writing.

This outcome was confusing in that those subjects with severe sleep problems and no fatigue or those with severe fatigue performed worse than those with moderate fatigue, suggesting some type of compensation process when not severely impacted and yet still affected. It is well known that those diagnosed with an attention problem tend to compensate for attention symptoms and underscore the issue that ADHD is an attitude of learned avoidance, dislike of school, and reading comprehension problems. This would be consistent with the reason why medication as a sole intervention fails to resolve the impact of this disorder and that following a honeymoon period, individuals are apt to be once again struggling with symptoms of attention manifested more through their emotions than actual attention symptoms.

Adolescents were found to perform better on measures of distractibility and divided attention but worse than adults on tasks of sequencing and cognitive flexibility, which may relate to their ability to compensate for distraction but not for speed and the visuospatial component involved in these tasks. Whether it is the normative data that become less rigorous for adults or the ability to handle the speed and visuospatial analysis remains an unanswered question.

Those who reported no sleep problems but moderate fatigue performed worse than those who reported no fatigue or severe fatigue on a task of sustained attention, fast-paced input. This raises the question of the effect of moderate fatigue; that compensation occurs only in the presence of severe fatigue. Individuals may get used to moderate fatigue, living with the problem as opposed to mobilizing resources for compensation.

Comparison of sleep complaints for children, adolescents, and adults suggests that as ADHD individuals age, sleep quality declines. There were more sleep problems and greater indication of the number of sleep problems with age. The same was true for anxiety and fatigue.

Notable was the increased presence of emotionality when comparing children and adolescents on the same parent self-report measures. There were statistically significant changes in self-esteem, parent–child relations, peer relations, and arguments over homework. There were decreased arguments over bedtime, likely the result of parents choosing their battles and being more upset with homework and poor grades than bedtime issues. When compared to children, the friends of adolescents had better grades than they did. Adolescents had become more involved with peers committing delinquent activities. Adolescents reported more negative self-esteem, more suicidal actions, as well as increased depression and anxiety symptoms. The escalation of anxiety creating more sleep problems especially with sleep onset may be a cyclical spiral associated with ADHD inattentive type.

This matches clinical experience whereby anxiety is generalized and genetic, seen in the family history evolving over time to become more significant as school becomes more difficult, and there is increased avoidance and procrastination leading to more anxiety and less sleep.

For the children, trouble getting to sleep and poor sleep were the most problematic sleep problems reported. In adolescents and adults, the most common sleep problem was nonrestorative sleep, trouble getting to sleep, waking up a lot at night, and restlessness, suggesting that sleep problems were becoming more pervasive.

In the adolescent population, more males reported having one to three sleep problems, while more females reported having either no sleep problems or having four to seven or more sleep problems. Almost 39% of the parents of children reported sleep problems (one to two problems) compared to parental report for adolescents of 62% and adult self-report at almost 60% reporting sleep problems. Two percent of the children were reported with three to four sleep problems compared to 12% for the adolescents of four to seven sleep problems and 20% of the adults (reporting four to seven sleep problems). Over 60% of the children were found to have no problems with fatigue compared to 43% of the adolescents and 53% of adults suffering from reported fatigue.

Anxiety increased to the point where 60% of the adults reported feeling irritable or nervous at least once per week. Statistically significant correlations were found between the frequency of sleep problems, anxiety, and fatigue in adolescents and adults.

Inattentive ADHD children performed worse than ADHD plus on a slow-paced verbal input task and better on measures of speed (Trail Making Tests) likely revealing the greater difficulty and pattern typically seen when there are additional issues beyond ADD; these tests were affected. In this regard, the problems of ADHD plus an additional disorder were seen as the result of executive reasoning deficits as opposed to visual–spatial producing more problems on these measures and a longer time to complete the task. The ADHD plus group may not have found the slow-paced task to be easier and boring as a result; thus, they performed better.

As expected with that seen clinically for all ages, inattentive ADHD subjects performed better than the ADHD plus group on tasks of divided attention, whole-brain functioning, cognitive flexibility portion of the trails, and paced addition task (likely the result of problematic working memory and/or speeded addition or math fluency).

CONCLUSIONS

1. Age is associated with increased sleep problems. Adults had more sleep problems than children or adolescents. Within the adult population, older age was associated with a higher number of reported sleep problems; that is, sleep problems were more frequent and occurred more often.
2. The presence of ADHD over time results in increased anxiety revealing the effect of age. Gender is another factor impacting this increase through time. This may be due to the impact of untreated anxiety over time, and/or the impact of attention is affecting anxiety as long-standing attention problems aggravate the individual and result in more anxiety symptoms.
3. The frequency of anxiety was found to be greater in those individuals diagnosed with ADHD than those diagnosed with ADHD plus an additional disorder. Anxiety in the ADHD plus population occurred at a frequency of either never or on a daily basis, suggesting the extreme of being highly problematic or no problem at all.
4. ADHD subtype has an impact. Those with the diagnosis of only ADD and not an additional disorder performed better on tasks of distractibility and divided attention, whole-brain functioning (with factors of speeded processing, short-term memory, and visual scanning), and cognitive flexibility (ability to switch sets). Contrary to this finding was the measure of slow-paced verbal input where the plus group (with an additional disorder) performed better, possibly the result of more difficulty with the task; hence, it was not boring. Another explanation would be increased perfectionism in reaction to their awareness of more cognitive problems.
5. Attention symptoms as well as anxiety over the years may be contributing to the increase of sleep problems. Compensation for attention symptoms may decrease with age and further compromised status via age, sleep, and anxiety.
6. Report of fatigue and number of sleep problems are separate issues and play different roles. Moderate fatigue presents more of a challenge. Individuals were seen as having more

problems with moderate fatigue than severe fatigue. It is hypothesized that individuals become used to moderate fatigue and do not employ compensatory mechanisms, whereas with severe fatigue, there is greater awareness and employment of coping strategies.

7. When severity of sleep problems and severity of fatigue were examined in relation to a task of whole-brain functioning, individuals with no sleep problems and no fatigue performed better than those with no sleep problems but reporting moderate or severe fatigue. Severe sleep problems were seen as having a significant impact on this task even when fatigue was not present.

8. Fatigue affected the slow-paced verbal input task revealing better performance when only moderate fatigue was present and no sleep problems. In fact, those with moderate and severe sleep problems as well as moderate and severe fatigue performed better than no sleep problems, suggesting either the presence of compensation on this boring task similar to that seen for the ADHD plus group and/or their ability to complete this task due to the slow pace.

9. There is some impact related to moderate fatigue that does not allow the degree of compensation seen when there is severe fatigue. On a task of fast-paced nonverbal input of information, those who reported a moderate level of fatigue even without sleep problems had worse performance than those who reported no sleep problems and no fatigue or severe fatigue.

10. Gender relates to sleep problems in adults. ADHD subtype (ADD versus ADHD plus) and gender were associated with increased frequency of sleep problems.

11. Adolescent findings suggested that more males than females report experiencing sleep problems on a nearly daily basis. Females may have better coping mechanisms or strategies to reduce sleep problems, and/or the stress of adolescent life may be contributing to more sleep issues in males.

12. In the adult population, males were found to experience fatigue more often than females indicating being tired during the day on a nearly daily basis. This again suggests that either the females are more equipped to handle fatigue and/or males are more affected by fatigue.

13. Fatigue affects adolescents and adults to an extensive degree, with 50% of subjects reporting feeling tired during the day. As individuals age, fatigue plays a greater role revealed by increased report of daytime fatigue.

14. Overall progression through the life span affects symptoms of ADHD, suggesting the complexity of this disorder as symptoms vary depending upon gender, sleep, and anxiety.

FOUR ABSTRACTS COMPLETED BASED UPON THE DATA

1. Gender differences across the lifespan in neuropsychological testing performance in ADHD population from the years 1991 to 2008 (Fisher et al., 2011b).

   Differences were found between males and females when comparing the test data of 673 adults, and adolescents from the age of 15–73 years were included in the study. There were 419 males and 254 females, and all subjects were diagnosed with ADHD (inattentive type). Excluded were those individuals who had any additional issues related to brain injury. The following neuropsychological tests were analyzed: PASAT, Trail Making Tests, Stroop task, and the Symbol Digits Modalities task (written) (SDMT-W). Results revealed that females of all ages performed worse than males on all four trials of the PASAT. On the Stroop task, a significant interaction of depression and gender was found with females without depression performing better than males without depression, while there were no gender differences for subjects with depression. Also depressed females performed worse than nondepressed females, while for males there was no difference. Males and females did not differ in performance on the SDMT and the two Trail Making Tests. Findings indicated that gender differences are present across the life span on tasks of information processing, as seen on performance on the PASAT. Additionally, depression serves as a moderating factor in performance on tasks assessing distractibility, as seen on the Stroop task to a greater degree for females than males. Significant gender differences do not occur systematically in performance on tasks such as the SDMT and Trail Making Tests, which involve speeded performance and whole-brain functioning.

2. Cognitive and behavioral differences between ADHD populations (inattentive type versus ADHD plus) using neuropsychological testing and self-reported symptoms in diagnosed population from the years 1991 to 2008 (Fisher et al., 2011a).

The goal was to investigate the relationship between inattentive type ADHD and ADHD plus using neuropsychological tests, self-reported anxiety, and hyperactivity in a clinic population.

Testing was analyzed for 1332 adults referred for ADD/ADHD testing (15–50 years, 831 males), 74% with diagnosed ADHD (inattentive type) and 24% with ADHD plus additional disorder (i.e., sleep apnea; brain dysfunction excluded). Neuropsychological tests included Trail Making Tests (A and B) and SDMT-W. Self-report measures assessed hyperactivity and anxiety on different self-report measures (PPCA, PHCA, PBC, PCC). The results suggest that hyperactivity and anxiety were frequently seen with no significant difference between ADHD and ADHD plus. We found a significant relationship between hyperactivity and anxiety. Individuals who reported yes to one or both anxiety items had higher hyperactivity scores than those who said no to both items. Those adults identified with ADD plus performed worse on all neuropsychological tests. Findings indicate that ADHD (inattentive type) and ADHD plus can be differentiated on cognitive measures but not on self-reported symptoms of anxiety and hyperactivity as these comorbid factors are highly prevalent in both populations.

3. Effect of reported sleep and attention symptoms on neuropsychological testing perfor-mance in adult diagnosed ADD/ADHD population from the years 1991 to 2008 (Fisher et al., 2011c).

The purpose of this abstract was to investigate the influence of sleep and attention-related symptoms on neuropsychological testing performance in a diagnosed ADD/ADHD population. There were a total of 1262 adults age 15–80 years included in the sample anal-ysis. There were 802 males and 451 females, 935 of which were diagnosed with ADD and 305 of which were diagnosed with ADD plus an additional disorder (affecting sleep and/or impact to brain function). A neuropsychological test battery was utilized to assess atten-tion variables, and self-report measures were employed to assess sleep and other health factors. The self-report measures included the Personal Problems Checklist for Adults, Personal History Checklist for Adults, Patient Behavior Checklist for ADHD Adults, and Physical Complaints Checklist for ADHD Adults. Neuropsychological test measures included Stroop Color Word Test, Symbol Digits Modalities Test (written), and the PASAT. Results revealed that those individuals diagnosed with only ADD (versus ADHD plus an additional disorder) performed better on most of the test measures. Females performed worse than males on all of the PASAT, paced addition trials. Sleep disturbances did not influence task performance, but tiredness had a significant interaction on the test measures, and the effect of tiredness was stronger for females.

4. Self-reported sleep problems and neuropsychological performance in ADHD (Fisher et al., 2011d)

The goal of this study was to explore the impact of self-reported sleep problems (disturbed sleep and hypersomnia/sleepiness) on neuropsychological performance in subjects with ADHD without a diagnosed sleep disorder. This was a retrospective chart review of 607 adults and adolescents (15–73 years, 229 females, 378 males) with diagnosed ADHD (inattentive type) and without diagnosed sleep disorder or brain injury/insult. Neuropsychological tests used the Trail Making Tests, the Stroop test, and the SDMT-W.

Self-reported problems initiating or maintaining sleep (sleep disturbance) and hypersomnia or sleepiness were extracted from the Personal History Checklist for Adults. Self-reported sleep problems were found to have no influence on performance in the Trails Making-B, Stroop test, or SDMT-W. Subjects with self-reported problems initiating or maintaining sleep performed worse on the Trail Making-A. Self-reported sleep problems in ADHD had an impact only on a speeded sequencing measure. There was no impact seen on a measure of whole-brain functioning that is also dependent upon speed. Similarly, there was not an influence seen on a task of divided attention measuring distractibility or a task of cognitive flexibility that assesses executive function when controlling for age, gender, depression, anxiety, and premorbid intelligence. While we have found that more ADHD subjects report sleep problems, these problems were found to influence performance on only one of the test measures assessed, which is a task highly dependent upon speed.

REFERENCES

Fisher, B.C. et al. (2011a) Cognitive and behavioral differences between ADHD populations (inattentive type versus ADHD plus) using neuropsychological testing and self-reported symptoms in diagnosed population from the years 1991 to 2008, presented as an abstract at the *ANA Annual Conference*, San Diego, CA, September 2011, United Psychological Services, Max Planck Institute of Psychiatry, Munich, Germany.

Fisher, B.C. et al. (2011b) Gender differences across the lifespan in neuropsychological testing performance in ADHD population from the years 1991 to 2008, presented as an abstract at the *ANA Annual Conference*, San Diego, CA, September 2011, United Psychological Services, Max Planck Institute of Psychiatry, Munich, Germany.

Fisher, B.C. et al. (2011c) Neuropsychological testing performance in adult diagnosed ADD/ADHD population from the years 1991 to 2008, presented as an abstract at the *APSS Annual Conference*, Baltimore, MD, June 2011, United Psychological Services, Max Planck Institute of Psychiatry, Munich, Germany.

Fisher, B.C. et al. (2011d) Self-reported sleep problems and neuropsychological performance in ADHD, presented as an abstract at the *WASM Conference*, Quebec, Canada, September 2011, United Psychological Services, Max Planck Institute of Psychiatry, Munich, Germany.

Fisher, B.C., Garges, D.M., Yoon, S.Y.R., Maguire, K., Zipay, D., and Gambino, M., Gender differences in neuropsychological testing performance across the lifespan in a diagnosed ADD/ADHD population from the years 1989 to 2009 (in preparation).

Yoon, S.Y.R., Fisher, B.C., Garges, D.M., Maguire, K., Zipay, D., and Shapiro, C.M., Sleep disturbances and executive function in adults with attention-deficit (in preparation).

13 Review of the Research for ADHD

A large survey study found ADHD symptoms in 9.2% of the population studied with a male/female ratio of 2.28:1 (Ramtekkar et al., 2010). In 2000, ADHD was the most common behavior disorder among children comprising 3%–7% of all school-age children. By 2007, there had been an increase to 9.5% for parent report of the presence of ADHD diagnosis for the age range of 4–17 years (Center for Disease Control and Prevention, 2010). Studies of college students and adults suggest an adult prevalence rate at 4%–5% (American Psychological Association, 2000; DuPaul et al., 2001). Kessler et al. (2006) reported a prevalence rate of 4.4%.

The number of children diagnosed with ADHD has steadily increased through the years as opposed to those diagnosed with a learning disability whose numbers have remained fairly stable. Children diagnosed with ADHD were more likely to have had contact with a mental health professional, to use prescription medication, and to have frequent health-care visits, while children with LD (or a learning disability) were more likely to use special education services. Children with Medicaid coverage were more likely than uninsured children and privately insured children to have a diagnosis of ADHD or LD (Pastor and Reuben, 2008).

Through our research, we have determined specific time periods when ADHD is more likely to be diagnosed. They are preschool and kindergarten (usually related to behavioral problems of hyperactivity and impulsivity), third grade (usually related to poor performance and reading comprehension difficulties), seventh grade (the result of uncompleted assignments, low motivation toward academic work), and high school (poor grades due to lack of effort). We also find to a lesser degree that diagnosis may occur after or during the first year of college (when academic probation is a primary reason for evaluation).

CONTROVERSY ABOUT TESTING FOR ADD/ADHD: SELF-REPORT MEASURES VERSUS NEUROPSYCHOLOGICAL TESTING

A literature review by Davidson (2008) suggests that a valid and reliable assessment should be comprehensive, including the use of symptom rating scales, clinical interview, neuropsychological testing, and corroboration of patient reports.

Neuropsychological testing for ADD/ADHD has brought forth many contradictory studies given the focus upon executive reasoning deficits as opposed to attention. Primary symptoms of executive reasoning are perseveration (getting stuck), selective attention (attending to everything and inability to attend to anything for long as a result), poor sequential analysis, problem solving, and integration (seeing the whole perspective). One of the problems is the lack of consensus in the field as to how to test for ADD/ADHD related to the lack of agreement of what this disorder truly is or means in the real world.

Reliance upon self-report measures yields different data than the neuropsychological testing. This is seen in the drug manufacturer's contention that newer nonstimulant medications such as Intuniv and older medications like Strattera help to alleviate ADD/ADHD symptoms. In our research, neuropsychological testing reports no differences in the effects of either of these medications on attention symptoms. Testing on and off of medication showed no differences compared to robust differences seen with the stimulant medications over the years. The problem with using self-report measures as the entire basis for diagnosis is that these symptoms can be seen with many disorders not just ADD/ADHD.

Klenberg et al. (2010) used an inventory addressing the executive reasoning deficits typically seen accompanying the ADHD combined disorder (symptoms of both inattention and hyperactivity–impulsivity). Gender differences were noted on this inventory with boys having a consistently higher rating of executive reasoning problems. Executive function (EF) issues were seen as related to the regulation of behavior in complex cognitive and social situations, comprising a wide range of regu-latory, attention, and memory functioning problems including response inhibition and interference control as well as deficits in working memory. Gender differences were seen as the result of better coping strategies and/or lower symptom levels in girls than boys. Similarly, Reddy et al. (2011) reported ADHD as a neurodevelopmental disorder involving EF using the BRIEF (Behavior Rating Inventory of Executive Function Parent Form for children) inventory with ADHD and matched con-trols. They found ADHD youth to display more symptom impairment in EF behaviors than controls. According to the authors, the Behavioral Regulation Index made the most significant contribution as the discriminating factor consistent with arguments that response inhibition is the primary deficit in ADHD. The problem is that these findings are based upon self-report measures and could be due to other undiagnosed disorders. Barkley et al. (2002) completed a study examining the persistence of ADHD into young adulthood using hyperactive children evaluated at ages 19–25 years finding that previous studies relying upon self-report may have substantially underestimated the persistence of ADHD into adulthood.

A recent study found slowness as a contributing factor to learning difficulties, similar to what we have characteristically seen with the inattentive type ADD such as the problem of slow speed on timed assessment. Slowness is seen as a core symptom of ADHD (contrary to the focus upon inattention and hyperactivity/impulsivity). Children with ADHD made more errors than children in the control group. While the problem decreased with age, children with ADHD were slower and exhibited greater response time variability than control children, which may explain the variation during the daytime of attention capacities in ADHD (Bourel-Ponchel et al., 2011).

In our research, a large population of clinically identified children with normal intelligence (886 children) were compared to a control group on tasks of learning, attention, graphomotor, and processing speed scores. While results revealed nonsignificant differences between the two groups for the diagnosis of emotional/behavioral disorders (anxiety, depression, and opposi-tional defiant disorder), there were significant differences seen for ADHD and autism diagnostic groups. Control children performed better than children with ADHD and autism in all areas. Children with ADHD and autism did not differ from one another except that children with ADHD had greater learning problems. Attention, graphomotor, and speed weaknesses are likely comorbid factors to the majority of children with autism and ADHD contributing significantly to the prediction of poorer academic achievement (Mayes and Calhoun, 2007). Individuals diag-nosed with ADHD combined disorder were found to have greater impulsivity than ADHD inat-tentive with the inattentive group revealing slower processing speed than the combined group (Mayes et al., 2009).

Simon et al. (2009) noted that the prevalence of ADHD in adults is seen as declining with age in the general population. The unclear validity of DSM-IV diagnostic criteria for this condition may have led to reduced prevalence rates as a result of underestimation of the prevalence of adult ADHD.

IMPACT OF ANXIETY AND OVERACTIVITY

Complicating the process further is the overlap between anxiety and overactivity. Females had significantly higher levels of symptoms of generalized anxiety than males when diagnosed with the combined subtype. Separation anxiety was significantly greater in girls diagnosed with the inatten-tive subtype. The ADHD combined subtype accounted for the majority of the comorbidity found (Klenberg et al., 2010).

CONTROVERSY ABOUT EXECUTIVE REASONING DEFICITS

There are researchers who maintain that ADD/ADHD is the result of executive reasoning deficits in a hard-wired brain regardless of other mitigating factors. Seidman et al. (2000) using siblings with ADHD as controls found greater impairment on measures of distractibility, verbal learning, and memory for those diagnosed as ADHD regardless of being on medication during the assessment. Siblings without ADHD were similar to controls on virtually all measures. ADHD status was associated with significant neuropsychological impairments not accounted for by psychiatric or cognitive comorbidity.

The change in diagnosis to all subtypes being labeled under the umbrella of ADHD (Fisher, 1998) has led to much confusion in the diagnosis of this disorder and accentuated the emphasis upon executive reasoning. Barkley (1997) proposed that ADHD comprises a deficit in behavioral inhibition. He proposed a theoretical model that links inhibition to four executive neuropsychological functions that appear to depend on it for their effective execution: working memory, self-regulation of affect–motivation–arousal, internalization of speech, and reconstitution (behavioral analysis and synthesis). The model predicts that ADHD should be associated with secondary impairments in these four executive abilities and the motor control they afford. Evidence was found to be the strongest for deficits in behavioral inhibition, working memory, regulation of motivation, and motor control in those with ADHD. Biederman et al. (2004) found an association between the presence of EF deficits and functional outcomes with ADHD. Those diagnosed as ADHD with EF deficits were more at risk for grade retention and a decrease in academic achievement relative to ADHD alone. No difference was found for social functioning. Children and adolescents with ADHD and executive deficits were found to be at high risk for significant impairments in academic functioning.

While it is clear that the ADD/ADHD population has cognitive and emotional problems, the question of executive reasoning deficits remains a more complicated area of study. Our perspective from testing this disorder for well over 20 years is that the executive reasoning deficits are present when there is an additional disorder, labeled as ADHD plus. The importance of this large study detailed in this book is to provide clinical research, suggesting that ADD is the true inattentive disorder and that executive reasoning deficits complicate the picture when there is a comorbid disorder.

Not all research is in agreement. Some studies using neuropsychological testing cite differences between the ADHD identified subtypes of inattentive, combined, and combined–hyperactive, while others see no differences and instead maintain that ADD is a neurodevelopmental disorder characterized by executive reasoning deficits. Perhaps one of the problems is medication. Studies reported testing while children were on medication, which would make a difference in the results, while the data reported in this book comprised testing completed while test subjects were not on medication, and often the children had never been on medication and were medication naive. Another problem is that different tests were used, tests for memory and executive reasoning, as opposed to a formal battery for attention that was consistently utilized across time. The difference in the research findings may be the result of the different measures assessed. Finally, the way that the different measures are analyzed becomes an issue in reporting research results. For example, the Stroop is a popular measure used by researchers and reported to be a measure of executive reasoning when it was designed to address divided attention.

O'Brien et al. (2010) found that boys and girls with ADHD revealed similar deficits on tests of executive reasoning excluding patterns that related to response inhibition and planning; girls had more of a problem with strategic planning and boys with inhibition. Findings highlight the multidimensional nature of executive reasoning and the need for diverse multiple methods of assessment (O'Brien et al., 2010). Motoric overflow (involuntary movement of the opposite hand that is voluntarily engaged in movement) was found to be more prominent in boys than girls with ADHD (MacNeil et al., 2011). The presence of mirror overflow was also found to be more prominent in the nondominant hand and seen more often with the diagnosis of ADHD than matched peers. This provides a window into the neuropathophysiology of ADHD. Mirror overflow was thought to result from impaired inhibition of involuntary synkinetic movements. Impairment of voluntary response inhibition is hypothesized to contribute to the core diagnostic features of excessive hyperactivity, impulsivity, and off-task behavior (MacNeil et al., 2011).

Hinshaw et al. (2007) performed a study prospectively following girls diagnosed with ADHD over a period of 5 years. Neuropsychological test measures examined attention skills, EFs, and language abilities. While finding moderate to large deficits in executive/attentional performance as well as rapid naming, they did not find differences for the ADHD subtypes. Girls diagnosed with ADHD during childhood continued to display significant deficits in comparison to matched controls but did not differ among the subtypes. When a similar study had been completed in 2002 without stimulant medication, all 10 variables of neuropsychological testing revealed significant subgroup differences. Neuropsychological deficits were more pronounced in girls with both ADHD and LD and in those without medications. ADHD was associated with modest, but significant, neuropsychological impairment. Seidman et al. (2006) found that girls with ADHD have neuropsychological deficits independent of psychiatric comorbidities and that those with comorbid learning disability have the most severe impairments.

Differentiating executive reasoning symptoms from the different ADHD subtypes has been confusing and less clear yielding different results leaving the question open as to whether executive reasoning deficits are the result of the ADHD diagnosis and/or the combined effect of comorbid disorders.

Young adults with ADHD were compared to controls on 14 measures of EF and olfactory identification, and the ADHD group performed significantly worse on 11 measures. No difference was found in the ADHD group as a function of ADHD subtype or comorbid oppositional defiance; comparisons between combined, hyperactive, and inattentive groups were not significant on any measure. Adults were found to demonstrate significant deficits in interference control, in response inhibition, and in sustained attention and working memory as well as being more impaired in olfactory identification, suggesting impact to the prefrontal brain region. Results suggest that the same pattern in childhood is represented in adulthood (Murphy et al., 2001).

Dual-process models of ADHD suggest that both EF and regulatory functions (processing speed) are involved and that EF weaknesses may be associated specifically with symptoms of inattention–disorganization but not hyperactivity/impulsivity. Inattention was associated with slower response speed and hyperactivity/impulsivity with faster output speed. Clear deficits in executive reasoning in the ADHD adult sample across several key measures were seen and noted on an aggregate composite EF factor. This EF deficit was largely related to symptoms of inattention/disorganization but not to hyperactivity/impulsivity. Speed emerged as a partially distinct neuropsychological factor related to both ADHD symptom domains. The overall finding was that EF is weakened in young adults diagnosed with ADHD similar to that observed in children (Nigg et al., 2005).

Aman et al. (1998) found that unmedicated ADHD boys exhibited performance deficits on tasks in both frontal and parietal domains compared to controls. Unmedicated ADHD boys appeared to be more severely impaired on the frontal tasks than on the parietal tasks. Medicated ADHD boys performed better in both task domains compared with unmedicated ADHD boys. Results support both theories of the frontal lobe and parietal lobe involvement, although the frontal lobe was more strongly supported.

Huang-Pollok et al. (2006) did not find any evidence for anterior or posterior system dysfunction for either subtype of ADHD. ADHD children with inattentive and combined subtypes had lower sensitivity to detect targets from nontargets on a visuospatial attention task. Performance for both subtypes decreased to a greater extent over time in a manner consistent with problems in sustained attention. Frazier et al. (2004) did not find support for the notion of a generalized executive reasoning deficit. They did find that overall cognitive ability was significantly lower among those diagnosed with ADHD. Academic measures of spelling and arithmetic skills were significantly more sensitive to ADHD than overall cognitive ability.

ADULT ADD/ADHD

ADHD is seen as a lifelong disorder, although there is an overall reduction in ADHD symptoms (decline of hyperactive–impulsive behavior and persistent inattention symptoms) as children grow into adolescence and adulthood. ADHD has been diagnosed in over seven million adults in the United States (only 33% had ADHD alone, the remainder had an additional comorbid disorder). Sixty-five percent of children diagnosed with ADHD continued to display behavioral problems and symptoms of this disorder into their adult lives with attention symptoms having a deleterious impact upon daily functioning. Only 25% had been diagnosed in childhood or adolescence. Of those who had not received a prior diagnosis, more than half had complained to other health professionals about ADHD symptoms (Adler, 2008; Reimherr, 2008). Lack of sleep, proper nutrition, overeating, and lack of exercise were seen as mimicking the presence of ADHD and/or increasing the severity of symptoms (Stein, 2008).

The variability in symptoms, severity, and functioning make assessing adult ADHD challenging. Many of the symptoms are nonspecific and common to many other disorders. Comorbidity is the rule rather than the exception in adult ADHD with 70%–75% having at least one comorbid diagnosis (Angold et al., 1999; Biederman, 2004). The rates for anxiety and depression among clinic-referred adults with ADHD are higher than would be predicted by chance (Fischer et al., 2002; McGough et al., 2005; Wilens et al., 2002). Substance abuse disorders are prominent with ADHD (Biederman et al., 1998; McGough et al., 2005).

In measuring memory consolidation gain on a task of motor skill acquisition, those diagnosed with ADHD were found to have a latent memory consolidation phase in motor sequence learning. This was evidenced as a delayed gain in speed as well as a greater delay in recovery of pretraining accuracy. Young adults were seen as having an atypical learning curve resulting in a gain in speed at the cost of accuracy (Adi-Japha et al., 2011). Burgess et al. (2010) hypothesized that there is working memory variability in the ADHD population. Young adults with combined-type ADHD were unable to maintain an appropriate task set, and this was associated with decreased activity in the left dorsolateral prefrontal cortex.

Another mainstay for testing for ADD/ADHD has been continuous performance testing. Research suggests that adults are able to provide a malingering or noncredible performance on continuous performance testing. This suggests the importance of considering other disorders that can affect continuous performance evaluation prior to the diagnosis of ADHD (Suhr et al., 2011).

A meta-analytic review was conducted by Hervey et al. in 2004 of the various research studies, suggesting that neuropsychological deficits are expressed in adults with ADHD across multiple domains of functioning with notable impairments in attention, behavioral inhibition, and memory depending upon the test utilized. Overall, there was a lack of consensus regarding the construction of a neuropsychological profile of adults with ADHD. When there was a comorbid condition involved, those adults performed worse on neuropsychological testing, suggesting that deficits may be exaggerated by the presence of another underlying disorder.

REFERENCES

Adi-Japha, E., Fox, O., and Karni, A., (2011) Atypical acquisition and atypical expression of memory consolidation gains in a motor skill in young female adults with ADHD, *Research in Developmental Disabilities*, 32, 1011–1020.

Adler, L.A., (2008) Best practices in adult ADHD: Special considerations, introduction, *CNS Spectrum*, (10 Suppl 15), 4.

Adler, L.A., (2008) Diagnosing and treating adult ADHD and comorbid conditions, *Journal of Clinical Psychiatry*, 69(11), e31.

Aman, C.J., Roberts, R.J., and Pennington, B.F., (1998) A neuropsychological examination of the underlying deficit in attention deficit hyperactivity disorder: Frontal lobe versus right parietal lobe theories, *Developmental Psychology*, 34(5), 956–969.

American Psychiatric Association, (2000) *Diagnostic and Statistical Manual of Mental Disorders*, 4th edn., Text Revision, American Psychiatric Association, Washington, DC.

Angold, A., Costello, E.J., and Erkanli, A., (1999) Comorbidity, *Journal of Child and Adolescent Psychiatry*, 40, 57–87.

Barkley, R.A., (1997) Behavioral inhibition, sustained attention, and executive functions: Constructing a unifying theory of ADHD, *Psychological Bulletin*, 121(1), 65–94.

Barkley, R.A., Fischer, M., Smallish, L., and Fletcher, K., (2002) The persistence of attention-deficit hyperactivity into young adulthood as a function of reporting source and definition of disorder, *Journal of Abnormal Psychology*, 111(2), 279–289.

Biederman, J., (2004) Impact of comorbidity in adults with attention deficit/hyperactivity disorder, *Journal of Clinical Psychiatry*, 65(Suppl. 3), 3–7.

Biederman, J., Monueaux, M.C., Doyle, A.E., Seidman, L.J., Wilens, T.E., Ferrero, F., Morgan, C.L., and Faraone, S.V., (2004) Impact of executive function deficits and attention-deficit hyperactivity disorder (ADHD) on academic outcomes in children, *Journal of Consulting and Clinical Psychology*, 72(5), 757–766.

Biederman, J., Wilens, T., Mick, E., Faraone, S.V., and Spencer, T., (1998) Does attention-deficit hyperactivity disorder impact the developmental course of drug and alcohol dependence? *Biological Psychiatry*, 44, 269–273.

Bourel-Ponchel, E., Querne, L., Moing, A.G.L., Delignieres, A., and deBroca, P.B., (2011) Maturation of response time and attentional control in ADHD: Evidence from an attentional capture paradigm, *Official Journal of the European Paediatric Neurology Society*, 15, 123–130.

Burgess, G.C., Depue, B.E., Ruzic, L., Willcutt, E.G., Du, Y.P., and Banich, M.T., (2010) Attentional control activation relates to working memory in attention-deficits/hyperactivity disorder, *Biology Psychiatry*, 67, 632–640.

Center for Disease Control and Prevention, (2010) Increasing prevalence of parent-reported attention-deficit/ hyperactivity disorder among children—United States, 2003 and 2007, *Morbidity and Mortality Weekly Report*, 59(44), 1439–1443.

Davidson, M.A., (2008) Literature review ADHD in adults: A review of the literature, *Journal of Attention Disorders*, 11, 628–641.

DuPaul, G.J. et al., (2001) Self-report of ADHD symptoms in university students: Cross-gender and cross-national prevalence, *Journal of Learning Disabilities*, 34, 370–379.

Fischer, M., Barkley, R.A., Smallish, L., and Fletcher, K., (2002) Young adult follow up of hyperactive children: self-reported psychiatric disorders, comorbidity and the role of childhood conduct problems, *Journal of Abnormal Child Psychology*, 30, 463–475.

Fisher, B.C., (1998) *Attention Deficit Disorder Misdiagnosis; Approaching Add from a Brain-Behavior/ Neuropsychological Perspective for Assessment and Treatment*, CRC Press, Boca Raton, FL.

Frazier, T.W., Demaree, H.A., and Youngstrom, E.A., (2004) Meta-analysis of intellectual and neuropsychological test performance in attention-deficit/hyperactivity disorder, *Neuropsychology*, 18(3), 543–555.

Hervey, A.S., Epstein, J.N., and Curry, J.F., (2004) Neuropsychology of adults with attention-deficit/ hyperactivity disorder: A meta-analytic review, *Neuropsychology*, 18(3), 485–503.

Hinshaw, S.P., Carte, E., Fan, C., Jassy, J.S., and Owens, E.B., (2007) Neuropsychological functioning of girls with attention-deficit/hyperactivity disorder followed prospectively into adolescence: Evidence for continuing deficits? *Neuropsychology*, 21(2), 263–273.

Huang-Pollok, C.L., Nigg, J.T., and Halperin, J.M., (2006) Single dissociation findings of ADHD deficits in vigilance but not anterior or posterior attention symptoms, *Neuropsychology*, 20(4), 420–429.

Kessler, R.C. et al., (2006) The prevalence and correlated of adult ADHD in the United States: Results from the National Comorbidity Survey Replication (NCS-R), *American Journal of Psychiatry*, 163, 716–723.

Klenberg, L., Jamsa, S., Hayrinen, T., Lahti-Nuuttila, P., and Korkman, M., (2010) The attention and executive function rating inventory (ATTEX): Psychometric properties and clinical utility in diagnosing ADHD subtypes, *Scandinavian Journal of Psychology*, 51, 439–448.

MacNeil, L.K., Xavier, P., Garvey, M.A., Gilbert, D.L., Ranta, M.E., Denckla, M.B., and Mostofsky, S.H., (2011) Quantifying excessive mirror overflow in children with attention deficit/hyperactivity disorder, *Neurology*, February 15, 76, 622–628.

Mayes, S.D. and Calhoun, S.L., (2007) Learning, attention, writing and processing speed in typical children and children with ADHD, autism, anxiety, depression and oppositional-defiant disorders, *Child Neuropsychology*, November, 13(6), 469–493.

Mayes, S.D., Calhoun, S.L., Chase, G.A, Mink, D.M., and Stagg, R.E., (2009) ADHD subtypes and co-occurring anxiety, depression, and oppositional -defiant disorder: Differences in Gordon diagnostic system and Wechsler working memory and processing speed index scores, *Journal of Attention Disorders*, May, 12(6), 540–550.

McGough, J.J. and Barkley, R.A., (2004) Diagnostic controversies in adult attention deficit hyperactivity disorder, *American Journal of Psychiatry*, 161, 1948–1956.

Murphy, K.R., Barkley, R.A., and Bush, T., (2001) Executive functioning and olfactory identification in young adults with attention deficit-hyperactivity disorder, *Neuropsychology*, 15(2), 211–220.

Nigg, J.T., Stavro, G., Ettenhofer, M., Hambrick, D.Z., Miller, T., and Henderson, J.M., (2005) Executive functions and ADHD in adults: Evidence for selective effects on ADHD symptom domains, *Journal of Abnormal Psychology*, 114(3), 706–717.

O'Brien, J.W., Dowell, L.R., Mostofsky, S.H., Denckla, M.B., and Mahone, M.E., (2010) Neuropsychological profile of executive function in girls with attention deficit hyperactivity disorder, *Archives of Clinical Neuropsychology*, 25, 656–670.

Pastor, P.N. and Reuben, C.A., (2008) *Diagnosed Attention Deficit Hyperactivity Disorder and Learning Disability: United States, 2004–2006*, Vital and Health Statistics, Series 10 No. 237, Data from the National Health Interview Survey, U.S. Department of Health and Human Services, Hyattsville, MD.

Reddy, L.A., Hale, J.B., and Brodzinsky, L.K., (2011) Discriminant validity of the behavior rating inventory of executive function parent form for children with attention-deficit/hyperactivity disorder, *School Psychology Quarterly*, 26(1), 45–55.

Reimherr, F.W., (2008) Comorbidity and diagnosis of ADHD, *CNS Spectrum*, 11(10 Suppl 11), 7–9.

Seidman, L.J., Biederman, J., Monuteaux, M.C., Weber, W., and Faraone, S.V., (2000) Neuropsychological functioning in non-referred siblings of children with attention deficit/hyperactivity disorder, *Journal of Abnormal Psychology*, 109(2), 252–265.

Seidman, L.J., Biederman, J., Valera, E.M., Monuteaux, M.C., Doyle, A.E., and Faraone, S.V., (2006) Neuropsychological functioning in girls with attention-deficit/hyperactivity disorder with and without learning disabilities, *Neuropsychology*, 20(2), 166–177.

Simon, V., Czobor, P., Balint, S., Meszaros, A., and Bitter, I., (2009) Prevalence and correlates of adult attention deficit hyperactivity disorder; meta analysis, *British Journal of Psychiatry*, 194, 204–211.

Stein, M.A., (2008) Medical mimics and differential diagnosis in adult ADHD, *CNS Spectrum*, (10 Suppl 15), 14–16.

Suhr, J.A., Sullivan, B.K., and Rodriguez, J.L., (2011) The relationship of non-credible performance to continuous performance test scores in adults referred for attention deficit/hyperactivity disorder evaluation, *Archives of Clinical Neuropsychology*, 26, 1–7.

Wilens, T.E., Biederman, J., and Spencer, T.J., (2002) Attention deficit/hyperactivity disorder across the lifespan, *Annual Review of Medicine*, 53, 113–131.

14 Review of the Comorbid Research and ADHD

DEPRESSION

One of the primary comorbid disorders for ADHD is depression. A review completed by Daviss (2008) suggested the presence of a significantly higher rate of depression in youths diagnosed with ADHD. A more severe course of psychopathology and higher risk of long-term issues (suicide) were evidenced in the combination of ADHD and depression as opposed to either disorder as a singular entity. Depression as a disorder typically emerged several years after the onset of ADHD symptoms, suggesting both the overlap of symptoms as well as the additive factors of chronic ADHD over time. The authors suggest the need to target environmental adversities and impairment in youth with ADHD with the goal of preventing the onset of comorbid depression (Daviss et al., 2009). Comorbid anxiety and depression were factors found to increase sleep problems whereas Oppositional Defiant Disorder did not increase sleep problems (Mayes et al., 2009).

The question is whether these are two overlapping genetic disorders that emerge through time starts with ADHD or begins with depression. Depression is seen more commonly in females and ADHD in males. Major depression in females with ADHD was associated with an earlier age at onset, greater than twice the duration and more severe depression and associated impairment, higher rate of suicide, and greater likelihood of requiring psychiatric hospitalization than the controls. A severe comorbidity was suggested (Biederman et al., 2008). Smoking was identified as a possible self-medication for ADHD or depression given the indirect effects of nicotine on the intrasynaptic dopamine level (Pinkhardt et al., 2009).

More cognitive (thoughts) depressive traits were seen in females with the combination of ADHD and learning disability (LD) than ADHD alone or males with ADHD and LD (McGilivray and Baker, 2009).

LEARNING DISABILITY

A national health study (Pastor and Reuben, 2008) found that in the ADHD population, 5% of the children studied had ADHD without LD, 5% had LD without ADHD, and 5% had both conditions. Children diagnosed with ADHD were more likely to have contact with a mental health professional, to use prescription medication, and to have frequent health-care visits, while children with LD were more likely to use special education services. Children with Medicaid coverage were more likely than uninsured children and privately insured children to have ADHD or LD.

ASPERGER'S SYNDROME/AUTISM SPECTRUM

The ASD (high-functioning autism or Asperger's syndrome) group plus ADHD symptoms had clear deficits in inhibitory performance compared to the ASD group without additional attention symptoms. Children with ASD and comorbid ADHD were found to have more of a speed than a comprehension problem in planning, working memory, or flexibility tasks. Significant differences were noted separating the ADHD children from controls on a task of inhibition showing deficits of ADHD children on tasks of inhibition as well as working memory. Children with ASD were found to be more impaired in planning and flexibility (Sinzig et al., 2008). Another study comparing

ADHD and high-functioning autism suggested the involvement of frontoparietal (executive reasoning and spatial) attention networks and subcortical arousal systems as primary in the pathology of ADHD. Prefrontal cortex dysfunction (executive reasoning processes) was seen as primary for the high-functioning autistic group. The ADHD group showed deficits in response inhibition and sustained attention through higher errors of commission and omission. The high-functioning autism group showed no sustained attention deficits but did show dissociation in response inhibition performance (Jonson et al., 2007).

A personality disorder profile was detected using self-ratings and clinical interviews. This confirmed that childhood onset neuropsychiatric disorders are reflected in difficult temperaments, deficits in character maturation, and personality disorders. A patient population diagnosed with ADHD reported high novelty-seeking and high harm-avoidance behavior. Those diagnosed with autism spectrum disorders reported low novelty seeking, low reward dependence, and high harm avoidance. ADHD and autism spectrum disorders were seen as associated with specific temperament configurations and an increased risk of personality disorders and deficits in character maturation (Anckarsater et al., 2006).

RACE

African Americans diagnosed with ADHD were less likely to report a family history of ADHD and were more likely to have longer periods between visits for treatment (Hervey-Jumper et al., 2006).

ADULT STUDIES

Of the ADHD cases diagnosed in over 7 million adults in the United States (as reported by the National Comorbidity Study), only 32% were ADHD alone without an additional disorder. The Multimodal Treatment Study of ADHD reported that 29% had ADHD plus oppositional defiant disorder and/or conduct disorder, 14% had ADHD plus anxiety or depression, and 25% experienced all three disorders (Reimherr and Frederick, 2008). Sixty-five percent of children diagnosed with ADHD continue to display behavioral problems and attention symptoms into their adult lives. ADHD has been found to have a deleterious impact upon the daily functioning of adults diagnosed as children demonstrating functional impairments in multiple domains (educational performance, occupation, and relationships) with the majority exhibiting at least one comorbid psychiatric disorder. The concept that ADHD worsens with time is demonstrated in the fact that only 25% of the adults diagnosed with this disorder had been diagnosed in childhood or adolescence. So is this the result of being able to cope until life became more complicated with added stressors? Among patients who had not received a prior diagnosis, more than half had complained about ADHD symptoms to other health professionals without being diagnosed (Adler, 2008).

Adult ADHD symptoms may often be hidden by other conditions, which similarly manifest in attention symptoms. The importance of identifying, which symptoms are representative of a primary disorder, becomes imperative when treating ADHD symptoms and/or ruling out other disorders affecting sleep. Mimics are important to identify because a different treatment regimen is often needed (e.g., absence seizures, hypothyroidism, sleep deprivation, bipolar disorder, obsessive–compulsive disorder, sleep apnea, and phenylketonuria are not treated with stimulant medications). Lack of sleep, proper nutrition, overeating, and lack of exercise may indicate the presence of ADHD and/or manifest as attention symptoms unrelated to a genetic disorder. It is well known that sleep can increase the severity of ADHD symptoms and daily life impairment (Stein, 2008).

Adults diagnosed with ADHD show significant comorbidities with depressive disorders, anxiety disorders, substance use, oppositional defiant disorder, personality disorders, sleep problems, and learning disabilities. Symptoms that result from ADHD such as moodiness or emotional lability are often mistaken for the existence of separate and distinct comorbid disorders. Comorbidity with ADHD impacts treatment compliance, treatment response, and patient insight. Insufficient data on the interaction between ADHD and comorbidities impede proper diagnosis and treatment.

Up to 50% of patients with ADHD have a complicating mood or anxiety disorder. Comorbidity may be a secondary outcome of living with ADHD, and adults may be more difficult to treat quickly as a result (Newcorn et al., 2007).

Levy (2004) proposed a biologically based theory of comorbidity of anxiety in the ADHD population, suggesting the impact of the dynamics of mesolimbic dopamine systems that results in impulsive fearless responses when impaired. A dual theory incorporating long-term tonic/phasic mesolimbic dopamine relationships and secondly impairment of prefrontal cortex and hippocampal inputs to synaptic gating of anxiety at the accumbens has implications for comorbidity in ADHD as well as for possible pharmacological interventions.

Adults aged 18–37 completed a neuropsychological test battery. The ADHD group had weaker performance than did the control group on both executive and speed measures. Symptoms of inattention/disorganization were uniquely related to executive functioning. Inattention was associated with slower response speed and hyperactivity–impulsivity with faster output speed (Nigg et al., 2005).

GENDER

Examination of gender in ADHD symptoms with comorbid symptoms of oppositional defiant disorder, conduct disorder, separation anxiety disorder, generalized anxiety disorder, and speech therapy and remedial reading in children showed significant differences between males and females. Significant differences between groups were found for inattention and hyperactive/impulsive symptoms with higher rates of oppositionality and conduct disorder (CD) in males and higher rates of separation anxiety disorders in females. Females were seen as having more internalizing symptoms compared to the externalizing symptoms of males. Children without ADHD consistently had few symptoms, while those with the combined subtype consistently showed more comorbid symptoms revealing a strong relationship between high rates of externalizing and internalizing symptoms.

Comorbidity was not seen as differing greatly for gender and symptoms, but instead related to severity, assuming that ADHD symptoms are more severe in the combined subtype. Gender differences were noted for separation anxiety disorder, which was more apparent in girls, and the inattentive subtype in boys with the combined subtype, suggesting immaturity in both groups. Females had significantly higher levels of symptoms of generalized anxiety than males when diagnosed with the combined subtype. The ADHD combined subtype accounted for the majority of the comorbidity found (Levy et al., 2005).

There was a gender difference seen in speech therapy, which was only significant for children who did not have the diagnosis of ADHD. Reading problems were significantly higher in the inattentive and combined subtypes than in the hyperactive/impulsive subtype with no difference between the genders (Levy et al., 2005).

. Boys with ADHD plus reading problems exhibited specific impairment on linguistic output tasks. Difficulties on neuropsychological tasks that required planning or controlled motor output could not be singularly explained by either ADHD or comorbid conditions (Nigg et al., 1998). Willcutt and Pennington (2000) reported a stronger association between reading disability and externalizing or antisocial psychopathology seen more often in boys. For girls, there was a significant relationship between reading disability and internalizing symptoms.

Examining the comorbid ADHD plus CD group, there was a finding of verbal deficits and lower verbal IQ not present in the pure ADHD group. Other neuropsychological impairments did not differentiate the two groups. Authors suggested that findings may be consistent with a developmental progression in which problems with hyperactivity/inattention emerge in development in early childhood (ages 4–6) before the emergence of antisocial behaviors, which usually occurs in middle childhood leading to the diagnosis of comorbid disorders and/or combined subtype. The emergence of subtle neuropsychological problems may be part of a developmental chain contributing to an antisocial behavioral outcome. The emergence of antisocial behavior once ADHD was diagnosed was unrelated to neuropsychological deficits and only to lowered Verbal IQ (Nigg et al., 1998).

Bae et al. (2010) addressed the question of morningness (lark, early morning) or eveningness (owl, late night) preference, gender, and adult ADHD. A questionnaire was completed and gender differences seen. Only attention in the female subjects was associated with the morningness–eveningness scale. Eveningness was strongly associated with inattention of adult ADHD and may be associated with hyperactivity and impulsivity behavior in adult male ADHD subjects (Bae et al., 2010).

Gender differences were seen across both self-report measures and neuropsychological test measures in our research presented in this book.

HEALTH BEHAVIORS AND OBESITY

Kim et al. (2011) found that, generally, children diagnosed with ADHD engaged in less physical activity, organized sports, and reading than their same age peers. Medication was seen as a protective factor for obesity. Children diagnosed with ADHD who were on medication had a higher prevalence of depression than those not taking medication. Depression emerged as a stand-alone diagnosis as the odds of being depressed remained significant after controlling for obesity. Health promotion and obesity prevention programs targeting children with ADHD should take gender and medication use into consideration. The odds of being obese were higher among girls than boys with nonmedicated ADHD compared to those without ADHD. Girls with no medication were found to have higher media time, which was associated with higher odds for obesity. Other health behaviors such as not participating in organized sports and lack of sleep were associated with obesity in boys with ADHD on medication. All children with ADHD were less likely to be physically active. Conclusively, the study illustrated that ADHD children are less likely to engage in physical activity regardless of gender and medication use compared to children without ADHD, whereas their odds of being obese was dependent on gender and medication status.

REFERENCES

Adler, L.A., (2008) Epidemiology, impairments and differential diagnosis in adult ADHD: Introduction, *CNS Spectrums*, 13, 8(Suppl 12), 4–5.

Anckarsater, H. et al., (2006) The impact of ADHD and autism spectrum disorders on temperament, character and personality development, *American Journal of Psychiatry*, 163, 1239–1244.

Bae, S.-M., Park, J.E., Lee, Y.J., Cho, I.H., Kim, J.-H., Koh, S.-H., Kim, S.J., and Cho, S.-J., (2010) Gender difference in the association between adult attention deficit hyperactivity disorder symptoms and morningness-eveningness, *Psychiatry and Clinical Neurosciences*, 64, 649–651.

Biederman, J., Ball, S.W., Monuteaux, M.C., Mick, E., Spencer, T.J., McCreary, M., Cote, M., and Faraone, S.V., (2008) New insights into the comorbidity between ADHD and major depression in adolescent and young adult females, *Journal of the American Academy Child and Adolescent Psychiatry*, April, 47(4), 426–434.

Daviss, W.B., (2008) A review of co-morbid depression in pediatric ADHD: Etiology, phenomenology, and treatment, *Journal of Child Adolescent Psychopharmacology*, December, 18(6), 565–571.

Daviss, W.B., Diler, R.S., and Birmaher, B., (2009) Associations of lifetime depression with trauma exposure, other environmental adversities and impairment in adolescents with ADHD, *Journal of Abnormal Child Psychology*, August, 37(6), 857–871.

Hervey-Jumper, H., Douyon, K., and Franco, K., (2006) Deficit in diagnosis, treatment and continuity of care in African-American children and adolescents with ADHD, *Journal of the National Medical Association*, 98(2), 233–238.

Jonson, K.A. et al., (2007) Dissociation in performance of children with ADHD and high functioning autism on a task of sustained attention, *Neuropsychologia*, 45(10), 2234–2245.

Kim, J., Mutyala, B., Agiovlasitis, S., and Fernhall, B., (2011) Health behaviors and obesity among US children with attention deficit hyperactivity disorder by gender and medication use, *Preventive Medicine*, 52, 218–222.

Levy, F., (2004) Synaptic gating and ADHD: A biological theory of comorbidity of ADHD and anxiety, *Neuropsychopharmacology*, 29, 1589–1596.

Levy, F., Hay, D.A., Bennett, K.S., and McStephen, M., (2005) Gender differences in ADHD subtype comorbidity, *Journal of American Academy Child Adolescent Psychiatry*, April, 44, 4.

Mayes, S.D., Calhoun, S.L., Bixler, E.O., Vgontzas, A.N., Mahr, F., Hillwig-Garcia, J., Elamir, B., Edhere-Ekezie, L., and Parvin, M., (2009) ADHD subtypes and comorbid anxiety, depression and oppositional-defiant disorder: Differences in sleep problems, *Sleep Diagnosis and Therapy*, 4, 134–140.

McGilivray, J.A. and Baker, K.L., (2009) Effects of comorbid ADHD with learning disabilities on anxiety, depression and aggression in adults, *Journal of Attention Disorders*, May, 12(6), 525–531.

Newcorn, J.H., Weiss, M., and Stein, M.A., (2007) The complexity of ADHD: Diagnosis and treatment of the adult patient with comorbidities, *CNS Spectrums*, 12(8 Suppl 12), 1–16.

Nigg, J.T., Hinshaw, S.P., Carte, E.T., and Treuting, J.J., (1998) Neuropsychological correlates of childhood attention-deficit/hyperactivity disorder: Explainable by comorbid disruptive behavior or reading problems, *Journal of Abnormal Psychology*, 107(3), 468–480.

Nigg, J.T., Stavro, G., Ettenhofer, M., Hambrick, D.Z., Miller, T., and Henderson, J.M., (2005) Executive functions and ADHD in adults: Evidence for selective effects on ADHD symptom domains, *Journal of Abnormal Psychology*, 114(3), 706–717.

Pastor, P.N. and Reuben, C.A., (2008) *Diagnosed Attention Deficit Hyperactivity Disorder and Learning Disability: United States, 2004–2006*, Vital and Health Statistics, Series 10 No. 237, Data from the National Health Interview Survey, U.S. Department of Health and Human Services, Hyattsville, MD.

Pinkhardt, E.H., Kassubek, J., Brummer, D., Koelch, M., Ludolph, A.C., Fegert, J.M., and Ludoph, A.G., (2009) Intensified testing for attention-deficit hyperactivity disorder (ADHD) in girls should reduce depression and smoking in adult females ant the prevalence of ADHD in the long term, *Medical Hypotheses*, April, 72(4), 409–412.

Reimherr, F., (2008) Comorbidity and diagnosis of ADHD, *CNS Spectrum*, 11, 10 (Supp 1), 7–9.

Sinzig, J., Morsch, D., Schmidt, M.H., and Lehmkuhl, G., (2008) Inhibition, flexibility, working memory and planning in autism spectrum disorders with and without comorbid ADHD-symptoms, *Child and Adolescent Psychiatry and Mental Health*, 2(4), 1753–2000.

Stein, M.A., (2008) Medical mimics and differential diagnosis in adult ADHD, *CNS Spectrums*, 13, 10(Suppl 15), 14–16.

Willcutt, E.G. and Pennington, B.F., (2000) Psychiatric comorbidity in children and adolescents with reading disability, *Journal of Child Psychological Psychiatry*, 41, 1039–1048.

15 Review of the Research for Sleep and ADHD

SLEEP DISORDERS AND ADHD

Sleep problems have been clinically reported in an estimated 25%–50% of children and adolescents diagnosed with Attention Deficit Hyperactivity Disorder (ADHD) (Owens, 2005). There is a two- to threefold higher prevalence of sleep problems in children with ADHD compared to controls, which includes difficulty falling asleep, frequent night waking, and increased tiredness upon awakening (Cohen-Zion and Ancoli-Israel, 2004). Parents of ADHD children have reported more sleep problems themselves (Kaplan et al., 1987). ADHD children had more sleep-related breathing disorder symptoms, enuresis, sleep talking, bruxism, as well as parasomnias (night terrors and sleepwalking) than control groups (Corkum et al., 2001). Children with ADHD were found to have significantly reduced sleep duration and increased number of stage shifts (Miano et al., 2006).

The presence of unidentified and untreated sleep disorders is widespread in the ADHD clinical population. Wiggs et al. (2005) found that only 8 of the 71 children were devoid of a sleep disorder in the clinical setting sample. The type of sleep disorders and disturbances seen more often was sleeplessness, symptoms of a sleep-related breathing disorder, and abnormal sleep-related movements. However, a large proportion of the sample of the clinical group failed to meet the research criteria for ADHD based upon DSM-IV criteria despite having received this diagnosis from their treating professionals. Parents reported a wide range of frequently occurring sleep disturbances in their children, although actigraphy did not document abnormalcy and there was poor correspondence between parent report and actigraphy (Wiggs et al., 2005).

Adolescents with a childhood diagnosis of ADHD were more likely to have current and lifetime sleep problems and sleep disorders (insomnia, sleep terrors, nightmares, bruxism (teeth grinding), and snoring). The presence of at least one psychiatric comorbid condition increased risks for the diagnoses of insomnia and nightmares (Shur-Fen Gau and Chiang, 2009).

Walters and colleagues (2008) completed a review of the literature of sleep, ADHD, and its relationship to movement disorders. Recent evidence reveals that the sleep of individuals diagnosed with ADHD is disrupted in a nonspecific way as well as the disorder having an increased association with simple sleep-related movement disorders such as restless legs or periodic limb movements in sleep, Rhythmic Movement Disorders (RMDs) (body rocking and headbanging), parasomnias, and disorders of partial arousal (sleepwalking, sleep terrors, and confusional arousals). There is increased comorbidity reported for ADHD and hypersomnia disorders (such as narcolepsy and sleep apnea) as well as circadian rhythm disorders such as Delayed Sleep Phase Syndrome (DSPS).

ADHD symptoms are seen accompanying specific sleep disorders and the impact of the sleep disorder affects attention. Symptoms of inattention are common in narcolepsy. The diagnosis of ADHD seems to be more common in RMD and RMD seems to be more common in ADHD. ADHD is related to sleep onset problems, which are often more characteristic of DSPS. However, the sleep disruption from delayed sleep onset was insufficient to explain the daytime symptoms of inattention and hyperactivity, which is characteristic of ADHD (Walters et al., 2008).

Restless Legs Syndrome (RLS)/Periodic Limb Movement Syndrome (PLMS) and ADHD symptoms may co-occur in children and in adults. Children diagnosed with PLMS on a sleep study were found to have a greater propensity for an ADHD diagnosis (44%). A circular relationship exists between RLS and ADHD with RLS exacerbating or leading to ADHD through the mechanism of sleep disruption; daytime drowsiness or fatigue from sleep disruption could increase or exacerbate the motor restlessness of RLS. The daytime manifestation of RLS symptoms may lead to ADHD diagnosis/symptoms, and both RLS and ADHD may be manifestation of a common central nervous system (CNS) disease sharing dopaminergic deficits. Obstructive Sleep Apnea (OSA) can cause mild inattention or hyperactivity similar to the impact of even a low level of Sleep Disordered Breathing (SDB) on sleep variables and cognitive tasks. Disorders of partial arousal appear to be prevalent in ADHD and emerge with chronic sleep deprivation resulting in more sleep fragmentation due to multiple arousals (Walters et al., 2008).

It is well known from a clinical perspective that ADHD and sleep are related. However, there are many studies presenting opposing points of view and objectively assessing the sleep problems reported by parents has been difficult. This raises the question of whether this is a reflection of the ability to accurately measure the symptoms reported by the parents or if the parents are reporting more symptoms than are actually there.

Research supports the comorbidity of ADHD and various sleep disorders such as OSA, SDB, periodic limb movements, restless legs, and narcolepsy. The quality of sleep in the ADHD population is separate from the presence of an actual sleep disorder and whether there is a preponderance of poor sleep having an impact upon daytime symptoms. On our checklists, parents frequently reported overall poor sleep quality in their child. Studies using the overnight sleep study or polysomnographic (PSG) did not always find robust differences to support this parental reporting, raising the question of either parental overreport or more subtle sleep problems insufficient to document using this type of objective measurement.

In a research review completed in 2003, O'Brien noted that studies using objective measures have not shown consistent evidence of the differences in sleep between ADHD and controls. Other studies reported varied and contradictory findings on sleep problems of short sleep duration, decrease in REM, and decreased REM latency (REM onset) between ADHD and controls.

ADHD, SLEEP, AND EMOTIONS

Choi et al. (2010) assessed sleep characteristics in children diagnosed with ADHD using PSG recordings and parental report of sleep problems. PSG evaluation was performed in 27 children (7–12 years) diagnosed with ADHD and compared to healthy controls. The ADHD group had significantly higher scores on the sleep onset delay, sleep duration, night waking, parasomnias, daytime sleepiness, and total sleep disturbance factors. However, there were no differences seen between the ADHD group and the healthy controls on the PSG variables of sleep structure, arousals, spontaneous arousal index, periodic limb movements, and respiratory disturbances. Parental report of sleep disturbance was significantly associated with almost all of the subscales from the Child Behavior Checklist (CBCL) as well as the total CBCL score. Conclusions were that the majority of sleep problems reported by the parents of ADHD children were not verified through the use of PSG, raising the possibility that some of the reported sleep problems in ADHD may be more related to disturbing emotional behaviors, which often characterize children with ADHD (Choi et al., 2010). The suggestion is that the sleep problems in the ADHD population are more subservient to ADHD symptoms. What seems to remain consistent in the research is the correlation of attention symptoms with sleep disorders and poor sleep.

Correlation analyses of the relationships between behavioral problems and sleep variables reported by parents on checklists indicated that sleep onset delay and sleep duration objectively measured on the PSG were significantly correlated with social and attention problems. Night waking had positive correlations with almost all emotional variables of the CBCL. Daytime sleepiness was highly correlated with social and attention problems and aggressiveness. Parasomnias had positive correlations with withdrawn and anxious/depressed symptoms. Total sleep disturbance was significantly associated with almost all subscales of the CBCL total behavioral problem score. Parents of children with ADHD complain of hyperactive and aggressive behaviors that occur all day long indicating the continuation of these behaviors to bedtime as the most likely explanation for the higher probability that parents of children with ADHD may overreport sleep problems.

Sleep problems can emerge from the comorbid disorder(s), which then creates attention symptoms. It is a well-known fact that poor sleep creates attention problems. Anxiety and inattention are covariables that were well established in our study. Anxiety alone leads to poor sleep.

Ninety percent of children diagnosed with some form of an anxiety disorder had at least one sleep-related problem and 82% had two or more sleep problems. Sleep problems did not differ for age range (6–18 years) or gender. A strong association was found between sleep-related problems and the number of anxiety disorders establishing a high co-occurrence and predictive relationship (Chase and Pincus, 2011).

ATTENTION AND MOVEMENT DURING SLEEP

Another issue is movement during sleep and its impact upon attention. Movement was found to be a predictor of impaired vigilance, verbal, and memory skills in children diagnosed with an SDB problem. Children with adenotonsillar hypertrophy or large tonsils, suspected of having an obstructive SDB problem, were studied with 6 days of actigraphy and a PSG or overnight sleep study. Their performance was measured on selected cognitive testing. Slower reaction time found on a measure of alertness and vigilance correlated with more movements (higher sum of all movements during time in bed) and greater time spent moving during sleep (higher number of minutes with greater than 5 movements per night). Lower scores on tests of defining words (vocabulary) and verbal concept formation (similarities) and memory (General Memory Index from the WRAML) correlated with less movement (more consolidation of movements, consecutive minutes with >5 movements). Other cognitive or behavioral scores were not correlated with actigraphy or PSG. Authors suggested that detecting movements during time in bed can help to predict children at risk for impaired function. Frequent movements during time in bed may be reflective of transient brain activation that impairs sustained vigilance to unstimulating tasks such as reaction time but does not impair tasks involving more substantial stimulation such as vocabulary or similarities. Significant movement consolidation or less movement was seen as reflective of more sustained nervous system activation that impairs tasks that involve more substantial stimulation. The apnea–hypopnea index was associated with more consolidation of movements (Suratt et al., 2011).

ADHD AND SDB

An SDB problem often results in more arousals and poor sleep. It is well known that the presence of SDB problems results in attention problems in the general population and creates more attention problems in the ADHD population. The prevalence of SDB is high with reports of up to 34.5% in children. The sleep of children (7–12 years) with SDB problems was examined using overnight sleep studies. Children were classified into four groups of primary snoring, mild OSA, moderate to severe Obstructive Sleep Apnea Syndrome (OSAS), and controls. Cognitive function was measured with an intellectual assessment (Wechsler Abbreviated Scale of Intelligence), achievement assessment (Wide Range Achievement Test), memory measure (Rey Complex Figure), and measure of verbal fluency (Controlled Oral Word Association Test). There was lower general intellectual ability in all children with an SDB problem regardless of severity. Higher rates of impairment were noted on measures of executive and academic functioning, and neuropsychological deficits were found to be common in children with SDB regardless of disease severity. Researchers felt that these difficulties may be present in children in the community who snore but are otherwise healthy. Research has shown that a combination of repeated episodes of hypoxia and sleep disruption contributes to cognitive impairment. In the past it was felt that only severe SDB created significant problems;

however, recent studies are finding that even mild SDB is having an impact. More children in the primary snoring group received impaired scores on a measure of academic functioning than in controls (Bourke et al., 2011).

In another study, ADHD children when evaluated with the overnight sleep study (PSG) revealed no evidence of sleep apnea or leg movements although there was a somewhat longer time to get to REM as well as a decreased percentage of REM sleep (Sangal et al., 2005). Only the hyperactive ADHD subtype diagnosis was associated with increased likelihood of chronic snoring. Sleep quality was poorer among children with ADHD than controls, although significant differences in sleep quality were not seen. Daytime sleepiness was greater in children with ADHD especially the hyperactive type (LeBourgeois et al., 2003).

There is a significant body of research pairing the association of snoring with inattention and hyperactivity, suggesting that SDB is clearly a causal factor of inattention and hyperactivity in children. The suggestion is that the child who snores and has been diagnosed with ADHD could potentially have ADHD symptoms reduced if the SDB problem was effectively treated. Improvement was seen in children 1 year post tonsillectomy in variables of inattention, hyperactivity, and daytime sleepiness (Chervin et al., 2006).

Hyperactivity behavior was found to be common among children referred for suspected SDB regardless of the presence or severity (Chervin and Hedger-Archbold, 2001).

Beebe (2006) examined research studies documenting the relationship between childhood SDB and neurobehavioral functioning. The result was strong evidence that childhood SDB is associated with deficits in behavioral and emotional regulation, scholastic performance, sustained attention, selective attention, and alertness. There is minimal association with a child's typical mood, expressive language skills, visual perception, and working memory. Findings were insufficient to draw conclusions about intelligence, memory, and some aspects of executive functioning. Clinical symptoms of chronic snoring remained one of the best predictors of morbidity. Failing to treat SDB appears to leave children at risk for long-term neurobehavioral deficits.

ADHD AND RLS

On a large-scaled cross-sectional study, using 65,554 women free of diabetes, arthritis, and pregnancy, mothers of children with ADHD were found to have an increased risk of having RLS (Nurses' Health Study II, female registered nurses age 25–42 years). This study suggests that ADHD and RLS could share some common genetic components and may exist across generations. There was a significant association between the presence of ADHD in the children and the risk of having RLS. Women who reported having a child with ADHD were more likely to be past smokers, to use antidepressants, and to have more deliveries during their lifetime. This is consistent with previous studies that report the co-occurrence of RLS and ADHD (Gao et al., 2011).

In a large-scaled cross-sectional study, a high prevalence of children or adolescents meeting the diagnostic criteria for definite RLS (14.8% among 8–11-year-olds and 17.6% among 12–17-year-olds) also met the criteria for ADHD/ADD. In a study including 18 children and adolescents with RLS, 13 of them were found to have ADHD and 10 with both ADHD and a family history of RLS. ADHD symptoms were more common in RLS patients than in patients with insomnia or controls. In diagnosed RLS adult patients, 26% met the criteria for ADHD (completed using neuropsychological evaluation) compared to only 6% of those diagnosed with insomnia or 5% of the control population. RLS leg discomfort or poor quality of sleep can potentially lead to daytime manifestation of hyperactivity and lack of concentration. RLS and ADHD may also be the result of dopamine deficiency. Review of the literature suggested that up to 44% of subjects diagnosed with ADHD have been found to have RLS or RLS symptoms and up to 26% of subjects with RLS were found to have ADHD or ADHD symptoms (Cortese et al., 2005, Gao et al., 2011, Wagner et al., 2004). In a double-blind study of dopaminergic therapy in children diagnosed with RLS/PLMS and ADHD, improvement was seen in the RLS symptoms but not the ADHD symptoms. This was a small sample and there were baseline differences in the severity of the ADHD symptoms (England et al., 2011).

Common genetic determinants are the following: BTBD9 is a potential candidate associated with decreased serum ferritin concentration and iron deficiency is suggested as risk factor for RLS. Other potential candidate genes include the protein tyrosine phosphatase gene and nitric oxide synthase 1 (found to be associated with the risk of both ADHD and RLS; both ADHD and RLS were reported in patients with Tourette's syndrome [TS]). A recent study of three RLS-related BTBD9 single-nucleotide polymorphisms was found to be significantly associated with TS risk (Gao et al., 2011).

Inattention and hyperactivity were associated with symptoms of PLMS and RLS in a study assessing 866 children (Chervin et al., 2002).

A population of adults already diagnosed with ADHD revealed that 20% had RLS. The adults diagnosed with RLS had more severe ADHD symptomatology, suggesting that symptoms of RLS can worsen daytime symptoms of ADHD (Zak et al., 2009).

Adult ADHD patients showed increased nocturnal motor activity (as indicated by heightened indices of PLMS), which was significantly correlated with reported total sleep time. Similar to the children, when total sleep time was objectively measured, there was increased time. However, subjective ratings continued to document impaired sleep quality and less sleep time. Other sleep variables did not differentiate ADHD from controls. Similar to children, adults with ADHD show increased nocturnal motor activity. The PLM index was significantly correlated with the number of arousals in total sleep time as well as with a decreased subjective report of total sleep time. The result was a lack of correlation between objective and subjective sleep parameters, suggesting the tendency to misinterpret sleep quality in those diagnosed with ADHD (Philipsen et al., 2005).

ATTENTION AND RESTRICTED SLEEP

Studies on sleep show the impact of restricted sleep on attention in the general population. There was a 20% prevalence of restricted sleep (6 h or less) in adolescents (ages 11–17 years) seen on a large study of 4175 youths. Chronicity was noted in 17% still having restricted sleep at follow-up on 3134 adolescents 1 year later. Data suggested that perhaps one in five or one in four youths get only two-thirds of the hours of sleep needed for optimal functioning with restricted sleep being more of the norm rather than an anomaly (Roberts et al., 2011). Assessment of attention of middle school students provided with the opportunity for one additional hour of sleep in the morning (by delaying school starting time) was compared to the control group who received no additional sleep time. Students who slept longer (average of 55 min for five nights for total of 275 min) performed better on measures of attention assessed on a mathematics continuous performance test and the d2 Test of Attention. There was a better performance in attention level, impulsivity, and rate of performance. Several studies have documented that the duration and efficiency of sleep impact the cognitive performance of attention, memory, learning, and concentration. The students who slept longer performed better than the control group on tests requiring attention (Lufi et al., 2011).

In children, experimental sleep restriction has been reported to be associated with ADHD like behavior and poor cognitive achievements. ADHD adult subjects reported impaired sleep quality, less restorative value of sleep, more fatigue and negative mood in the evening, and more psychosomatic symptoms such as palpitations, even myalgia, or leg movements during sleep onset (Philipsen et al., 2005).

Performance of children with ADHD following sleep restriction deteriorated from subclinical levels to the clinical range of inattention on two-thirds of the Continuous Performance Test outcome measures. Experimental design used sleep restriction to mimic changes in everyday life while assessing sleep in the home environment on consecutive nights. Cumulative reduction of 40.7 minutes of sleep was associated with detectable deterioration in most of CPT variables measuring vigilance and sustained attention. Deterioration for ADHD children led to the diagnostic change from subclinical to clinical ADHD (Gruber et al., 2011).

STIMULANT MEDICATION AND ADHD

Parents report sleep disturbances when their children are taking stimulant medication (Day and Abmayr, 1998). Children given methylphenidate for ADHD had prolonged sleep onset latency, reduced sleep efficiency, and shortened sleep. A study compared 27 children diagnosed with ADHD (6–12 years) to healthy controls. Findings were that of a more prolonged sleep onset by an average of 29 min, shortened sleep by 1.2 h, reduced sleep efficiency by 6.5%, and decreased REM sleep by 2.4% (Gruber et al., 2009).

Medicated children had greater difficulty falling asleep than unmedicated children in a study completed using parent report for 681 children (diagnosed with ADHD combined type or ADHD inattentive type with or without comorbid oppositional defiant disorder [ODD]), anxiety, or depression) compared to a control group. Children with ADHD inattentive type alone (no comorbid disorder) had the fewest sleep problems and did not differ from controls. Children with ADHD combined subtype had more sleep problems than controls and inattentive ADHD. Comorbid anxiety and depression variables increased sleep problems, whereas ODD did not. However, the presence of daytime sleepiness was greatest in the inattentive type whose sleep was greater than the control population (Mayes et al., 2009). Whether the daytime sleepiness was a precursor of an undiagnosed sleep problem remains in question.

Children with ADHD experienced significant improvement on some measures of vigilance performance when given stimulant medication but only if their sleep efficiency was poor. Improvement following administration of stimulant medication was seen as a result of increased arousal level, which facilitated vigilance performance (Gruber et al., 2007).

Medication with methylphenidate appeared to have beneficial effects on sleep parameters in adults diagnosed with ADHD resulting in improved sleep efficiency and sleep onset. Nonmedicated ADHD adults displayed reduced sleep efficiency with longer sleep onset and more nocturnal awakenings. Additionally there was an altered sleep architecture with a higher percentage of stage 1 (lightest stage of sleep) and reduced percentage of REM sleep. ADHD adults not on medication showed a trend toward a reduced total REM density and elevated percentage of wakefulness after sleep onset. Sleep architecture and number of PLMS with and without arousal did not change with medication. Suggested is that medication results in better adjustment during the day, which has a beneficial effect on sleep at night, and/or that stimulants influence chronobiological brain function (Sobanski et al., 2008).

Shur-Fen Gau and Chiang (2009) found that use of methylphenidate was not associated with further increased risk of sleep problems except in the case of bruxism. Other than a higher rate of nightmares in girls and snoring for boys, there were no sex or gender differences. The contribution of psychostimulants to sleep problems and disorders in adolescents with ADHD appeared to be relatively slight (Shur-Fen Gau and Chiang, 2009).

Several studies have indicated greater daytime sleepiness in ADHD children. This may explain the benefit of stimulant medication. A study was completed using the Multiple Sleep Latency Test (MSLT), consisting of a series of nap opportunities and yielding a nap score documenting daytime sleepiness. Those diagnosed with ADHD were significantly sleepier during the day than the control group seen on the mean MSLT score. Fifteen percent of the children had PLMD during sleep versus none in the control group. Children without SDB or PLMD had the lowest nocturnal sleep efficiency and total sleep time (Golan et al., 2004).

SLEEP HYGIENE

The degree that parents influence the sleep problems they predict in their child was assessed using a diagnosed ADHD population where 73% reported significant sleep difficulties. Parent stress was correlated with their report of sleep difficulties in their children. Parenting stress predicted child sleep anxiety. The lack of bedtime routine was found to be associated with greater bedtime resistance, resulting in increased parent–child conflict and reduced quantity and quality of sleep. The implementation of consistent routines, especially those related to bedtime, may be a key factor in facilitating sleep among children who display ADHD behaviors. Lower-income parents who may be more stressed were found to implement less consistent daily routines. Suggested is that the relationship between parenting stress and child sleep difficulties is mediated by household routines. Daily life routine was not a significant predictor of total sleep problems but was the only significant predictor of bedtime resistance after accounting for child and family characteristics as well as parental report of internalizing and externalizing symptoms (Noble et al., 2012).

REFERENCES

Beebe, D.W., (2006) Neurobehavioral morbidity associated with disordered breathing during sleep in children: A comprehensive review, *Sleep*, 29(9), 1115–1134.

Bourke, R. et al., (2011) Cognitive and academic functions are impaired in children with all severities of sleep disordered breathing, *Sleep Medicine*, 12, 489–496.

Chase, R.M. and Pincus, D.B., (2011) Sleep related problems in children and adolescents with anxiety disorders, *Behavioral Sleep Medicine*, 9, 224–236.

Chervin, R.D. and Hedger Archbold, K., (2001) Hyperactivity and polysomnographic findings in children evaluated for sleep disordered breathing, *Sleep*, 24(3), 313–320.

Chervin, R.D., Archbold, K.H., Dillon, J.E., Pituch, K.J., Panahi, P., Dahl, R., and Guilleminault, C., (2002) Associations between symptoms of inattention, hyperactivity, restless legs and periodic leg movements, *Sleep*, 25(2), 213–218.

Chervin, R.D., Ruzicka, D.L., Giordani, B.J., Weatherly, R.A., Dillon, J.E., Hodges, E.K., Marcus, C.L., and Guire, K.E., (2006) Sleep disordered breathing, behavior, and cognition in children before and after adenotonsillectomy, *Pediatrics*, 117(4), 769–778.

Choi, J., Yoon, I.Y., Kim, H.W., Chung, S., and Yoo, H.J., (2010) Differences between objective and subjective sleep measures in children with attention deficit hyperactivity disorder, *Journal of Clinical Sleep Medicine*, 6(6), 589–596.

Cohen-Zion, M. and Ancoli-Israel, S., (2004) Sleep in children with attention-deficit hyperactivity disorder (ADHD): A review of naturalistic and stimulant intervention studies, *Sleep Medicine Review*, 8, 379–402.

Corkum, P., Tannock, R., Moldofsky, H., Hogg-Johnson, S., and Humphries, T., (2001) Actigraphy and parental ratings of sleep in children with attention deficit hyperactivity disorder (ADHD), *Sleep*, 24, 303–312.

Cortese, S., Konofal, E., Lecendreux, M., Amulf, I., Mouren, M.-C., Darra, F., and Dalla Bernardina, B., (2005) Restless legs syndrome and attention-deficit hyperactivity disorder: A review of the literature, *Sleep*, 28(8), 1007–1013.

Day, H.D. and Abmayr, S.B., (1998) Parent reports of sleep disturbances in stimulant medicated children with attention deficit hyperactivity disorder, *Journal of Clinical Psychology*, 54, 701–716.

England, S. et al., (2011) VmL-Dopa improves Restless Legs Syndrome and periodic limb movements in sleep but not Attention-Deficit-Hyperactivity Disorder in a double-blind trial in children, *Sleep Medicine*, 12, 471–477.

Galland, B.C., Tripp, E.G., and Taylor, B.I., (2010) The sleep of children with attention deficit hyperactivity disorder on and off methylphenidate: A matched case control study, *Journal of Sleep Research*, June, 19(2), 366–373.

Gao, X., Lyall, K., Palacios, N., Walters, A.S., and Ascherio, A., (2011) RLS in middle aged women and attention deficit/hyperactivity disorder in their offspring, *Sleep Medicine*, 12, 89–91.

Golan, N., Shahar, E., Ravid, S., and Pillar, G., (2004) Sleep disorders and daytime sleepiness in children with attention deficit hyperactive disorder, *Sleep*, 27(2), 261–266.

Gruber, R., Grizenko, N., Schwartz, G., Bellingham, J., Guzman, R., and Joober, R., (2007) Performance on the continuous performance test in children with ADHD is associated with sleep efficiency, *Sleep*, August 1, 30(8), 1003–1009.

Gruber, R., Wiebe, S., Montecalvo, L., Brunetti, B., Amsel, R., and Carrier, J., (2011) Impact of sleep restriction on neurobehavioral functioning of children with attention deficit hyperactivity disorder, *Sleep*, 34(3), 315–323.

Gruber, R., Xi, T., Frenette, S., Robert, M., Vannasinh, P., and Carrier, J., (2009) Sleep disturbances in prepubertal children with attention deficit hyperactivity disorder: A home polysomnography study, *Sleep*, 32, 343–350.

Kaplan, B.J., McNicol, J., Conte, R.A., and Moghadam, H.K., (1987) Sleep disturbance in preschool-aged hyperactive and nonhyperactive children, *Pediatrics*, 80, 839–844.

LeBourgeois, M., Avis, K., Mixon, M., Olmi, J., and Harsh, J., (2003) Snoring, sleep quality, and sleepiness across attention deficit hyperactivity disorder subtypes, *Sleep*, 27(3), 520–525.

Lufi, D., Tzischinsky, O., and Hadar, S., (2011) Delaying school starting time by one hour: Some effects on attention levels in adolescents, *Journal of Clinical Sleep Medicine*, 7(2), 137–142.

Mayes, S.D., Calhoun, S.L., Bixler, E.O., Vgontzas, A.N., Mahr, F., Hillwig-Garcia, J., Elamir, B., Edhere-Ekezie, L., and Parvin, M., (2009) ADHD subtypes and comorbid anxiety, depression, and oppositional–defiant disorder: Differences in sleep problems, *Journal Pediatric Psychology*, April, 34(3), 328–337.

Miano, S., Donfrancesco, R., Bruni, O., Ferri, R., Galiffa, S., Pagani, J., Montemitro, E., Kheirandish, L., Gozal, D., and Pia, Villa, M., (2006) NREM sleep instability is reduced in children with attention-deficit/ hyperactivity disorder, *Sleep*, 29(6), 797–803.

Noble, G.S., O'Laughlin, L., and Brubaker, B., (2012) Attention deficit hyperactivity disorder and sleep disturbances: Consideration of parental influence, *Behavioral Sleep Medicine*, 10, 41–53.

O'Brien, L.M. et al., (2003) Sleep and neurobehavioral characteristics of 5–7 year old children with parentally reported symptoms of attention deficit hyperactivity disorder, *Pediatric Research*, 54, 237–243.

Owens, J.A., (2005) The ADHD and sleep conundrum: A review, *Journal of Developmental Behavioral Pediatrics*, 26, 312–322.

Philipsen, A., Feige, B., Hesslinger, B., Ebert, D., Carl, C., Hornyak, M., Lieb, K., and Voderholzer, R.D., (2005) Sleep in adults with attention-deficit hyperactivity disorder: A controlled polysomnographic study including spectral analysis of the sleep EEG, *Sleep*, 28(28), 877–884.

Roberts, R.E., Roberts, C.R., and King, Y., (2011) Restricted sleep among adolescents: Prevalence, incidence, persistence and associated factors, *Behavioral Sleep Medicine*, 9, 18–30.

Sangal, B.R., Owens, J.A., and Sangal, J., (2005) Patients with attention deficit hyperactivity disorder without observed apneic episodes in sleep or daytime sleepiness have normal sleep on polysomnography, *Sleep*, 28(9), 1143–1148.

Shur-Fen Gau, S. and Chiang, H.-L., (2009) Sleep problems and disorders among adolescents with persistent and subthreshold attention-deficit hyperactivity disorders, *Sleep*, 32(5), 671–679.

Sobanski, E., Schredl, M., Kettler, N., and Alm, B., (2008) Sleep in adults with attention deficit hyperactivity disorder (ADHD) before and during treatment with methylphenidate: A controlled polysomnographic study, *Sleep*, 31(3), 375–381.

Suratt, P.M., Diamond, R., Barth, J.T., Nikova, M., and Rembold, C., (2011) Movements during sleep correlate with impaired attention and verbal and memory skills in children with adenotonsillar hypertrophy suspected for having obstructive sleep disordered breathing, *Sleep Medicine*, 12, 322–328.

Wagner, M.L., Walters, A.S., and Fisher, B.C., (2004) Symptoms of attention-deficit hyperactivity disorder in adults with restless legs syndrome, *Sleep*, 27(8), 1499–1504.

Walters, A.S., Silvestri, R., Zucconi, M., Chandrashekariah, R., and Konofal, E., (2008) Review of the possible relationship and hypothetical links between attention deficit hyperactivity disorder (ADHD) and the simple sleep related movement disorders, parasomnias, hypersomnias, and circadian rhythm disorders, *Journal Clinical Sleep Medicine*, December, 15, 4(6), 591–600.

Wiggs, L., Montgomery, P., and Stores, G., (2005) Actigraphic and parent reports of sleep patterns and sleep disorders in children with subtypes of attention deficit hyperactivity disorder, *Sleep*, 28(11), 1437–1445.

Zak, R., Couvadelli, B.V., Fisher, B., Moss, N.M., and Walters, A.S., (2009) Preliminary study of the prevalence of restless legs syndrome in adults with attention deficit hyperactivity disorder, *Perceptual and Motor Skills*, 108, 759–763.

16 Review of Research on Inattention and ADHD

Children with ADHD predominantly inattentive type and reading disorders were found to share similar symptomology that influences RAN (Rapid Automatized Naming) outcomes such as slower processing speed and semantic processing problems. RAN has been a significant predictor of reading fluency and indicated as a mediator of the relationship between inattention and reading fluency. It is seen as a predictor of reading performance and core difficulty among children with reading disorders due to the timing demands and required integration of phonological and lexical processes. RAN relies upon continuous responding and sustained attention to stimuli for accurate performance. Parent and teacher ratings of inattention predicted RAN speed and oral reading fluency after controlling for gender, working memory, and estimated IQ. Suggested was the need to consider attentional variables when assessing reading performance even among normally developing children (Pham et al., 2011).

Willcutt and Pennington (2000) reported a stronger association between reading disability and externalizing or antisocial psychopathology seen more often in boys. For girls there was a significant relationship between reading disability and internalizing symptoms.

A gender difference was evidenced in speech therapy and was only significant for children who did not have the diagnosis of ADHD. Reading problems were significantly higher in the inattentive and combined subtypes than in the hyperactive/impulsive subtype with no difference between the genders (Levy et al., 2005). This is contrary to the report by Levy in 1996 of the strong association between ADHD and reading and speech problems finding more symptoms in males than females.

Boys with ADHD plus reading problems exhibited specific impairment on linguistic output tasks. Difficulties on neuropsychological tasks that required planning or controlled motor output could not be singularly explained by either ADHD or comorbid conditions (Nigg et al., 1998). On a study using neuropsychological evaluation, boys with ADHD plus a reading problem exhibited specific impairment on linguistic output tasks (Nigg et al., 1998).

REFERENCES

Levy, F., Hay, D.A., McLaughlin, M., Wood, C., and Waldman, I., (1996) Twin sibling differences in parental reports of ADHD, speech reading and behavior problems, *Journal Child Psychological Psychiatry*, 37, 569–578.

Levy, F., Hay, D.A., Bennett, K.S., and McStephen, M., (2005) Gender differences in ADHD subtype comorbidity, *Journal of American Academy Child Adolescent Psychiatry*, 44(4), April, 368–376.

Nigg, J.T., Hinshaw, S.P., Carte, E.T., and Treuting, J.J., (1998) Neuropsychological correlates of childhood attention-deficit/hyperactivity disorder: Explainable by comorbid disruptive behavior or reading problems, *Journal of Abnormal Psychology*, 107(3), 468–480.

Pham, A.V., Fine, J.G., and Semrud-Clikeman, M., (2011) The influence of inattention and rapid automatized naming on reading performance, *Archives of Clinical Neuropsychology*, 26, 214–224.

Willcutt, E.G. and Pennington, B.F., (2000) Psychiatric comorbidity in children and adolescents with reading disability, *Journal Child Psychological Psychiatry*, 41, 1039–1048.

17 Summary and Conclusions
The Take Home Message

A wealth of data has been presented in this book based upon the examination of 2531 children, adolescents, and adults over 20 year period using the same neuropsychological evaluation and self-report measures. This is the largest clinical population for this purpose studied over the longest period of time. The result is the emergence of ADHD Inattentive Type as the real ADD, seen most often and consistently across time.

What was abundantly clear in the self-report measures is the presence of more inattention (than hyperactive or impulsive) and anxiety symptoms manifested in various forms. Anxiety affects sleep, and creates a more emotional individuals. Neuropsychological testing over this extensive period of time provided consistent test profiles documenting the presence of a genetic attention disorder and differentiating it from additional issues labeled as ADHD plus (ADD plus an additional disorder). Those with ADHD plus performed worse on the testing than the ADD or ADHD Inattentive Type. Neuropsychological testing provides confirmation of the cognitive symptoms of a genetic attention disorder and accompanying self-report measures that primarily reveal symptoms of inattention.

Thus, using a scientific method through time to diagnose ADHD, our finding is not that of hyperactivity, nor that of impulsivity, but instead the presence of the combined issues of anxiety and attention. Anxiety by itself and combined with another disorder involving the brain or sleep can look like ADHD Hyperactive or Impulsive or combined subtypes.

In comparing individuals over time, it can be seen how anxiety manifested in ADD children looks different in ADD adolescents as well as ADD adults. Anxiety in children is seen in restlessness (during the day or night) fidgeting behaviors and continual shifting of movement. Anxiety in adolescents is seen in the avoidance of any activity that appears to be difficult. Anger can be a method of avoidance, and depression can be the consequence of the cyclical pattern of avoidance and more avoidance. Adolescents had more emotions than children, increased depression, and suicidal thoughts. Friends and social skills were more problematic in childhood than in adolescence; however, by the time of adolescence, friends were getting better grades and there was an increased tendency to associate with individuals involved in delinquent activities. Family relationships deteriorated from childhood to adolescence as a consequence of increased avoidance of school work. Arguments over bedtime in childhood morphed into arguments over homework in adolescence.

Sleep problems increased from childhood to adulthood as well as daytime fatigue. Sleep onset was more problematic in adolescence extending into adulthood. Anxiety in adults affected sleep; sleep onset or maintenance insomnia. By the time of adulthood, goals and dreams had been altered by the pervasive avoidance of difficult tasks.

Of concern is the depression of the adolescents and the increased emotional symptoms seen in the adults suggesting that the primary issue while initially involving cognitive deficits of inattention, over time, is related to the consequences of continually struggling to read, feeling less than competent, and learning to avoid rather than confront problematic issues in one's life. The result is a change in values, goals, and desires to live a life that one thinks one can accomplish regardless if this is consistent with the reality of what one can actually achieve.

The goal is to catch attention problems while in childhood. The goal is to make a difference with cognitive training, to make a difference in their belief in themselves, to make a difference in their response to tasks being more difficult, and to make a difference in reading and study habits. We are losing the potential of bright individuals who are not maximizing themselves and lowering their standards to remain comfortable in life.

The answer is not the band aid of medication, although medication when used correctly as a short term (as opposed to a lifetime) intervention can be helpful. During the difficult times of childhood, we seem all too ready as a population to medicate this disorder. This is one of the few disorders that we rely upon only a minimal amount of information to prescribe. Once on medication, the natural tendency is to continue to try different medications looking for that singular time when it initially made a difference which was usually when first used. Once the novelty wears off, the medication is a band aid and like any band aid eventually it falls victim to overuse and no longer works.

Evaluation provides information and guidance for treatment. If you believe that ADD is a brain behavior disorder, you are going to use brain behavior neuropsychological test measures to assess this disorder. Testing determines if there is an attention disorder, how severe it is, and allows the ability to make an informed decision to medicate or not medicate.

We have been using a cognitive training program for almost 15 years as a treatment course for our ADD/ADHD patients. Using the same measures that were used to diagnose ADD/ADHD, testing before and after the program is completed (pre- and post testing) reveals differences in attention functioning that can be life changing. Everyone shows a difference on testing; the difference being more or less depending upon the presence of additional issues complicating ADD (ADHD plus) and if they have been addressed and treated.

Therefore, medication may be a good short-term (not long term) treatment solution, used to make a difference in specific, as opposed to the general symptoms of ADD. Re-testing on medication can determine whether it is working or not as well as evidence changes in their daily life at school or work. Testing and observation (or self-report measures) are jointly needed to provide accurate information on whether the medication is actually making a difference. We see the nonstimulant medications making a difference in anxiety but not in attention symptoms when measured on testing.

The goal is to approach ADD/ADHD in a scientific manner, identifying the coexisting additional factors that present a different picture of ADD providing clarity as to what ADD is as well as what it is not.

Index

Printed in the United States
by Baker & Taylor Publisher Services